MEDICINE AT THE MARGINS

POLIS: Fordham Series in Urban Studies
Edited by Daniel J. Monti, Saint Louis University

POLIS will address the questions of what makes a good community and how urban dwellers succeed and fail to live up to the idea that people from various backgrounds and levels of society can live together effectively, if not always congenially. The series is the province of no single discipline; we are searching for authors in fields as diverse as American studies, anthropology, history, political science, sociology, and urban studies who can write for both academic and informed lay audiences. Our objective is to celebrate and critically assess the customary ways in which urbanites make the world corrigible for themselves and the other kinds of people with whom they come into contact every day.

To this end, we will publish both book-length manuscripts and a series of "digital shorts" (e-books) focusing on case studies of groups, locales, and events that provide clues as to how urban people accomplish this delicate and exciting task. We expect to publish one or two books every year and a larger number of "digital shorts." The digital shorts will be 20,000 words or fewer and have a strong narrative voice.

Medicine at the Margins

EMS WORKERS IN URBAN AMERICA

Christopher Prener

FORDHAM UNIVERSITY PRESS   NEW YORK   2022

Fordham University Press also publishes its books in a variety of electronic formats. Some content that appears in print may not be available in electronic books.

Visit us online at www.fordhampress.com.

Library of Congress Cataloging-in-Publication Data available online at https://catalog.loc.gov.

Printed in the United States of America

24 23 22 5 4 3 2 1

First edition

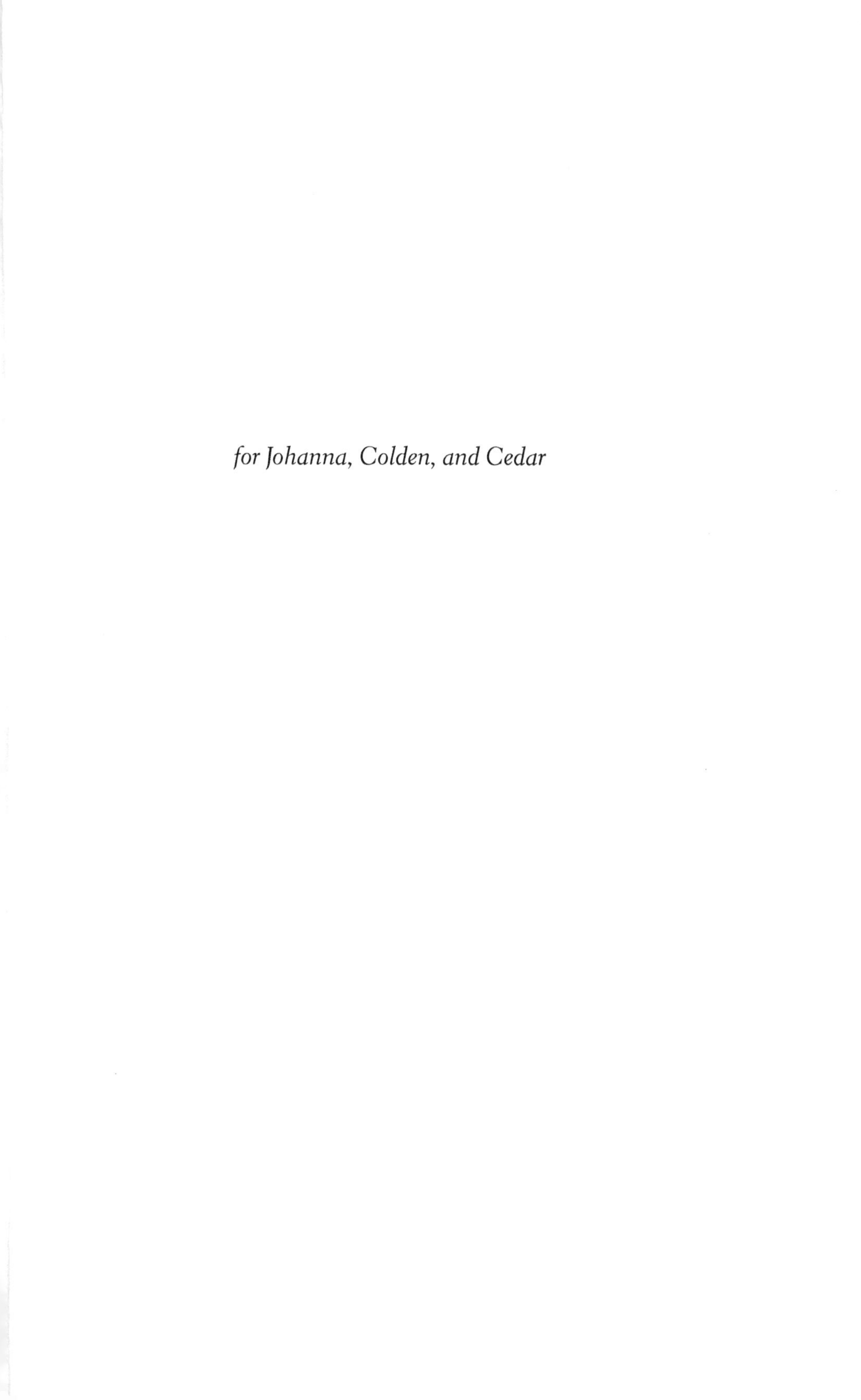

for Johanna, Colden, and Cedar

Contents

Preface

I have always enjoyed how emergency lights, whether they are on a police car, fire apparatus, or ambulance, reflect off buildings in the dark. They seem to dance back and forth, providing a brief illumination of the city as the emergency vehicle drives on toward its destination. In many ways this feels like an apt metaphor for emergency medical services itself. In short bursts, emergency medical technicians (EMTs) and paramedics flash into peoples' lives. Like other health-care providers, they are privy to aspects of their patients' lives that may not be shared with others. Like other first responders, they witness the material conditions in which their patients live. In the process, they gain an intimate understanding of cities. From the cab of the ambulance as they crisscross dark cities, lights illuminating the buildings and passing cars, they sit at a unique vantage point for viewing the urban landscape. EMS providers *see* the city in a unique way, refracted through their institutional lenses.

When we imagine these calls they respond to, we think of the most serious medical tragedies that might befall us. As Josh Seim (2020) has found, and as we shall see here, these types of emergencies certainly happen. People die, are injured, or sustain violent illness. Far more often, however, ambulances are summoned for a host of other reasons. Providers' views of the city are not just a prism through which we can view urban space itself, but through which we can see the contemporary consequences of age-old problems: substance use, poverty, and mental illness.

In 1851, English journalist Henry Mayhew collected more than a decade's worth of reporting in a three-volume work called *London Labour and the London Poor* (Mayhew 1861). Three decades before London's first ambulance service began operating and more than 160 years before I would step into the world of Private Ambulance half a world away, Mayhew's reporting brought working peoples' London to life. Just as many of the patients I saw with Private Ambulance used alcohol, Mayhew's working-class Londoners used snuff, gin, whiskey, and tobacco to dull the crushing experiences of poverty surrounding them. "They'll rather have a penn'orth of gin, or half a pint of beer with the chill off, under shelter," one street seller told Mayhew about his counterparts (Mayhew 1861). These same residents told Mayhew about their experiences. One of Mayhew's confidants told him that "the police drive us about like dogs, not gentleman's dogs, but stray or mad dogs" (Mayhew 1861).

In the space between 1840s Manchester and London and twenty-first-century Chapman exists nearly two centuries of social-science research about the people living at the margins of cities and the institutions nominally charged with addressing urban suffering. This is a thread connecting seminal works by early sociologists like W. E. B. Du Bois (Du Bois and Eaton 1996; Morris 2017) and Jane Addams (Knight 2010), the Chicago School (Bulmer 1986), William Julius Wilson (2011, 2012), Loïc Wacquant (1993, 2008), and Robert Sampson (2012) among the many contemporary sociologists invested in better understanding urban life.

Despite this research legacy, urban suffering remains common, though not always as visible as in London in the 1840s. For every person sleeping in an alcove or drinking on a park bench, dozens of others live in shelters, in apartment complexes, on friends' couches, and try to squeeze out an existence. Like Philippe Bourgois and Jeff Schonberg's *Righteous Dopefiend* (Bourgois and Schonberg 2009), Forrest Stuart's *Down, Out, and Under Arrest* (Stuart 2016), and Teresa Gowan's *Hobos, Hustlers, and Backsliders* (Gowan 2010), some of the best recent social science helps peel back the curtain on these spaces.

For EMS providers in American cities, viewing this type of suffering is an everyday part of the job. EMS providers and the other first responders with whom they work regularly find themselves in the alleys and apartments that generations of social scientists have sought to uncover. EMS providers are also products of the same economic forces; they are working-class health-care providers whose work so often revolves around treating the health consequences of inequality and marginality. The EMS system is therefore an unparalleled prism through which we can see the forces shaping health-care institutions, medical work, and the social problems endemic in cities.

The Sociologist in the Ambulance

Unlike other health-care contexts, sociologists have tended to gloss over EMS work. The world of EMS work sometimes appears fleetingly in urban sociologists' accounts of cities, not unlike sirens passing on a nearby block, here one moment and gone the next. Michael Corman's *Paramedics On and Off the Streets* (2017) and Josh Seim's *Bandage, Sort, and Hustle* (2020) are some of the only contemporary accounts of modern EMS work. Both were critical reads for me as I developed this book, though each left unanswered questions: how did the EMS system end up this way? How do we explain just how tedious EMS work can be? Where do space and place fit into our understanding of EMS?

Unlike Corman and Seim, I come to EMS work and these questions not as a researcher first but as a practitioner.[1] In Rochester, New York's, suburbs, where my family had moved from the Baltimore-Washington corridor when I was eight, local "third service" agencies utilizing volunteers were the norm. In the fall of 2000, I joined Perinton Ambulance's "Explorer" program. Nominally a part of the Scouting movement, explorer organizations provide high-school-aged youth the opportunity to experience different careers. Explorers provide a recruiting avenue and, at times, necessary personnel to staff events for EMS agencies and fire departments.

My first real opportunity to staff an event came the following summer, after monthly training sessions throughout the school year. Eight years before I first arrived at Private Ambulance, the agency home to *Medicine at the Margins*, I sat in the sun along Main Street in the suburban village of Fairport, New York. Like many canal towns in upstate New York, Fairport hosts a street festival each year. "Canal Days" is a mixture of artisan stalls, food vendors, and concerts. The influx of attendees presents a logistical challenge for Perinton Ambulance and an opportunity for Explorers to see EMS work firsthand. I do not remember much from my first Canal Days. The Explorers staffed a blood-pressure screening station, and I remember feeling awkward talking to people who stopped by that I did not know. I also remember riding in golf carts with EMTs and the feeling of wearing a uniform in public.

At Perinton Ambulance, I became an ambulance dispatcher and a New York State Certified First Responder when I turned sixteen. Two years later, I was a New York State Emergency Medical Technician, treating patients by myself. I spent the next four years alternating between summers at Perinton Ambulance and school years away at college, where I was part of my university's EMS squad. I can still vividly remember my first cardiac arrest and the eyes of the little girl who had stopped breathing in the arms of her father. I remember car accidents, the little boy who fell about twenty-five feet out of a tree, the man who jumped through a second-story window while high, and the woman with bilateral compound fractures to her arms after falling downstairs amid an ice storm. At university, I remember working the search for a missing fellow student, the numerous calls for intoxicated peers, and the close friend we dragged back from the grave in a dark common room.

By the time I arrived at graduate school, thinking I wanted to study violent conflict in Northern Ireland, I had spent eight years on ambulances, including four as an EMT. All of that seemed in the past, however. I had no designs to study EMS or health. After my future advisor, Alisa K. Lincoln, Ph.D., came to speak to my first-year cohort about her research on psychiatric emergency rooms, I pulled her aside. We should talk, I told her. I have seen all the things you are interested in but from a different perspective. Like always, EMTs had been in the background of Alisa's work: the people who came to take psychiatric patients away. It was time to foreground them in sociology, we decided.

Studying EMS was not my original plan for graduate school, but at the time, it felt right. Thus, during the summer of 2009, I walked into Private Ambulance to start "riding third." I brought my experience as an EMS provider, though my goal was to do as little patient care as possible. Those experiences helped me be a better field researcher and know how to fit in; sociologists call this "peripheral membership." I had never worked in urban EMS, however, and I had a lot to learn. This book is the culmination of those experiences at Private Ambulance beginning in 2009. Several years later, I spent most of the summer and fall of 2013 riding with providers before returning to interview them in early 2014. This fieldwork formed the basis of *Medicine at the Margins*. It is the story of providers at Private Ambulance that I am fortunate enough to pass on and share. The daily-grind EMS work in an American city's heart is a story about our failings as a society. It is also a story about the people who try to step into the void, sometimes reluctantly, to attempt to clean up the wreckage.

A Note on Names and Places

All names used in *Medicine at the Margins*, including the City of Chapman, neighborhoods within it, Private Ambulance, and the names of providers and patients, are pseudonyms. Early in my fieldwork, I agreed to keep Private Ambulance's name confidential as I conducted and later reported on my research. This was a pragmatic decision, motivated by my identity as a relative outsider attempting to gain access to Private Ambulance. The world of EMS is a small one, and I also worried that it would be easy to identify my participants or even some patients if I gave away key details about where this work had taken place. It is impossible to identify Chapman without making it immediately obvious what Private Ambulance's actual name is, and so the location of this work must remain confidential as well. Other data points, like patient names, were never collected. As other researchers of EMS settings have noted, getting patient content for research in the midst of a 9-1-1 call is a deeply problematic effort. Writing about place and space without being able to disclose the research site is a challenging one, and since I began my fieldwork in 2009, there have been conversations among qualitative sociologists about our default position to grant confidentiality to research participants. However, I continue to believe that the fieldwork presented here would not have been possible without guaranteeing Private Ambulance's owners as well as their providers themselves a degree of confidentiality.

Abbreviations

ALS	Advanced Life Support, practiced by paramedics
BLS	Basic Life Support, practiced by EMS personnel
EMS	Emergency Medical Services
EMT	emergency medical technician
IFT	interfacility transfer

MEDICINE AT THE MARGINS

Introduction

Shit Work on Urban America's Front Lines

"They smell like booze." (Riley)

The smell of fecal matter was overwhelming for the EMS providers. The patient, in the words of one of the EMTs, had "shit themselves." Imagine a smell so overpowering that it causes vomit to rise into the throat slowly. Mix in a week or more's worth of accumulated body odor and the stench of stale alcohol. Then allow it to fester in a small, enclosed van. When the side door of the ambulance opened into the chilly, clear night, the smell rushed out into the ambulance bay. It was physically, brutally appalling, the kind of smell that lingers in the nostrils long after the first breath of fresh air.

The ambulance crew had been sitting in the dimly lit ambulance bay at the side of Chapman Hospital's emergency department (ED), swapping war stories. The "ambulance bay" is a dedicated entrance for arriving "trucks" (individual ambulances) to park at and drop off patients destined for the ED, separate from the public entrance to the hospital. After calls, crews from various services often linger, cleaning their ambulances, filling out a record of their last patient on a tablet computer, smoking, or napping in the cab of their truck. That night, they were the only ambulance there. In the dark and separated from the street by a concrete wall, it was like a little oasis, immune from the bustle of nurses and fluorescent glare of the ED's lights as well as the humming of Chapman in late evening: cabs honking, drunk college students screaming, the neon lights of restaurants and bars.

When ambulance B6 pulled in,[1] the EMT driving the van-like vehicle frantically waved over the crew I sat with, a mix of horror and disgust written on his face. The side door opened immediately, and the other EMT, who was in back with the patient, nearly fell out gasping for air. One of the providers I was riding with went and got a wheelchair, covered it with a crisp off-white flat sheet, and helped B6's crew move their patient into it. The sheet, in this case, worn from innumerable uses and washings in the hospital, preserved some semblance of cleanliness for the wheelchair. The patient, his few belongings, and his walker were whisked into the ED by one of the EMTs with the ambulance doors left open to air the patient compartment out. I stood by while the crew I was with chatted with B6 afterward, describing in detail the patient's unkempt state and how badly the ambulance smelled.

Intellectually, we can contextualize the EMTs' responses to this patient. In the preeminent sociologist Erving Goffman's language (Goffman 2009), characteristics like body odor become discrediting characteristics that both underscore the sometimes extreme physical suffering of homelessness and stigmatize individuals in the eyes of others.[2] The EMTs' responses that night bear out this stigmatization, a point we will return to throughout this book.

As a group, however, those providers do not speak the language of Goffman. They live in what they consider the "real world," as a paramedic reminded me one afternoon as we sat and talked about the Affordable Care Act. Their world is not the EMS work of the movies, prime-time dramas, or the public eye. That night for B6's crew was no critically ill patient. No pulse-raising, blood-soaked, adrenaline-infused drama. No "big save," no glamor, no heroism. The crew had driven with their lights and sirens to the hospital, but only to ease their path through a city pulsing with late-evening activity. Indeed, the pungent gut check this patient offered represents an entirely different kind of reality. EMS work not as imagined but as providers experienced themselves: often dull, sometimes dirty work.

The Ambulance as a Prism

Sociologists have developed a lexicon for describing work like what B6 engaged in that night. Alternatively referred to as "dirty work," "shit work," or "scut work," these jobs have an air of contamination buried in the very language we select to describe them.[3] The call B6's crew experienced embodies this sense of perceived impurity of the work itself. Moreover, it draws attention to the core argument of *Medicine at the Margins*: pre-hospital emergency medical care is a critical piece of our medical infrastructure, yet it remains at the periphery. This sense of marginality, I argue, captures the distinct institutional role of the EMS system, is a defining feature of the experience of EMS work, and is a statement about the patient population urban EMS providers care for daily.

Stuck amid this marginality are EMS providers themselves. When B6's crew rolled their patient into the emergency department, they brought with them volumes of contextual knowledge about him. They develop this knowledge over the course of their employment, meaning that their way of "seeing the city" is a product of their institutional position. How providers view Chapman relies on how they view their work itself in the city, emergency work more generally, and the relative worthiness of Chapman's citizens to receive clinical services from Private Ambulance. If we want to develop an understanding of how individual perceptions of place develop, then, we must understand the institutional perspective these individuals bring with them to their work.

We, in turn, benefit from coming to understand this distinct institutional role. Not only do EMS providers see the city in particular ways, but through their experience we can gain an understanding of our collective failure to manage chronic health and social challenges. Providers reject this work as "bullshit," characterizing patients as falling outside of their mandate. Like the public hospital, then, the EMS system is a key but misunderstood part of our system of last resort. They are the epitome of the "little Dutch boy," holding back floodwaters by jamming a finger into a leaking dike.

Therefore, the story of EMS providers and urban EMS work is much more significant than EMS itself. It is a story about structural changes in how we deliver care to our most vulnerable neighbors and how changing conditions in cities' neighborhoods leave behind residents who lack stable housing and struggle with substance use. It is also a story of work we do not fully value as a society, despite the demands we place on the EMS system to be available at a moment's notice, anywhere they are needed. Much of this is not visible to outsiders, who may only catch a glimpse of this world for fleeting seconds as an ambulance speeds past toward some unseen crisis. In this world of the emergency medical technician and paramedic, we find a unique prism through which urban social problems, the health-care system, and the struggling social safety net refract and intersect in largely unseen ways.

The Imaginary Ambulance

At the outset, it is essential to understand that though we often speak of the "Emergency Medical Services system," this is a misnomer in the United States. We have a patchwork of local agencies that provide a mix of emergency or 9-1-1 work as well as medical transit for patients who require specialized transportation between appointments or medical facilities. Some of these agencies are private, some are public, and some are a part of the fire service. Many but not all the private agencies are for-profit, with the largest of these also being publicly traded. American EMS, therefore, differs significantly from its counterparts in other countries. Systems in most other developed nations tend to be state-run, centralized organizations. In contrast, American EMS is far more balkanized and privatized, meaning that while some aspects of EMS work are similar across national borders, the institutional context within which prehospital medicine operates varies dramatically. *Medicine at the Margins* is meant to capture life at a busy, urban, private EMS agency in all its drudgery, dirtiness, and occasional intensity.

Across this varied and segmented system, more than 32 million patients are treated by EMS providers each year.[4] Indeed, for its many structural flaws, the EMS system occupies a unique corner of the health-care system. It is nearly ubiquitous in America. Pick up a phone in nearly any part of the United States, dial 9-1-1, and *someone* will be able to respond to treat whatever medical crisis has befallen you. The response times may vary, particularly in remote parts of the American West and Alaska, but the system is in place, something no other part of the American health-care system can boast.[5]

The system itself consists of a set of interlinked parts. There is the telecommunications system present in most American communities, popularly known as the "9-1-1" system, which matches callers with call takers who can dispatch resources to the caller's location. These call takers, or telecommunicators, are not merely emergency receptionists. Instead, they are the first link in the Emergency Medical Dispatch (EMD) system, which involves a highly structured series of questions designed to provide an initial clinical assessment of the seriousness of the illness or injury.

Once recorded, information about the call is passed on to dispatchers. These individuals are critical links for EMS providers in the field, providing them with the locations of emergency calls, updates passed on from telecommunicators, and access to the broader network of first responders. In some communities like Chapman, the implementation of the EMD system means that police officers, firefighters, and EMS providers are all alerted to the presence of a medical emergency. The telecommunicator's initial assessment of the patient determines which institutions, and how many of their personnel, respond. Depending on the community, both the police officers and the firefighters may also have significant medical training that can even be on par with the training provided by the EMS providers themselves. It is the role of the EMS providers, however, to ultimately treat and transport the patient if necessary to a hospital emergency department.

Embedded in this system is a culture of openness. Unlike the rest of the health-care system, where demonstrating insurance coverage is often a precondition of care, there is generally no prescreening of patients for characteristics like insurance status or the ability to pay. A telecommunicator or EMS provider's first question will not be about how the patient intends to pay for the service being received but rather about the patient's clinical condition. The classic salutation for telecommunicators underscores this point: "9-1-1, what is your emergency?" Social class, income, and wealth are not essential parts of the trajectory outlined in this experience, though, as we will see, they operate in ways less immediately noticeable.

Such openness does not mean the system operates without billing patients, but it does mean the financial considerations that govern much of the interactions Americans have with their health-care system are absent at the outset of an encounter with an EMT or paramedic. A 2018 incident in Boston typifies this anomaly: when a woman fell between a subway car and the platform, cutting her leg open to the bone in the process, she begged bystanders not to call 9-1-1 because she was not sure if she could afford the bill. Interviewed afterward, the chief of Boston's ambulance system (known as "Boston EMS") noted that while costs could run between $1,200 and $1,900 for a critical patient, the individual's ability to pay was secondary:

> We just worry about taking care of people. . . . We don't want to cause them more stress. We just want to reassure them that nothing bad is going to happen to them because of their inability to pay.

It is difficult to imagine a similar statement from many hospital or physicians' group executives in the United States, where medical problems contribute to a significant number of bankruptcies each year (Austin 2014; Himmelstein et al. 2009). Thus, while there still may be market forces at work, at least some EMS agencies exercise discretion over how their billing practices impact patients.

Despite this openness and ubiquity, most of us may go years or even decades or a lifetime without ever setting foot in the back of an ambulance. Yet, ambulances are something we feel familiar with. We see them frequently, perhaps pulling over to allow one to pass on its way, we imagine, to some unseen crisis. If you live in an urban area the sound of sirens is a frequent one. Yet, as only a fraction of Americans experiences them with any regularity, what happens *inside* the ambulance is less well known.

Situating Emergency Medical Services Work

The Sisyphean task of providing emergency care in the pre-hospital setting is often assumed to be similar to work in an emergency department. Yet even acknowledging EMS providers is a rare phenomenon. In otherwise excellent books on social problems like homelessness, substance use, and the health consequences of poverty, they are often glossed over or ignored. EMS work, therefore, remains an understudied element of the health-care system, but one ripe for exploration. While most of what Freidson called "paramedical occupations" (Freidson 1988) suffer from a lack of autonomy, EMTs and paramedics stand out for the relative freedom within which they work. A physician does not stand over their shoulders or hover nearby, and the city itself is at their disposal when they are not treating a patient. This places them in a distinct position among low-prestige service workers where the very nature of their work bestows on them a degree of autonomy and independence often lacking in low-wage occupations.

Despite these unique and compelling features of EMS work, little time has been spent understanding pre-hospital medicine from the perspective of the EMS providers themselves. The limited literature on EMS work suggests they frequently work with patients whom providers find frustrating and who may have socially stigmatized conditions. The two seminal studies of EMS work are a pair of ethnographies capturing EMS in its infantile stages in the late 1970s and 1980s.[6] One, *Emergency Encounters* (Mannon 1992), is particularly relevant here. Mannon emphasizes the task of "street-level social work" as a significant yet informal aspect of EMS work. Being an EMT, in Mannon's early telling, was as much a structural intervention in the ills of society as it was a nascent critical-care service. Such a position is both a discrete occupational challenge and indicative of what was then a still evolving and ill-defined occupation.

This fundamental interest in "street-level social work" has remained a primary area of focus for the few social scientists looking at EMS care in the United States.[7] In particular, it shines through in two recent monographs about the American EMS industry. Ieva Jusionyte's *Threshold* (2018), for example, looks at cross-border emergency services between the United States and Mexico, focusing on the work first responders do to provide emergency care to migrants. In Jusionyte's work, the role of first responders in bandaging the bodies broken (in some cases literally) by the immigration system is the central focus. Likewise, in Josh Seim's *Bandage, Sort, and Hustle*,[8] the EMS system reluctantly bandages the bodies ravaged by the physical and emotional effects of poverty. This focus remains despite significant expansion of EMS providers' operational and clinical capacities (Institute of Medicine 2007; Prener and Lincoln 2015).

Seim's book, like Mannon's before him, delves into the world of what EMS providers call "bullshit." These are patients, problems, and situations providers themselves deem undeserving of attention from the EMS system. Such a focus on "bullshit" versus "legit" calls has strong roots in medical sociology's understanding of care provided in other health-care settings. It also overlaps with the calls Canadian EMS providers call "gooders" in Michael Corman's *Paramedics On and Off the Street* (2017), which is the third recent monograph on EMS work. Both Corman and Seim also share an interest in the ways management extracts labor power from EMS providers who, both in the U.S. (in Seim's work) and Canada (in Corman's), suffer from low wages and limited occupational prestige. Capital, in Seim's telling, structures EMS work both by creating a lumpen class of "bullshit" patients and precarity in the position of EMS providers themselves.

Each of the three books highlights essential and vital details about the state of EMS care. They capture EMS after several decades of maturation since Mannon's pioneering early research. There remain, however, critical gaps in our understanding of the fundamental work of EMS providers. Corman's book, for example, captures the very different institutional context of Canadian EMS. This book strives to address these gaps and differs from these recent texts in three key ways: history, time, and space. Whereas Seim sees "bullshit" calls through the lens of capital, I argue that the EMS's systems role as an underacknowledged part of the social safety net has less to do with profitability. Much of the EMS system in the United States is nonprofit, and the relations between these agencies and "capital" require a more nuanced view than Seim offers. In particular, I argue that the institutional path dependency that creates an EMS system full of "bullshit" patients has its roots in the 1950s and 1960s in the very beginnings of both the EMS system's development and in the parallel movement to deinstitutionalize the care of mental and behavioral illnesses.

I develop a theoretical model of EMS work to capture not just the fundamental work of EMS providers others have focused on, but how this work is stitched together both across space and time during shifts. Research on EMS has understandably focused on the "exciting" part, the adrenaline rush of emergency care, without reckoning seriously with significant time spent between calls. Seim again notes how supervisors, in pursuit of maximum labor value, rush providers outside of the informal break rooms at hospitals. Beyond this observation, however, "downtime" is mostly absent from our understanding of the world of EMS care.

So too is the flow of shifts across cities, both during downtime and in terms of the calls themselves. This focus on space foregrounds how "bullshit" work is not just a condition providers confront on-scene or in their ambulance, but how "bullshit" work occurs in neighborhoods providers begin to associate with the negative connotations they ascribe to patients. The rise of neighborhood stigma and the consequences it holds for patients who are assumed by providers to be malingering is critical for understanding not just the phenomenon of "bullshit" calls, but why they matter for all patients.

Marginality, Urban Life, and Emergency Medicine

This limited focus of social science on EMS is not only indicative of inattention on the part of the academy but part of something more fundamental at work. In this book, I argue that the defining feature of EMS work is not the high-adrenaline work we imagine paramedics to undertake but something else entirely. The experience of B6's crew encompassed this reality. The crew served as little more than a vector for a patient to get between places. Paramedics routinely recoil when called "taxi drivers" or "ambulance drivers" because both terms directly deskill their work. However, the complexity of EMS work is that often paramedics' skills are not well used. The patient they treated was not, in their eyes, critically ill or injured. His health problems were part of a broader constellation of social problems: housing instability, poor personal hygiene, and poverty. These are not problems the EMS system is set up to manage or treat. At EMS agencies around the United States, then, the defining feature of EMS work is its marginality and the marginality of the patients the EMS system serves, including those confronting the weight of mental illness, poverty, and addiction. Sparse attention from researchers fits into this broader narrative of marginality. The limited literature reflects the marginal nature of the institution and the relative importance attached to it by health-care scholars.

Theorizing Marginality

"Marginality" is a curious word within sociology and the social sciences. It is used with increasing frequency both within the discipline and more generally, as the results of a Google ngram search reveal (see Figure 1). It first appears in sociology in Robert Park's 1928 essay "Human Migration and the Marginal Man" (Park 1928). However, when researchers invoke marginality, it is often to make a passing reference to "marginalization" or "marginalized groups" without taking a more in-depth look at what exactly constitutes marginality in the first place. What results from this practice is the informal use of the term in contemporary scholarship without a critical lens on what it means and represents.

Defining marginality is, therefore, a critical yet overlooked task. Marginality implies a lack of centrality to a social process or conversely a sense of being pushed aside, overlooked, or ignored. Vivek Chibber criticizes academia's overreliance on the term: "The key category in the last twenty-five years has been

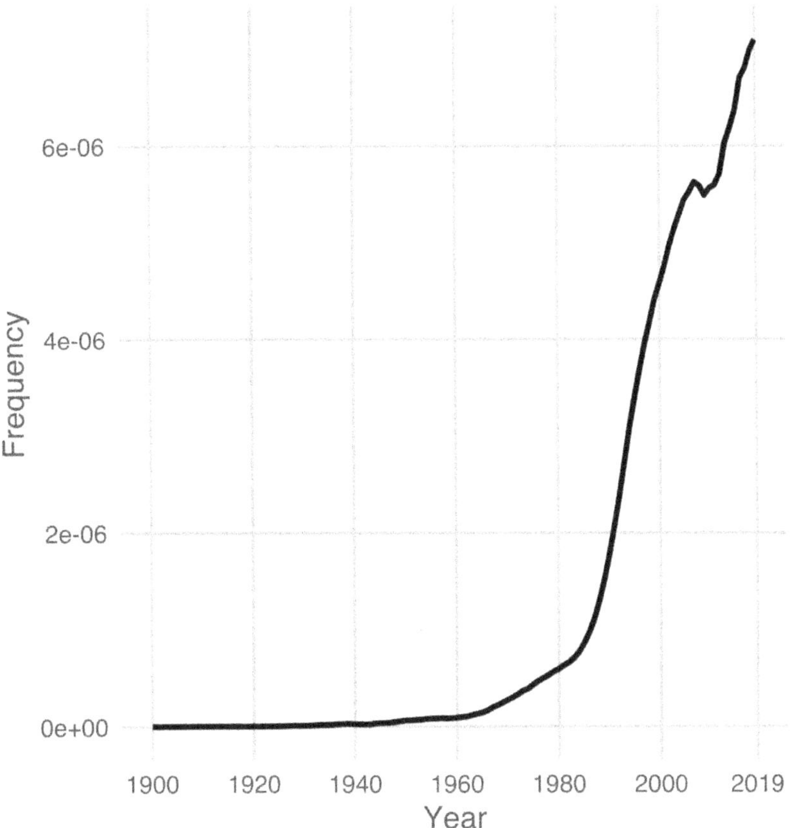

Figure 1. Frequency of the Term "Marginality"

the margins: marginality, embracing the margins, advocating for the margins, being the margins" (Chibber 2017). In the context of left-leaning politics, Chibber argues, we need to focus on the core of power structures in society. Moreover, we also recognize that some of the groups and institutions we frame as marginalized are central to those processes. Chibber uses the example of the working class, whom he frames as essential to the exploitation of wage labor within capitalism. They are not ignored, he implies, they are the most important aspect of capitalism after capital itself (Chibber 2017). This echoes, for example, Hebert Gans's description of the "positive functions" of poverty, which he argues is critical to the development of jobs that engage dirty work and, in the state of being poor, creates entire industries that exist to serve or profit from impoverished communities (Gans 1972). Likewise, James C. Scott eloquently illustrates the power that supposedly marginalized peasant groups can wield (Scott 1985).

In the context of EMS work, this tension between centrality and marginality plays out on a daily basis. If you call 9-1-1, the ambulance that responds is central to the experience that you have. In fact, the EMS system is a critical aspect of our health-care system that ensures a certain group of patients can get to and from hospitals efficiently. In this power relationship with patients, especially those who have unstable housing or active substance use, EMS providers are in the privileged position. Yet at the same time, EMS providers are powerless to control the flow of their work and do not work as full members of the health-care system. For all the centrality of the EMS system, however, it is marginalized institutionally, and the work itself is often challenging and austere. This tension reveals the way in which "marginality" does not mean "unimportant" or "powerless." Rather, marginality is situational and depends concretely on whom or what something is marginalized from. At Private Ambulance and in Chapman, marginality functions in several distinct ways: institutional marginality, occupational marginality, and work with marginalized populations.[9] Each of these three marginalities results in a distinct set of consequences for the overall practice of EMS work. In turn, they influence how providers' perceptions of the city are socially constructed.

Marginal Institutions

The first of these marginalities represents the structural position of EMS providers.[10] For EMTs and paramedics, who fall outside of the traditional division of labor for health-care practice, structural marginality describes many facets of their daily work. For example, in Chapman, EMS providers do not need anything more than a high school degree to practice, and the socioeconomic status of providers reflects this. Lawmakers and bureaucrats set these policies at the state level, and so there is some variation nationally, particularly for paramedics.

EMTs and paramedics have the lowest compensation rates among first responders (see Table 1). Using median weekly earnings data for 2018, EMTs make 82 percent of the median weekly compensation for police officers and 79 percent of the same for firefighters. Likewise, they make significantly less than allied health professions. The providers they interact with most closely, registered nurses in the emergency departments, physician assistants, nurse practitioners, and physicians, all make significantly more in terms of median weekly income. The statistics for EMTs and paramedics are most comparable

Table 1. Median Weekly Earnings (2018)

Occupation	All	Men	Women
EMTs and Paramedics	$894	$943	$764
Other First Responders			
Police Patrol Officers	$1,092	$1,131	$816
Firefighters	$1,126	$1,133	*not available*
Other Health-Care Providers			
Licensed Practical Nurses	$757	$936	$743
Miscellaneous Health Technologists	$873	*not available*	$791
Clinical Laboratory Technicians	$893	$819	$911
Dietitians	$967	*not available*	$940
Registered Nurses	$1,167	$1,271	$1,156
Physician Assistants	$1,752	*not available*	$1,646
Nurse Practitioners	$1,894	*not available*	$1,891
Physicians	$2,001	$2,513	$1,677

Note: Data via the Bureau of Labor Statistics' Current Population Survey. Weekly earnings estimates broken down by gender are not available for all occupations because of the small numbers of men or women working in particular fields.

to other relatively low-prestige health-care occupations, like lab technicians, miscellaneous health technologists, and dietitians. In terms of power, providers occupy a particular clinical niche where standing orders and protocols allow them significant discretion when it comes to intervening with patients. Though they provide care under a physician's medical direction, and an on-call medical control system exists for providers to receive guidance in the field, in practice these power structures feel far removed from EMS care as it is delivered. Despite lower socioeconomic status, then, providers have significant autonomy.

More generally, the EMS system remains divorced from the broader health-care system not only because EMS providers do not receive the traditional signifier of health-care workers, a college degree, but because the policymaking apparatus for EMS care sits in the Department of Transportation at the federal level in the United States. The historical path dependency that produced this outcome has left a residue of separation. EMS providers are not always clearly acknowledged as first responders, but they also are not integrated into the broader world of health care as an institution. These significant degrees of separation capture the essence of institutional marginality: the lack of power and socioeconomic status at the individual and institutional levels gives rise to a form of disenfranchisement.

Marginal Work

Beyond this institutional level, providers' work itself is marginalizing, and there is a certain "lack of fit" providers experience relative to other health-care providers and first responders.[11] For example, EMS providers as a group perform what sociologists refer to as "dirty work." Though they have significant autonomy, in practice their professional standing belies this, with other health-care providers sometimes referring to them as "ambulance drivers" or "transporters," implying EMS care is little more than a taxi service. Such framing is the essence of "dirty work," work that is either discrediting or discreditable. For EMS providers, their discreditability comes both from their lack of formal educational credentialing and from a lack of understanding among other health-care providers as to what EMS work entails. It therefore is easy to treat EMS work as deskilled, rudimentary work involving little more than moving patients from one place to another.

Another related facet with "dirty work" is the work's repetitive nature. For EMS providers, though each call has its unique elements, most share a few common features. Despite the idea of the EMS system as one that responds to critically ill patients, much of urban EMS work falls into the category of non- or sub-acute patients. These patients do not fully challenge providers' skill sets, and there can be a certain monotony to these calls. Such challenges are particularly true for EMS providers who do large amounts of what they refer to as "transfer work," providing transportation between medical facilities for patients who require additional assistance. This work comes perilously close to the idea of EMS work as taxi work and unsurprisingly has a negative connotation among providers.

That these calls do not challenge providers' skill set is indicative of another related idea: EMS work is often dull. The calls themselves may not be challenging, and downtime is often a significant portion of shifts for providers. Providers at agencies like Private Ambulance lack station houses or precincts to return to and may spend the bulk of their shifts in their ambulance cabs when not on calls. Lacking a physical station or base means they continually confront small challenges like finding parking and public restrooms and catching catnaps throughout their shifts. Of course, the work during these shifts can also be literally dirty. The vignette at the beginning of the chapter captures this. Providers regularly come into contact with bodily fluids like blood, urine, and fecal matter and sometimes confront patients who pose a danger to themselves or the EMS providers. Overlapping constructs like "shit work," for example, have been used to describe other occupations with similar types of exposures. In the context of "dirty" work, it is not fit within the broader group that is problematic, but how that group relates to a broader occupational structure. In this case, the work differs fundamentally from physicians and even other first responders, and it therefore carries a particular stigma of impurity.

Marginalized Populations

The third facet of the EMS system's marginality is the socially and culturally devaluated status of the communities they serve.[12] For EMS work, this is less about themselves, as Bureau of Labor Statistics data suggest EMS work is dominated by white men (see Table 2). Instead, it is indicative of the patients they find themselves treating. Though the EMS system as an institution prioritizes providing critical care, the patient population is far more diverse both clinically and in terms of acuity. Agencies who dig into their patient-care records find a significant share of calls come from a small set of patients for whom responses for psychiatric illnesses and behavioral health problems are common. These agencies also find that many of their patients are not seriously ill.[13]

People living with mental illnesses, substance-use disorders, housing instability, and the physical and mental health consequences of poverty form the very types of communities cultural marginality is meant to capture. These are all identities we can fit into Goffman's classic conception of stigma (Goffman 2009) for whom significant barriers exist in American society.[14] EMS workers' significant set of interactions with patients who are part of these spaces in social life are therefore a third significant facet of marginality for the pre-hospital medical system. Their identification of patients as "homeless," "mentally ill," or "alcoholics" can serve to label them, a key component (Link and Phelan 2001) of the stigma process. EMS providers' responses to these patients are part of what has been referred to as the "packaged deal" of stigma and mental health (Link et al. 1997), where patients potentially gain access to resources by being labeled, but those labels in turn can provoke stigmatized responses from health-care providers (Desai et al. 2002; Druss et al. 2002; Link, Mirotznik, and Cullen 1991).

It is not just patients who have mental illnesses, however, who are relevant to this form of marginality of EMS providers. Rather, it is a broader slice of Americans who find themselves as outcasts in urban America. Marginality in this context refers more expansively to those who rely on safety-net services because of poverty and racial discrimination. This *advanced marginality* that sociologists have come to recognize as part and parcel of the urban experience is a structural one. So, while our qualitative responses as a society to individuals who have mental illnesses, use illicit substances, or do not have stable

Table 2. Gender and Racial Diversity in First Responder Occupations

Occupation	% Women	% White	% African American
EMTs and Paramedics	33.9%	84.3%	11.9%
Firefighters	5.1%	87.1%	8.9%
Police Patrol Officers	15.4%	81.7%	12.7%

Note: Data via the Bureau of Labor Statistics' Current Population Survey.

housing fit the scope of cultural marginality, there is a vast set of structural forces shaping these experiences. It therefore makes sense to come full circle and view the patient populations common in urban EMS work as simultaneously representative of dueling forms of cultural as well as structural marginality.

Moreover, the marginality of these communities complicates earlier treatments of marginality. Though some scholars have recoiled from viewing these marginalities as connected continuums, the work of Loïc Wacquant, for example, calls us to look at their points of intersection. In Wacquant's telling of the experience of the American ghetto and French *banlieue*, it is the simultaneous experiences of cultural and structural marginality at work (Wacquant 2008). The current "hyperghetto," for instance, cannot be separated from hundreds of years of "ethnoracial" exclusion in the United States. It makes sense to understand marginality not as a strictly cultural or structural phenomenon but rather as a process that is part and parcel of broader cultural and structural trends.

The Social Construction of Neighborhood Stigma

Marginality is not only something patients and providers experience in its various forms but also an idea that is actively applied by providers to neighborhoods. For EMS providers, there is a keen sense of place in their work. EMS work is not unique in its spatiality. Indeed, there is a sense within the social sciences that *everything* is located in some sense not just spatially but temporally, culturally, and historically.[15] Emergency department work in twenty-first-century America, for example, is a product of particular temporal and historical processes creating not just EDs as distinct units within hospitals but also a social construction of the ED as a place of last resort for a broken safety net. Moreover, EDs are *located* physically within hospitals and spatially within cities and regions. Such an idea of physical place is an abstracted notion, however. Particularly within the windowless ED, place seems to melt away. There is a constant rhythm to ED work inside the hospital while, outside and out of view, the day passes into night and people go about their lives on a continuous cycle.

For EMS work, though, the spatial boundaries are different and more immediate. EMS work happens within concretely defined districts. Private Ambulance serves a particular geography, the city of Chapman. Within the city, there are neighborhoods and regions where providers are asked to "cover."[16] Dispatchers transmit calls to ambulance units with spatial information in the form of street addresses or intersections and perhaps additional place details (like a building name or description) to go along with it. For the emergency department, space and place are abstracted. For EMS workers, space and place are immediate and (sometimes literally) concrete.

Additionally, space and place are *part* of the EMS experience, not just in a sense that the EMS providers must pass *through* parts of a city to get to a call, but because each call is a part of space as well. EMS providers get to see patients on their commute or out while they run an errand, at play, and in their homes. This observation is obvious, perhaps, but it brings with it additional information other health-care providers typically never get to see. An emergency department physician may know in the abstract that the patient lives on the street, but providers get to see and feel the patient's reality when they transport a patient from a shelter, encampment, park bench, or stoop. Paramedics and EMTs see patients' homes, their college residence halls, their offices, restaurant kitchens, and a thousand other places where injury and illness manifest themselves.

Since calls happen regularly and providers spend their downtime in the same neighborhoods where they treat patients, providers also develop generalizations of place over time. Providers develop a sense of how particular patient populations are situated spatially, revealing both evident and subtle patterns to cities that belie demographic patterns, the physical geography of social problems, and the hidden worlds certain social groups inhabit. These impressions of space and place may be positive or negative and embody their value judgments about the world they inhabit.

Such a set of judgments is not unique to EMS providers, as we all develop a keen sense of what "good" and "bad" places and neighborhoods are.[17] These frames reflect where we feel safe when we navigate a city or a town and where we feel less comfortable. Intuitively, we can carve up space in ways that reflect our priorities, prejudices, preferences, and preconceptions. In this way, when we define a neighborhood or region as "bad," we apply stigma to place just as we apply it to mental illnesses. Stigma here parallels Goffman's notion of discrediting and discreditable (Goffman 2009). Negative perceptions of space are discrediting for individuals whom paramedics find in such places and discreditable if they must disclose that they live there to health-care providers. From a social-science perspective, however, we know relatively little about *how* neighborhood stigmas are constructed and utilized.[18] For EMS providers, it is the clustering of patients that is the most salient feature of space. There are neighborhoods with college students who are perceived to drink too much or present with problems that seem minor to the paramedics who privilege their own life experience and hold it in high regard. There are neighborhoods with wealthy people, poor people, substance users, and individuals living on the street. When an ambulance responds to a particular location, providers compare the dispatch information against these heuristics and anticipate what they will find when they arrive on the scene. Neighborhood stigmas, a place with a large homeless population, for example, become tools for coloring between the lines of often vague dispatch information.

Moreover, I argue that these perceptions become a means for reproducing marginality. When providers pair dispatch information with location and construct a notion of the call they are likely to see, there are two crucial possible outcomes. First, if their notion is confirmed and providers find the expected patient, it reifies their view that a neighborhood contains a particular clinical population or social group of patients. However, the second possible outcome is that they risk creating a framework resistant to information they receive through updates or once they arrive at a call. Their term for this, "getting burned," encapsulates the risk that they overlook critical signs and symptoms of illness. The threat here, I argue, is the first outcome, when it occurs repeatedly, that increases the probability of the second outcome. Neighborhood stigma is itself a kind of marginalization of place and space, and therefore represents a way in which marginality creeps into the practice of EMS work by providers.

Modeling Marginality in Urban EMS Work

At first blush, the connections between marginalized institutions, work, and populations may seem indirect. There have been several attempts among sociologists to draw geometric parallels between work on the shop floor (Burawoy 1982) or in service-work settings (see Figure 2). Each element of both the two-sided model of industrial work and the three-sided model (also known as the "service triangle") captures a key workplace constituency.[19] The connecting arrows represent both the interactive nature of the work itself and the power dynamics existing among labor, management, and customers when they are present.

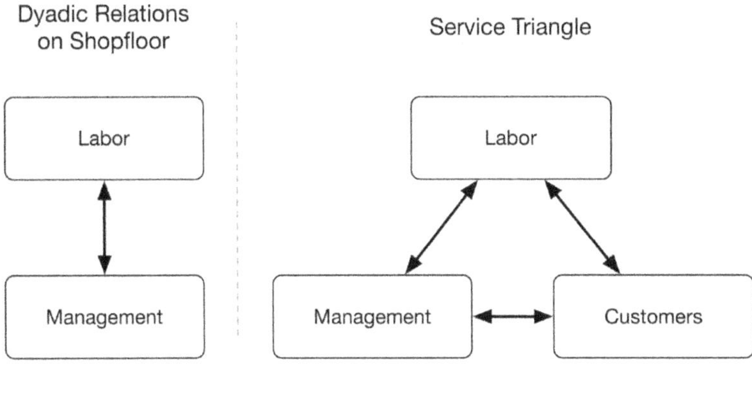

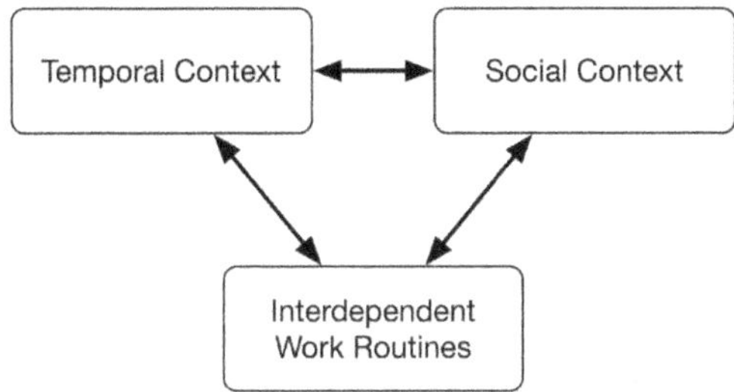

Figure 2. Geometric Models of Work in Sociology (graph by author)

A similar dynamic exists in the "sociology of work time" (Perlow 1999), which captures the dynamics leading to time pressure in white-collar workplaces. The different constituencies present in the service triangle appear under the label "interdependent work patterns." These routines are affected, Perlow argues, by the social context within which work occurs and the temporal context. The social context refers to norms and practices influencing work routines, while the temporal context refers to the pace and timing of work activities affecting how these work patterns unfold.

Seim's book on EMS work has grappled with both the idea of interdependent work routines and, to a lesser extent, the social context within which EMS work takes place (Seim 2020). His book offers a model of EMS work that highlights some of the relationships providers enter into as they provide emergency care, particularly with administration, law enforcement, and hospital staff. Seim also details two institutions, capital and systems of protocols, that each affect the social context of EMS work.

All three of these models, the "service triangle," Perlow's model of work time, and Seim's model of EMS work, present incomplete snapshots of EMS work and mobile service work generally. Each chapter of this book, while elucidating essential elements of urban EMS work, also *locates* these elements in a theoretical model designed to extend these prior efforts to model service work. This emergent model of EMS work incorporates elements from all three past models but does so intending to develop a model of EMS work that applies not just to urban, for-profit EMS work, but also to public or volunteer EMS agencies.

Using Perlow's model as a base, the emergent model presented here illustrates the social and temporal context EMS work occurs in. Since "social context" refers not only to the specific norms and practices in Perlow's work, but also the wider model itself, I change this node's label to more specifically refer to "workplace norms and practices." I also expand the "interdependent work routines" node, using the "service triangle" literature as a basis for presenting a more sophisticated understanding of the relations providers must navigate during shifts. These two models sit within a broader *spatial* context. Crucially, it is not just when and how work takes place, but where work takes place that is critical for understanding EMS care. This spatial context sits in turn within an even broader cultural context affecting all facets of EMS care. This cultural context, which in particular includes cultural stigmas toward mental illness, substance use, and homelessness, informs how providers view their work and the neighborhoods where this work takes place.

Exploring Marginality in Urban EMS Work

The exploration of multiple forms of marginality forms the core of the remaining parts of this book. In "The Scene," I introduce Chapman and its EMS system, which revolves around Private Ambulance. I also describe how most providers come to know Chapman from the institutional position of EMS providers. Next, the book unfolds over three pairs of interrelated chapters followed by a final concluding chapter that ties together the various strands of EMS work explored into a contextual understanding of emergency medicine and safety-net institutions more generally. The technical details of how the data featured here were collected are included in an extensive Appendix at the back of the book.

Part I, "EMS as a Marginal Institution," begins with a macro-level view of EMS as a marginal institution among both health-care workers and the first-responder community. In Chapter 1, I describe the historical development of EMS from its nascency during the nineteenth century to its formal birth in the 1960s and early 1970s in the United States. This historical analysis supports the core argument of this section: that the EMS system developed and exists separately and apart from the health-care and public-safety systems in the United States. With this foundation established, I segue into a discussion of the manifest function of the EMS system, as it is understood both in the popular press and in public-policy circles, to respond to "real emergencies." Providers have unsurprisingly bought into this idea, and I use their views to illustrate how EMS providers construct the idea of "real emergencies" and the cognitive dissonance existing for providers between these "real emergencies" and the "bullshit calls" that seem to dominate their shifts. These findings reinforce earlier work on EMS (Seim 2020; Mannon 1992; Metz 1981) and strongly affirm Seim's (2020) recent findings, albeit in a different organizational context. However, by locating providers' dissonance at the end of a set of historical processes, I am better able to contextualize the point from which their frustration emanates.

As a consequence of the institutional development discussed in Chapter 1, EMS providers find themselves continuously having to navigate a complex set of interactions as they deliver patient care. In Chapter 2, I draw on and subsequently offer critiques of theories from the sociology of work for understanding how power is distributed in everyday workplace interactions. For EMS providers, their regular interactions with other first responders, hospital staff, EMS management, and patients themselves are constant sources of conflict and contestation.

Emblematic of this struggle is the constant framing of EMS providers not as skilled clinicians but as "ambulance drivers," the equivalent of a medical taxi service for shuttling patients to hospitals. I connect this framing to interfacility transfer work, which prior EMS research has ignored by focusing instead almost exclusively on emergency calls. Patients and other health-care providers both engage in this framing of EMS work, and EMS managers reinforce it with the constant technological surveillance used to monitor the work practices of EMS providers in the field. The construction of EMTs and paramedics as "ambulance drivers" complicates the narrative of "real emergencies" and creates a space that other institutions can exploit by shifting responsibility for social problems onto the EMS system. It also forces EMS providers to constantly re-legitimate their role, skills, and expertise to other health-care providers and even some patients. Negotiation is therefore a critical component of EMS care.

Part II, "EMS as Marginal Work," segues from an institutional perspective to a focus on the instrumental work of EMS providers themselves. In Chapter 3, "The Twenty-Four," I dive deeply into a single shift, "Shift 99," from the second round of fieldwork. It describes the flow between emergency calls and downtime, emphasizing how EMS is at once a clinical, social, and spatial activity. Shifts, including "Shift 99," have varying paces dictated by the frequency of calls, downtime activity, and the amount of driving they entail. After describing "Shift 99" in detail, this chapter expands on the spatial aspects of EMS work by describing more macro-level spatial trends in EMS work in "Chapman" with maps and statistical analyses of EMS work. Unsurprisingly, EMS work is neither evenly nor randomly distributed throughout the city, and its distribution does not follow predictable trends like race, poverty, or poor population health. Such spatial patterning provides the opening to interrogate the meaning of space in EMS work throughout the remaining chapters.

One of the key findings from "Shift 99" and the broader set of field observations is that providers spend nearly two-thirds of duty time not on emergency calls but on what I call "downtime." In Chapter 4, "Hurry Up and Wait," I take this two-thirds of shift time and describe it in detail using ethnographic and interview data. This downtime is spent doing paperwork, reading, watching movies on phones or tablets, socializing with other providers, and driving around "Chapman" merely killing time before the next call. Like EMS work as a whole, downtime is an inherently spatial activity. Specific neighborhoods lend themselves to downtime (with ample parking, a large number of restaurants, and clean public restrooms) while others do not. Neighborhoods are not equally welcoming to providers' presence. This chapter explores conflicts that emerged between local business and Private Ambulance, which ultimately resulted in the ejection of the paramedics from a particular neighborhood. This natural experiment reveals the critical ways in which space shapes (for better and worse) work environments and the experience of EMS providers as they wait for their next emergency call.

In Part III, "EMS in the Marginal City," we move from a view of EMS work itself as marginal to EMS work *on* marginalized patients. In Chapter 5, "The Daily Grind of Grunt Work," I compare the actual distribution of EMS calls with providers' perceptions of where work takes place. There is a wide gap between these objective and subjective measures, and I argue that this is driven by "grunt," "bullshit," or "shit" work that defines providers' views of their jobs. Areas with high concentrations of these types of calls, ones involving individuals who are homeless, substance users, the mentally ill, and the urban poor, come to dominate providers' perceptions of their work, leading them to overemphasize their work in certain areas and underestimate it in others. While there has been a small amount of research done on *where* EMS work takes place (Seim 2020; Seim, English, and Sporer 2017; Seim et al. 2018), we have little understanding of *how* EMS providers think about place and process spatial data. This chapter therefore provides a unique methodological approach to another understudied facet of EMS work.

In the final substantive chapter of *Medicine at the Margins*, I explore "grunt" work as an expressly spatial phenomenon. One neighborhood in particular, "Midtown," captures all the providers' frustrations with their work. Chapter 6, "Stigma and Space in Midtown," makes three arguments about why "Midtown" comes to dominate providers' views of their work. First, I argue that providers' emphasis on this neighborhood is the result of a subset of "Chapman's" homeless population who providers believe have comorbid mental and behavioral health issues. Second, I argue that the Midtown neighborhood itself becomes intertwined with the stigmatized views providers have about mental and behavioral health issues. The strong, shared views providers hold about these patients illustrate how institutions foster and reproduce stigmas. Finally, I argue that the intersection of social and spatial stigma has discrete consequences for both patients and providers. Providers take on an informal role in policing the use of space in "Midtown," helping to push patients who are street homeless toward more marginal spaces within the city. Providers also risk "getting burned" when they assume patients in the Midtown neighborhood are malingering and attempting to misuse the EMS system.

In the concluding chapter, "Marginality, Stigma, and the Future of Pre-Hospital Medicine," I synthesize how marginality functions in EMS work, reviewing the connections made throughout the manuscript between the EMS system as a marginalized institution, EMS work itself as subject to marginalization, and EMS work with marginalized, stigmatized patient groups. What is particularly fascinating about the case of EMS work in Chapman is that providers have been subject to the very same spatial exclusion processes they facilitate in the cause of individuals who are street homeless. These two examples of spatial exclusion underscore the importance of understanding how neighborhoods are defined not just spatially but also socially. They also illustrate how the EMS system does not just reflect all social processes at work in a city, but how it contributes to the reproduction of these same social issues.

The Scene

"I used to think it was a lot bigger of a place . . . now knowing it as well as I do, it just feels like a town. It doesn't feel big anymore." (Ben)

"They're Sending the Whole City"

At 05:55 hours, I met Bryson and Rob in Private Ambulance's oversized garage at the north end of Chapman. I was waiting in the garage because the crew of the "zero-six-hundred truck" who worked from six in the morning the previous day until six this morning was still asleep on the couches in the crew room upstairs. Bryson joined me first, and we talked about our previous shift when he was on a different truck from me. He said it must have been pretty quiet because he did not remember much about the shift. As we drove south toward Chapman's most densely populated parts, Bryson and Rob conferred in the cab about breakfast options. They decided they wanted breakfast from the Eaton Market. As we drove, the two providers talked about riding motorcycles and dirt bikes.

Parking for "the Market," a favorite location for Private Ambulance crews, was in a loading zone that was able to accommodate several ambulances. Parking there was not strictly speaking legal, since it was a tow-away zone. Nevertheless, it was a frequent haunt for Private's crews during the first few months of my fieldwork. Eaton Plaza was near the heart of the Old Quarter, which had a more upper-class profile than other neighborhoods in Chapman. As we walked up the street to the Market, we passed a car with a husky sitting in the driver's seat, wearing a neck pillow. Bryson could not help laughing hysterically and asked us if the dog was wearing a cervical collar (used to protect patients' necks if they may have suffered a traumatic injury). Rob shook his head, lamenting that he had no idea what was going on there. Such was life in the Old Quarter, which some providers loved during downtime for its people-watching opportunities.

Inside the Eaton Market, both Bryson and Rob ordered breakfast sandwiches. Rob and I also ducked across the street to a chain coffee and donut shop to buy coffees. Ordering coffee was an arduous process. The teenager behind the counter was barely awake, and another customer cut us in line. We talked as we waited, and Rob brought up "37-Delta" patients, often characterized as living on the street and having an alcohol use disorder. "They get seen all the time," he told me, and sometimes "if we see them too much and they're a burden on the system, they can lock them up for three months." One woman just got back to Chapman from a few months of being institutionalized, Rob told me, and Private had already transported her three times from Midtown "for being drunk."

After a detour, because I forgot a straw for my iced coffee, we got back in the ambulance, and Bryson and Rob started eating their sandwiches. As they ate, "fire alarm," the fire and EMS dispatchers in Chapman, came on the air with a reported structure fire. The two providers recognized the address, and we listened as the first-due engine company responded and confirmed a working fire. As the dispatchers sent additional resources, Bryson laughed that "they're sending the whole city." They both had a sense of where the different fire companies were coming from and recognized that they were the closest ambulance. As Bryson continued to laugh and Rob made fun of the dispatcher's thick local accent, they stowed their sandwiches and started toward the fire.

Chapman

Chapman is a mid-sized city in the Eastern United States that is part of a larger metropolitan area. Like many American cities, Chapman followed a trajectory beginning with nineteenth-century urbanization and industrialization. The new city was an amalgamation of several smaller agricultural villages and a rapidly expanding industrial site known as East Chapman. The neighborhoods that emerged from Chapman's incorporation had been filled first with Irish immigrants and, later in the nineteenth century, immigrants from Italy, Eastern Europe, and the Iberian Peninsula. These same immigrant groups also found housing to the north, away from the original villages and toward a marsh-filled area known as North Chapman. Here Irish immigrants labored in brickworks, steel mills, and railroad yards lining a stream known as Bullhead

Brook. This area was the last area of the city to see large-scale growth, which occurred during the early to mid-twentieth century.

The industrial base for the city in East Chapman and other neighborhoods in the southern and central parts of the city eroded sharply during the Depression and after World War II. These trends mirrored broader demographic and economic shifts in the United States (Bluestone and Harrison 1982). Downtown Chapman, in particular, was the focus of postwar urban renewal projects where public housing complexes rose on the footprints of demolished factories. Elsewhere, there was substantial mid-century development in North Chapman as suburbanization and highways provided new transit links into the city. The city's neighborhoods continued to retain some of their ethnic identities, though as the city's economy changed, so did its demographic profile. In particular, the city had transitioned away from manufacturing toward the service industry and the "knowledge economy" (Powell and Snellman 2004) over the last three decades.

The process of deindustrialization resulted in an overall population decline for the city of Chapman. However, the turn toward service work and the "knowledge economy" has resulted in a rebounding population, with over 100,000 current residents. Contemporary Chapman is racially and ethnically diverse, with a majority white population and substantial African American and Asian communities. These non-white communities are not segregated in "ghettoized" areas as they are in other cities, though much of West Chapman remains a primarily white neighborhood of the city.

EMS in Chapman

Three agencies, public and private, provide first-responder services to Chapman. The Chapman police and fire departments are both publicly operated first-responder organizations. The fire department, in addition to providing fire suppression services, also operates the City's Emergency Medical Services system in partnership with a private ambulance company. "Private Ambulance," as I call it here, is contracted by the city to provide medical transport services from emergency scenes to local hospitals. Private Ambulance receives emergency calls through the city's 9-1-1 center, which is colloquially known as "fire alarm."

The 9-1-1 process deserves some additional explanation because it is the source of the call data presented in subsequent chapters. Once a patient or bystander makes a call to the 9-1-1 center, a call-taker records information about the call and, for most medical calls, proceeds through the Emergency Medical

Dispatch (EMD) system. The EMD is a guided set of questions designed to help the call-taker determine the appropriate type and number of medical resources to send. The result of the EMD system is the creation of a determinant code that describes, roughly, the type of medical emergency the caller is reporting. Fire alarm will dispatch resources from the Chapman Fire Department, Police Department, and Private Ambulance based on this code. For higher-priority codes, known as "Charlie," "Delta," or "Echo" codes, Advanced Life Support resources, which consist of one of the engine companies, "the rescue," and two smaller vehicles known as "the squads," from the fire department respond along with the closest fire apparatus and an ambulance. For lower-priority codes, known as "Alpha" and "Bravo" codes, fire alarm will only dispatch a Basic Life Support ambulance along with, for some calls, the closest fire apparatus.

The terms "Basic Life Support" (BLS) and "Advanced Life Support" (ALS) refer to the qualifications of the providers who staff these units. Emergency medical technicians, commonly called EMTs, provide care at the BLS level. BLS care includes assessing and treating common sub-acute illnesses and injuries and a few more advanced interventions for critical patients. Patients who are extremely ill or injured, however, are typically attended to by ALS providers. Most ALS providers are paramedics ("medics"), who have at their disposal a far more extensive array of both physical and pharmacological interventions, as well as tools for more advanced diagnostics.[1]

Importantly, this response system is only the primary system for EMS response in Chapman. Private Ambulance also responds to calls made directly to them from various health-care facilities that it has signed operating agreements with for ambulance services. These calls are dispatched to ambulance units as if they were emergency calls, but Private Ambulance's crews do not have to keep the city's 9-1-1 center notified of their progress. Private also provides interfacility transfer services for both medical centers in the city: the "Muir" Hospital located in West Chapman and the "Mather Hospital" located on the city's eastern edge. Of the two, the "Mather" is the city's safety-net hospital operating under a public-private partnership between Chapman and a private health-care system.

If all of this were not complicated enough, other health-care facilities within the city, particularly several nursing and rehabilitation facilities, would contract with other EMS services to provide pre-hospital care to their clients. Chapman, therefore, mirrors much of the complexity that exists elsewhere in the United States when it comes to the delivery of pre-hospital care: multiple public and private agencies providing overlapping services within a single municipality with varying levels of clinical ability.

Private Ambulance

Private Ambulance's headquarters sits in a squat, gray warehouse off a secluded dead-end street on the north side of Chapman. Visitors must be buzzed in through the front door into the upper part of the headquarters, where classrooms and offices surround a cramped dispatch center. There are typically two dispatchers working during weekdays and one dispatcher during overnights and weekends. The dispatch office is a hub of activity. The dispatchers answer incoming phone calls for business related to the company and requests for ambulance responses from their various contract sites that contact Private directly rather than through the 9-1-1 system. Computer screens and a large bank of flat-screen TVs display information about the location of each of Private's ambulances. GPS units in the cab of each ambulance enable this tracking. The TVs also display historical call data so dispatchers can identify city areas that could be "hot spots" for calls given the historical call volume for the given day and time.

The dispatchers receive incoming calls from the 9-1-1 system through a Computer Automated Dispatch (CAD) system whose interface and courier font type evoke the early 1990s Microsoft DOS operating system. Calls pop up on the CAD terminals as the 9-1-1 center dispatches them, and then Private Ambulance's dispatchers send the closest appropriate ambulance. The exchange typically goes like this:

> DISPATCHER: M6 . . .
> M6: 6 . . .
> DISPATCHER: M6, respond to 123 Main Street for the man down. Call comes in through fire alarm.
> M6: 6 is responding.

Ambulances are each designated with a call sign. In the previous example, "M6" refers to both the level of care the ambulance can provide (Medic or "M") and the ambulance's identification number ("6"). Ambulances with "medics" always are staffed with one and often two paramedics. When a medic and an EMT are partners, Private Ambulance personnel refer to them as "MB" trucks, a designation that refers to both the paramedic ("M") and the EMT or "Basic" ("B") working onboard. Ambulances with only EMTs use similar call signs, except they replace the "M" designation in the previous example with a "B." Thus, "M6" is paramedic ambulance six while "B1" refers to EMT ambulance one.

Whether staffed with one or two medics, the medic trucks are box-like ambulances known within EMS as Type III ambulances (see Figure 3, Panel A).

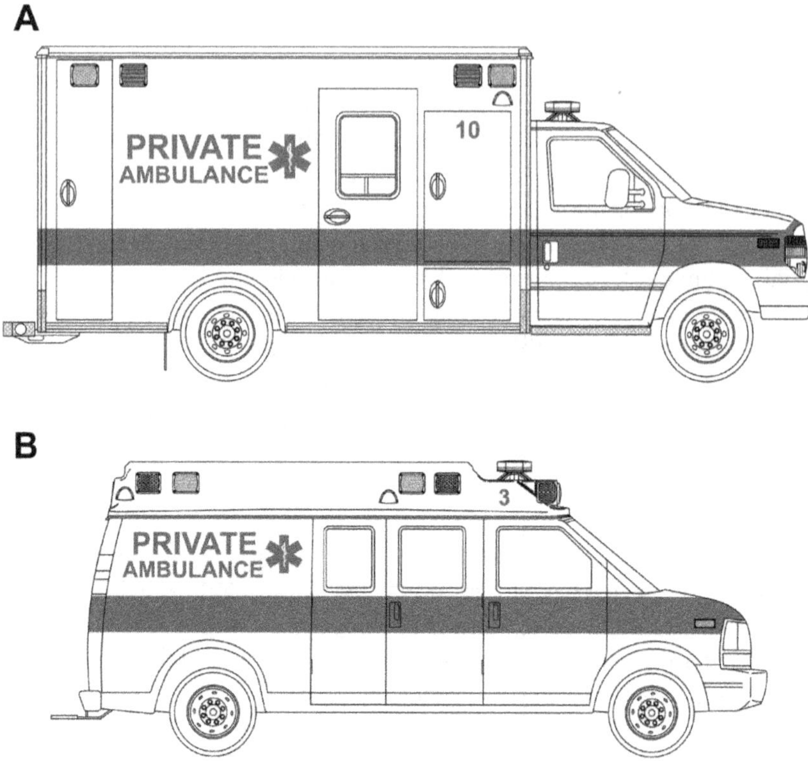

Figure 3. Private Ambulance Units: (A) is the larger design utilized by Paramedics ("Medic 10" or "M10") while (B) is the van design used by EMTs ("B3") (graph by author)

These ambulances have more storage room for equipment and additional room in the patient compartment. These are essential considerations for paramedics who carry more patient-care equipment and often have students or other providers in the back of the ambulance as they deliver patient care. The ambulances designated for the EMTs are Type II ambulances (see Figure 3, Panel B), which use a smaller van-style chassis. These have less room for storage and patient care and are slightly less comfortable to spend shifts in because of their smaller size.

EMS Shifts in Chapman

When providers arrive for their shifts, they visit the dispatch office and are assigned either a medic truck or van-style ambulance, based on their skills and who their partner is for the shift. On one wall of the dispatch center, portable radios sit in chargers, with two radios assigned to each ambulance. Providers will grab the pair of radios corresponding to their assigned ambulance and then walk downstairs to the oversized, two-story-high garage at the rear of Private's headquarters. Inside the garage are ambulances packed tightly together, several support vehicles, and personal vehicles for some members who choose to park inside (a perk during colder months). There is also storage for additional medical equipment and a locker room that includes a bathroom and showers. Several technicians work in the garage full-time, cleaning and restocking ambulances and performing basic maintenance tasks on the vehicles.

Once they are downstairs, they find their assigned ambulance, ensure it is in working order, and sign onto the tablet computer they use to complete patient-care reports. They will also quickly check their medical equipment to ensure their supplies and tools are in order before heading out on the road. There is often a push to get ambulances out "on the road" as soon as possible, so crews are available for calls and in a position to respond quickly. Occasionally, however, at the beginning of shifts, providers will be asked to run errands for the dispatchers, including taking the ambulances around the corner to a maintenance facility that provides service to Private Ambulance and other first responders in Chapman. Since Private's ambulances are on the road almost every day, they require frequent maintenance to keep them running. Once either the providers or the vehicle service technicians finish restocking and replacement, providers will notify their dispatcher that they are "on the air" (monitoring the appropriate radio frequency) and available for calls as they pull out of the garage.

For providers, being on the road means spending nearly their entire shift in their ambulances. Dispatchers will occasionally ask crews to return to base (Dispatcher: "M6, can you 60?"—with "60" being the radio code for returning to the headquarters). However, this is not the norm for most trucks on most shifts. What each shift is like for providers depends primarily on whether they are part of a medic or "MB" truck or are on a BLS ambulance.

Medics often work twenty-four-hour shifts ("twenty-fours") that begin at either "oh-six-hundred" or "oh-seven-hundred" hours (6 A.M. or 7 A.M. respectively; communication within EMS and the first responder world more generally occurs using a twenty-four-hour clock). Three ambulances are staffed each day for twenty-four hours, and these are all typically staffed with at least one medic. Additionally, some medics work shorter shifts, typically twelve-hour shifts ("twelves") that begin in the morning and end in the late evening.

EMTs working on a BLS ambulance for the day begin their shifts, which are between eight and twelve hours long, throughout the morning with start times staggered between 0800 hours (8 A.M.) and 1200 hours (noon). A typical day has four BLS ambulances routinely staffed, and there is also an extra BLS shift, which is only staffed on Fridays and Saturdays from 1400 hours (2 P.M.) until 0200 hours (2 A.M.) the next day.

The three medic trucks have two designations on twenty-four-hour shifts: a single "base" truck and two "city" trucks. The base truck returns to Private Ambulance sometime between 2300 hours (11 P.M.) and 0200 hours (2 A.M.) depending on call volume and whether it is a weekend; the weekend trucks remain on the road until 0200 hours (2 A.M.) or later. The providers assigned to this truck spend the night sleeping in one of two bunkrooms or on one of the two large couches in the "crew room," which contains TV trays for eating meals and a TV. Providers who are not working overnight but only have a few hours between shifts also sleep at the headquarters if they do not live nearby.

The "city" trucks do not return to the headquarters to sleep. Instead, they spend the night in a bunkroom at the Mather Hospital. This bunkroom contains two bunk beds with futons set up underneath, several TV trays, and a television. Crews are actively discouraged from using the crew room at the Mather during the day. Dispatchers will monitor their location and ask providers to "centralize" or post in particular parts of the city if they notice an ambulance lingering at the Mather hospital during the day. The exception is Sundays, when the atmosphere is more laid back, and providers will often spend the day lounging at the Mather, watching TV marathons or movies.

Learning Chapman from the Ambulance Cab

Most of the providers at Private Ambulance I interacted with came to know Chapman from the cab of their ambulances. Of the thirty providers I interviewed during the primary data collection phase in 2013 and 2014, most had never lived in Chapman (70 percent). A smaller majority (57 percent) had no familiarity with the city before working at Private Ambulance. For many providers, the deeper knowledge they gained through this work was the root of their mixed views about the city as a whole:

> BEN: It's a . . . I used to think it was a lot bigger of a place when I would come here to visit, the city was overwhelming, like "Oh my god, I'm in the city," getting on and off the [Regional Transit] like it was kind of overwhelming. I really felt like I was in the city. Now knowing it as well as I do, it just feels like a town. It doesn't feel big anymore. It's not intimidating anymore. . . . So in that sense I guess it's a positive and negative. I've learned a lot about the city, but a lot of the luster is gone. You see it for kind of what it is. The groups of people in certain

areas and it's just it's not as magical as what it was when you visit it as an outsider. And now I feel like I'm on the inside.

For Ben and other providers at Private Ambulance, seeing the city "for what it is" meant opening their eyes to the social problems endemic in Chapman and other cities, including substance use, violence, and poverty. It also meant the daily exposure to wealth and privilege that far exceeded the providers' circumstances.

New hires at Private Ambulance go through a field training program where they ride with more experienced providers. There is much to learn. For example, starting an IV or doing CPR in the classroom is one thing. Doing both in the back of a moving ambulance is another thing entirely. Aside from clinical skills, they also need to learn how to drive an emergency vehicle. Emergency medical technician or paramedic classes, which focus on clinical preparation, do not teach driving skills. Even if there is some basic training, providers need to acquire experience driving with their emergency lights and sirens activated. They also must learn to multi-task, since responding to emergencies requires driving as well as listening to their radio and navigating unfamiliar streets. Providers learn the quickest ways to major hospitals, where the best places to eat and spend downtime are, and what streets to avoid at certain times of the day. Learning the city, therefore, has a tactile feel. Longtime employees are not unlike London cabbies, who can navigate to and from emergency calls using just their memory of the street grid.

The exposure providers have to Chapman through the ambulance cab is not about generating that practical knowledge. Instead, they also develop perceptions of neighborhoods and the city itself. Asked to describe the city, Preston called it "a unique place." He continued, saying that:

> It's diverse. . . . We have some pretty substantial affluence mixed with some legitimate poverty . . . and everything in between. Umm very liberal city, very, you know now I wouldn't say hippy but it's certainly not the conservative place to be. But it's interesting. You meet a very wide-ranging group of people.

Other providers concurred with this perspective. They routinely discussed "diversity," as Preston did, in terms of the socioeconomic variation of the city and specifically in terms of particular neighborhoods as "poorer" or "wealthier." For example, one provider noted that the city Chapman is "diverse . . . could be, you can be in low-income housing one call, you could be in a shelter another call, or you could be in a mansion at another call up off of [Muir] Street [in the wealthier area of West Chapman] . . . so it's diverse." The socioeconomic diversity these providers identified presented both an interesting and sometimes challenging work environment.

Providers identified socioeconomic diversity as a particular challenge because it had consequences for the types of calls they experienced on their shifts and their interactions with bystanders and other members of the public. One downside providers expressed was a perceived entitlement or privilege among upper-class residents of the city.

> Pam: And I think a lot of people like to hear themselves talk in [Chapman]. . . . I think there's a lot of privileged people in [Chapman] and that's good and bad . . . lately with people being so nasty about where we're parking and everything [it] is definitely annoying. [And] there's a lot of physicians in [Chapman]. And they're not trained in anything emergency. So it's like they're like "give them Haldol." And it's like I don't have Haldol. Get away from me, you know what I mean?
>
> Cp: So these are physicians not that are part of the call necessarily?
>
> Pam: No. They're like they're bystanders or they're callers. And they mean well. I know they mean well, but it's definitely annoying. And you have to kind of be like, okay, thank you, sir, like we have this. Like I do this every day and a hundred times a day.

Like Pam, providers described Chapman's more affluent residents in largely disparaging terms. In particular, the providers singled them out as individuals who often did not understand the role of EMS providers, who interfered with patient care (despite their good intentions) or were confused about why ambulances are parking in certain parts of the city. This privilege, some providers believed, also meant that there were class differences in who accessed the EMS system:

> Jeffrey: There's a lot of different, broad spectrum of patients. . . . Students, because of [the] schools here. A lot of homeless people. Good amount of drugs, is all mixed in, some violence, a lot of rich people, too. But most of the time, you don't really see the rich people until they get really sick . . . because they can actually, know what they need to do. They have the right health care. They can go see a doctor and get it treated. But usually when you're finding the upper-class people, they're really sick and they need an ambulance.

Another provider concurred, stating that in Chapman, "you have the lowest of the lows and you have the highest of the highs. Like you'll have your [wet shelter] population, then you have your [Muir Street] population, which is like gorgeous, these million-dollar homes. So the spread of wealth in the city is huge." This association with social class and the EMS system is essential because many of the providers focused their attention during the interviews, as Jeffrey did, on patients who lived in public housing or who were homeless.

Institutions as Mediating Forces in Subjective Views of Place

The experience of most providers was that they learned how to negotiate Chapman from the cab on their ambulance after they began to work at Private Ambulance. Many learn about Chapman for the first time on the job, sitting in the cab of the ambulance as they roam the city in search of call locations, bathrooms, and easy parking for meals. For the minority of providers who know Chapman as a city on its terms, there is still a learning experience of the best driving routes and downtime locations for their specific institutional role. As we see in the opening vignette, knowing where to get breakfast, how to park there, who has the most desirable coffee, and where other first responders may be is all part of the spatial knowledge providers develop on the job. Even if you know the city generally, these are still institutionally specific sets of knowledge that providers adopt.

As we contemplate where neighborhood frames and stigmas originate, institutional actors do not often appear in our frameworks. However, at Private Ambulance, the instrumental work of EMS providers is inexorably linked to these understandings of place. Over time, they take these accumulated on-the-job experiences and use them to inform how they see their work:

> I asked Tim about seeing the [homeless] patient before. He said that he saw him a few weeks ago for the same reason but thought that he hadn't been "on the scene" very long. He noted that they didn't go to those types of patients very often in [Uptown]. He also noted that they see many of those patients in East [Chapman] and [Midtown], which are the most "inner city"; West [Chapman] is where the "money" is.

As they spatialize descriptions of their work, providers attach meaning to different neighborhoods and definitions of these neighborhoods themselves. In other words, they "see" the city in particular ways that we cannot separate from their clinical experiences. Their understandings of place, for example, revolve around a version of Chapman's geography that is, to a degree, unique to their institutional role. Places like "Midtown" are not official neighborhoods, for example. Instead, providers and other first responders give them meaning through their experiences responding to calls there.

Developing these mental frameworks is not the end game, however. Providers turn around to each other, other first responders, and other health-care providers and tell stories about the city to them. At Private's headquarters, in the ambulance, over meals, and in a dozen other places, storytelling is a vital part of how EMS providers relate to one another. Downtime often revolved around reminding each other of calls from yesterday, a prior week, or even long ago if the call was especially noteworthy. Telling stories about a place is just one variant of this practice. At hospitals, too, when providers transfer care, they include where the patient "was found" when they arrived on-scene. Through the specific medium of transferring care, they paint a picture of place for emergency department staff who otherwise exist in a windowless, fluorescent island for their shifts.

How EMS providers see the city, then, matters not only for their views but how they undertake their jobs. Thus, to understand EMS work and its relationship with place, we need to understand EMS's institutional location in the worlds of health care and first-responder work. In addition, understanding EMS work itself, its rhythms, the necessity of downtime, what life is like in the cab of that ambulance, and how providers understand emergency work, is also essential for developing a sense of how providers "see" the city. Marginality characterizes EMS work in each of these venues. In each subsequent chapter, we will revisit this topic to develop a sense of providers' relationships with urban space.

PART I
EMS as a Marginal Institution

The woman, "Loraine," had been crossing the street at a crosswalk in Chapman after leaving work. As she entered the crosswalk, she did not see a cyclist hurtling toward her until they collided. By the time Medic 1 arrived on-scene, both the woman and the cyclist had moved to the sidewalk. Andy parked the ambulance facing the wrong way against traffic, and he and his partner moved the woman onto a board EMS providers use to protect a patient's spine. Once Andy had placed the woman onto the ambulance's cot and moved into the patient compartment, it became clear that Loraine had retrograde amnesia, a condition caused by a traumatic event where short-term memory capacity is lost. Andy, concerned she had a head injury, asked his partner to quickly head for the trauma center.

These types of injuries are what Emergency Medical Services (EMS) providers call "real emergencies." They are what we imagine when we think of the role that the EMS system plays in the United States and elsewhere. However, many calls do not involve such acute patients. Moreover, the patients, first responders, and health-care providers that EMTs and paramedics work with regularly often misunderstand the clinical capacity of EMS providers. Providers must, therefore, negotiate and renegotiate their role in American health care on a call-by-call, shift-by-shift basis. This misrecognition and the emotional labor that providers must engage in to correct it are consequences of the EMS system's institutional marginality. Part I explores this marginality, first by exploring the idea of "real emergencies" and then through the lens of negotiation. These are common themes in the literature on EMS—and critically important ones—that are essential to understanding contemporary EMS work and ultimately how providers view urban life.

1
Dial 9-1-1 for Emergencies

"So in my mind, I think it is a poor use of the system." (Andrea)

Jello Molds

On a crisp, clear fall night in Chapman in a crowded performance space on a university campus, a performance was wrapping up. The opulently decorated performance hall had waist-high, richly stained decorative millwork on the walls. As the performance ended and the attendees filtered out, "Irina" tripped and fell to the floor, her forehead glancing off the millwork. The resulting gash in her head began immediately to bleed profusely. The staff rushed to her aid, finding towels and calling 9-1-1.

Meanwhile, the crew of Medic 11 was in Midtown, where Sanders had parked so he could meet up with his girlfriend, who was a nurse and was out with some friends drinking at a bar in the neighborhood. Miles turned the radio to hardcore rock and worked on run reports from prior calls on the ambulance's laptop while they waited for Sam's girlfriend to arrive. We all paused what we were doing when Medic 6 passed us, driving with its lights and sirens on through Midtown. When Sam's girlfriend arrived, they spoke with her about what bars she had been to and the calls we had been on so far that night. After a few minutes, she and her friends left for their next bar, and Sanders pulled the ambulance out to head up to the Old Quarter.

As we drove, Miles called his dispatcher to request an ambulance meet us with additional spinal immobilization supplies, since we were running low. Medic 6, who had passed us in Midtown a few minutes ago but was already back "in-service," was sent to meet us. We arrived to find Irina sitting in a chair near the front door, bleeding profusely. A university police officer was helping hold a towel to her head, and there was blood pooled in several places on the floor. Sanders and Miles went to work, trying to inspect the wound, but the volume of blood was so great they could not see the gash through Irina's matted hair.

With Medic 6's help, Sanders and Miles placed Irina on a backboard (used to keep a patient's spine safe when it might be injured). As they secured her head, their gloved hands came back coated in blood, which visibly stressed out one of Medic 6's paramedics. As we drove to the hospital, blood began to pool under the cot on the passenger side of the ambulance, where I was sitting on the bench seat. Miles handed me towels to place under the backboard and catch the blood and asked Sanders to call in a "trauma alert" so the Benton General Hospital staff were ready for our arrival.

When we arrived at the hospital, the triage nurses directed us immediately back to a trauma bay, where several doctors and nurses helped us move Irina to a hospital bed. When they slid the backboard over to the bed, several large blood clots were left behind. During the drive, blood had collected and clotted in the backboard's handles. The handles acted like a Jello mold, leaving congealed, dark red blood clots sitting on the cot, jiggling ever so slightly. As several senior attending physicians and a group of residents gathered around, one doctor removed the last bandage Sanders and Miles had applied. A spurt of blood traveled in an arc across the room, confirming the presence of an arterial bleed that the assembled trauma team worked to clear. This type of trauma injury was a serious threat to the patient's life (a "real emergency"), but also a textbook "good call," though not a particularly fun one to clean up the ambulance afterward; blood had spread throughout the back of the truck during our drive to the hospital.

The "Ultimate Patient"

Earlier in our shift, after another ambulance crew had brought me down to the Old Quarter to meet Medic 11, we were dispatched for the report of "difficulty breathing" for a female patient. When the call came in, Sanders became visibly angry. He told Miles and me that he thought the patient would be "Kathy" because of the reported age and the call's location. Sanders was angry that they were the crew assigned by the dispatcher to treat her. We arrived on-scene after a quick drive down to Midtown and met one of the Chapman Fire Department medic units, who was outside with the patient. Sanders was right. The patient was Kathy, just as he predicted.

Miles did not exit the driver's seat but rolled down the window and chatted with the firefighters while Sanders got out and ushered Kathy into the ambulance.

She jumped into the airway seat behind the cot and buckled her seatbelt immediately. Sanders asked her, "What is going on today?," and confirmed that she was reporting trouble breathing. He also asked if she had anything to drink that morning. Sanders identified signs of intoxication as Kathy kept asking Sanders for oxygen through her nose (apparently asking for a nasal cannula). Sanders tried to give her an oxygen mask, telling her, "It will be more fun" to use the mask. Kathy asked for oxygen only through her nose again, and Sanders laughed, opening a package containing a nasal cannula. She grabbed it from him, put it on correctly herself, and asked for the oxygen to be set to two, which was the correct dosage for that delivery route. Miles turned around and shouted, "Are you serious?" through the doorway. Sanders laughed again, turned the oxygen on, and checked Kathy's blood sugar as Miles drove to the hospital.

When we arrived at the Mather Hospital's ambulance bay, Miles found a wheelchair and helped Kathy into it while admonishing her. "It is too early to be seeing you," he told her, continuing that "if I have to see you again today, I'm going to be very upset." The nurses directed us to "the tank," a room in the ED reserved for patients who are intoxicated as well as patients who the hospital staff believe to be street homeless. The nurses asked Miles and Sanders about where they found Kathy, and they all laughed about her ability to put the nasal cannula into her nose correctly.

After Sanders and Miles transferred care to the nurses, I followed Miles to get Kathy registered. The staff member asked us why the patient was here, which was a standard question. Sanders replied that it was for intoxication and added that he was giving intoxication as the chief complaint to avoid getting into trouble "for not working up the most frequent of frequent fliers."[1] He paused, turned to me, and said, "That would suck." On the way back past the nurses' station, Sanders grabbed a sticker for pediatric patients that says, "ultimate patient," and has a Spiderman cartoon on it. Sanders gave the sticker to Kathy before we went back to the ambulance, where Miles was waiting for us.

Emergency Medical Services in the United States

The different ways Sanders and Miles responded to these two calls, one quite serious and the other that they immediately dismissed based on the gender, age, and location of the patient, speaks volumes about the state of EMS care in the United States. The call for the fall was a "real emergency" while the "ultimate patient" call was treated as what providers describe as "bullshit." This distinction in the worthiness of each patient reflects the broader EMS's systems priorities and the vision its providers have about what their jobs should entail.

What we recognize today as pre-hospital medicine had its roots in a relatively recent series of developments. The modern EMS system emerged during the 1960s in response to a growing recognition that automobile deaths and cardiac arrest were both glaring and preventable causes of morbidity and mortality (Institute of Medicine 2007; Pozner et al. 2004; Zink 2005). Whereas organized firefighting in the United States dates to the colonial era and modern policing dates from the early nineteenth century (Greenberg 2016; Monkkonen 2004), EMS is a far younger institution, preceded by nearly a century of ambulance services unable to do more than offer patients transport to a hospital. The fact that EMS developed well over a century after organized policing and firefighting in the United States, in vastly different social and policy environments, is critical for understanding the EMS system's own institutional marginality.

EMS prior to 1945

What we recognize today as pre-hospital medicine had its roots in the French *ambulance volant* of the late eighteenth century. Amidst the carnage of the Reign of Terror during the French Revolution, a Frenchman named Baron Dominique-Jean Larrey surveyed the dismal state of battlefield medicine and set out designing a new approach for treating wounded soldiers (Shah 2006). Instead of leaving the wounded, writhing in pain and soaked in blood, to rot on the battlefield, a system of wagons staffed by medical personnel would ferry the wounded to field hospitals (Pozner et al. 2004). Larrey called these *ambulance volant* ("flying ambulance"), units of over three hundred men supervised by a surgeon who would follow advancing infantry into battle (Haller 1990, 2011). This effort to stem the consequences of the carnage wrought on the French people by other French citizens marks the beginning of another era in human history, one in which we recognized we could save lives if only we had a way to get the wounded, sick, and dying to a hospital capable of providing long-term care for them.

The birth of EMS as an outgrowth of military necessity is unsurprising, given the wider social upheaval violent conflict can bring to societies. That the first role of the ambulance was to treat critically injured soldiers is essential not only as a historical fact but also because it prefigured what EMS would become. These soldiers, gravely wounded, became the first archetype of the deserving patient. The *ambulance volant* was not created for the people, broadly defined, but for those who had sacrificed themselves for France. This notion of deservingness rooted in the experience of the French Revolution remains as a critical tension for the EMS system. The adaption of this outlook on battlefield medicine in America was slow, however. Before the initial battles of the American Civil War, there was little in the way of medical organization in the American army. During the Mexican American War in the 1840s, seven times the number of soldiers died of disease as did those injured in battle. By the winter of 1861, when the American Civil War broke out, only a hundred or so surgeons were employed by the Medical Corps. Generals in both armies quickly recognized that they were overwhelmingly unprepared for the coming onslaught. The first battles between the two sides saw erratically organized wagon services designated to transport the wounded off the battlefield. Baron Larrey's *ambulance volant* inspired these efforts, but the governments in Washington and Richmond did not offer resources to support them early in the war (Pozner et al. 2004).

After tragedies like the Second Battle of Bull Run fought in Manassas, Virginia, just over a year after the war began, thousands of Union soldiers were left wounded on the battlefield for days. Fearing this result contributed to higher mortality rates than necessary, a Union major named Jonathan Letterman established a new system for ferrying the wounded off the battlefield based on Larrey's principles. This time, with the backing of the Union command, Maj. Letterman's efforts yielded real results and were eventually applied in other Union armies, as well (Haller 1990, 2011; Pozner et al. 2004). The ambulances of this era were sparse and utilitarian. They were often open-air wagons, like the Zouave ambulance pictured in Figure 4. Their singular purpose, like Larrey's flying ambulances of the 1790s, was to ferry wounded soldiers to field hospitals where field surgeons could give them care (Pozner et al. 2004).

After the war's conclusion, civilian organizations translated these military practices into the first municipal ambulance services in Cincinnati (1865) and New York City (1869) (Pozner et al. 2004). These first civilian services had the same goal of transporting citizens to hospitals without providing care to the sick or injured patient in the back of the wagon. Seventy years later, little had changed. Local ambulance assistance had, by the eve of the Second World War, propagated throughout the United States' cities and many of its suburbs.

However, local funeral homes operated more than half of these services. Like their nineteenth-century predecessors, the local ambulances were still staffed by attendants who lacked even basic first aid training (Pozner et al. 2004, 240). Many funeral homes did not have separate ambulance vehicles, opting as they did in Mound Bayou, Mississippi (see Figure 5), to have hearses double as ambulances when there was a need to transport a live patient instead of a departed community member. For many other communities, it was law enforcement that provided first aid and transportation (Edwards 2019).

For the early history of the ambulance in the United States, which we associate today with medical care, they were essentially demedicalized transport

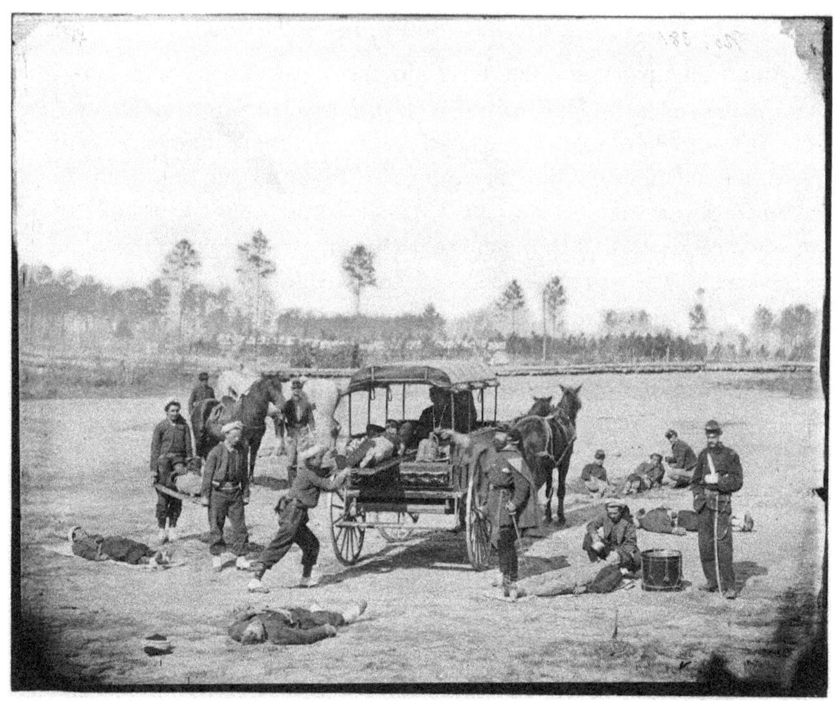

Figure 4. Union Army Zouave Ambulance Wagon during the American Civil War (Library of Congress; photographer unknown)

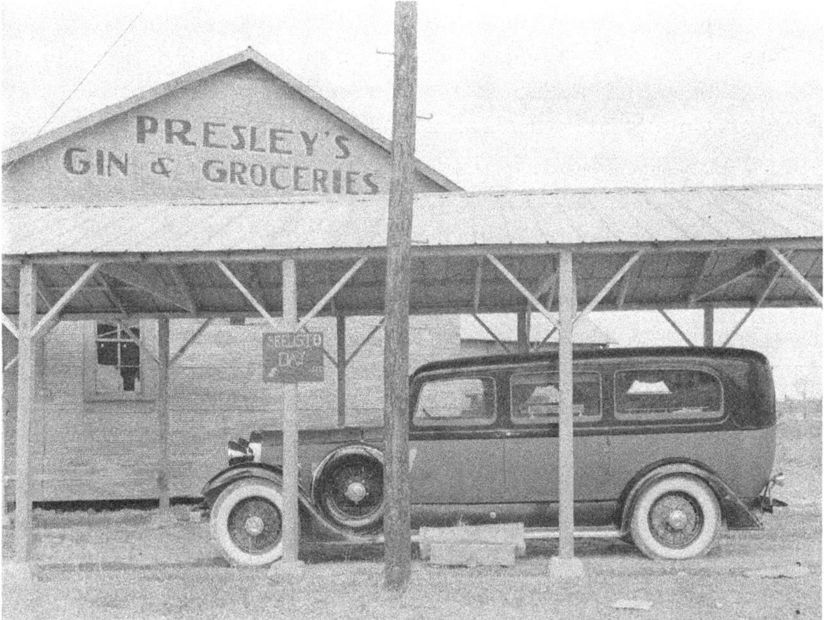

Figure 5. Funeral Home Ambulance in Mound Bayou, Mississippi (Library of Congress; photo by Russell Lee)

services. This suited a time period when a parallel set of services existed for many Americans to receive care in their homes. Before the Second World War broke out, an estimated 75 percent of physicians described themselves as general practitioners (Zink 2005). These "GPs," as they were known, were the front line of American medicine. Not only did they run a practice with regular hours and often maintain privileges at a local hospital, but they were available after hours, as well. As one physician from Michigan described it, "Nothing about medicine is as impressive to the layman as our willingness to get up and go out at midnight" (Zink 2005, 5). This twenty-four-hour commitment meant that ambulance services did not need to fill the same role they do today.

EMS between 1945 and 1966

On September 2, 1945, a delegation of Japanese officials boarded the battleship USS *Missouri*, then moored in Tokyo Bay, to formally surrender to the United States. Like the French Revolution 150 years prior and the American Civil War just eighty years beforehand, World War II would fundamentally reshape American medicine and emergency medical services. Physicians returning from military service, along with their newly minted colleagues, began to shift away from providing the always-on-call hours that had been the hallmark of prewar GPs: "The traditional family doctor was under siege and found he could not be a 24-hour-a-day, 7-days-a-week, 365-days-a-year bonesetter and pill roller to the thousands who rang his office phone" (Zink 2005, 5).

The allure of specialty work and its increasing financial rewards drew more significant numbers of young doctors away from general practice each year. Younger physicians were less inclined to go into general practice. By the mid-1960s, only 31 percent of physicians would do the work of the general practitioner. Many of those remaining GPs were less willing to make themselves available after hours, with many preferring to spend their increasing postwar pay on leisure activities instead (Zink 2005).

At the same time as American cities, towns, and villages steadily began to lose general practitioners, American medicine was also changing. More than a third of American physicians in practice in 1944 were in the army and the navy, and they returned to the American home front fresh from experiences in a vastly improved combat medicine system. Mortality rates for American soldiers were halved compared to World War I, driven by advances in both trauma care and the treatment of infectious diseases. A more integrated system of triaging, evacuating, and ultimately treating wounded soldiers also helped reduce the mortality rate among soldiers (Zink 2005, 7–8). These physicians were uniquely suited for a postwar society where traumatic injury would become a leading cause of death.

However, these lessons in battlefield medicine that evolved during World War II and the Korean War were slow to filter down to the civilian Emergency Medical Services. Physicians began to develop and staff emergency rooms in their hospitals, but these were small at first, often literally just a single room (Zink 2005). It would take American medicine until the early 1960s to begin to realize the evolution needed in pre-hospital medical care:

> In 1960, only 6 states had standard courses for rescuers, only 4 states regulated ambulance design specifications, and fewer than half of all EMS personnel had received even minimal training (e.g., American Red Cross first aid). A survey of 900 cities in 1965 found that only 23% regulated EMS service, and only 8% reported advanced EMS medical training, such as the American Red Cross advanced first aid course. (Shah 2006)

Meanwhile, physicians embroiled in yet another violent conflict, this time in Vietnam, quickly realized just how advanced military medicine had become relative to civilian trauma care: "We used to say that getting shot in Vietnam was like getting shot on the steps of the hospital. You could actually be in surgery in 20 minutes in a lot of these places" (Zink 2005, 68). That battlefield casualties in Southeast Asia had better access to care than many Americans back home underscored a need for evolution and was the first of three critical shifts during this era.

Importantly, this rapid access to trauma care was needed in the U.S. more than ever. Traumatic injuries were the leading cause of death for young Americans (Institute of Medicine 2007, 32–33), and automobiles were the leading cause of traumatic deaths—nearly 46 percent of the traumatic deaths in 1965 were caused by motor vehicle collisions. Rapid trauma care was not an abstract desire therefore, but an immediate necessity, painted as an "epidemic" by the National Academy of Sciences in their landmark 1966 report *Accidental Death and Disability* (Shock 1966). The recognition that American roads were taking a significant number of young lives each year spurred a second movement, particularly at the highest levels of American government, to address both road safety and the lack of trauma care available in many American communities.

The growing recognition of traffic safety's paramount importance and the reality that the nation's health-care system was not equipped to respond to this crisis spurred the Johnson administration to form the President's Committee for Traffic Safety. Its 1965 report *Health, Medical Care and Transportation of the Injured* (Safety 1965), combined with *Accidental Death and Disability* a year later (Shock 1966), suggested that systematic changes were needed. There were few standardized ways for constructing, outfitting, and staffing ambulances in the United States, and both reports identified these deficiencies as priorities for policymakers to address.

EMS after 1966

In the years immediately following the publication of *Accidental Death and Disability*, a movement began to develop around the state-level organization of EMS services. The Highway Safety Act of 1966, given the focus and attention of motor vehicle accidents, provided a major source of funding to build new EMS agencies as well as a bureaucratic apparatus for overseeing them. The focus on traffic safety meant that the task of developing the first educational curriculum for EMS providers would fall to the National Highway Transportation Safety Administration (NHTSA). The primary curriculum NHTSA developed was a seventy-hour training program for the nation's first official emergency medical technicians. Millions of dollars were allotted to states to develop programs for implementing this curriculum as well as to create standards for how ambulances should be built and supplied (Institute of Medicine 2007; Pozner et al. 2004).

Since the focus remained on traffic safety, it was left to the federal Department of Transportation to disperse the funds, giving the DOT a significant role in the early development of Emergency Medical Services in the United States. The natural federal agency to lead this effort, the Department of Health, Education, and Welfare (DHEW), was slow to insert itself into these early efforts (Zink 2005). Both the American Medical Association and the National Academy of Sciences also formed their standing committees on Emergency Medical Services, but it would remain the DOT's prerogative to lead much of the development of pre-hospital medicine.

The DHEW's high point of EMS involvement would come in 1973 when Congress passed the EMS Systems Act. This legislation gave DHEW access to $300 million in funds (equivalent to nearly $1.8 billion in 2018 dollars) to expand American's EMS system. These funds were used to expand elements of the system, including training, medical direction, planning, and the establishment of interagency cooperation agreements known as "mutual aid." These gave agencies access to additional resources, whether they were guidance from physicians in the form of medical direction or additional ambulances at a severe incident through the new mutual aid agreements put in place with these funds (Institute of Medicine 2007, 34).

The EMS System Act, however, created a wedge in federal involvement. The Department of Transportation remained in control of setting federal training guidelines, while the DHEW controlled the disbursement of funding for implementation in local communities. The act also oriented federal involvement narrowly on these communities (Institute of Medicine 2007, 34). While it did encourage interagency collaboration, the organization of EMS systems was primarily left to local efforts, meaning these developments were "driven by local needs, characteristics, and concerns" (Institute of Medicine 2007, 34). At both the local and federal levels, then, the EMS system began to be defined by its balkanization and patchwork nature.

At its outset, the clinical care this system provided was also limited. The early focus on trauma care did not embrace the new efforts to develop techniques for managing cardiac events in patients. The efforts to develop resuscitation techniques began in the 1960s with evaluations of what was called "external chest message." These efforts would evolve into cardiopulmonary resuscitation, or "CPR," well before the passage of the landmark EMS legislation in 1966 (Timmermans 2010). Out-of-hospital defibrillation also began to be tested before the legislation but was similarly not included (Pozner et al. 2004).

However, separate developments were occurring that would bring cardiac care into the fold of EMS work within a few years. First, President Lyndon Johnson spurred the development of Regional Medical Programs (RMPs) designed to address poor cardiac, stroke, and cancer outcomes (Shah 2006). While these were not specific to EMS care, the RMPs were instrumental in creating the initial workforce of EMS providers. They were used to train some of the initial emergency medical technicians and played a role in piloting some of the first Advanced Life Support care in the United States. In 1965 in Belfast, Northern Ireland, a cardiologist began staffing a mobile coronary-care unit (MCCU) and first reported it the next year (Pantridge and Geddes 1967). However, a physician was required to be present in these first MCCU ambulances. This service resulted in declining mortality for patients experiencing cardiac arrest in Belfast, and physicians began piloting it in Columbus, Ohio, Seattle, Washington, and New York City (Shah 2006). The Seattle program, named "Medic 1," was made possible by RMP funding.

Finally, physicians in Pittsburgh, Pennsylvania, dismayed with the lack of response the police-run ambulance service had for neighborhoods that Black residents were segregated into, began offering paramedic courses to residents of those neighborhoods. The result was the Freedom House Ambulance Service, which showed that with purposeful though limited training, paramedics could effectively deliver patient care in the community. Though Freedom House Ambulance itself was short-lived and eventually was subsumed into a wider EMS service for Pittsburgh, its first medics helped pave the way for future generations of providers (Edwards 2019).

All these projects demonstrated the abilities of EMS providers to deliver advanced clinical care pre-hospitally and laid the groundwork for the eventual introduction of paramedics as a formal piece of EMS care throughout the United States. The early history of EMS in the United States is one of development in dialogue with what Whalley and Barley (1997) described as the "amateur trappings" of its past. Despite now having an official curriculum for education and an official mandate at the federal level, the first ambulance providers were not trained to implement some of the most cutting-edge interventions like CPR. Even when EMS providers were trained to more advanced levels, physicians were slow to relinquish direct oversight over the provision of care.

EMS Today

EMS Oversight Today

These oversight and clinical divisions represent critical junctures for understanding the position of Emergency Medical Services today. The National Academy of Sciences heavily criticized DHEW's role in the oversight of EMS in a 1978 report, and by 1981 all interagency cooperation between DHEW and the Department of Transportation ceased, along with the funds allocated originally by the EMS System Act in 1973. The Department of Transportation was nominally left in charge of federal EMS policy but lacked the funding to support the local implementation of its efforts. EMS policy at the federal level, then, lacked significant recognition and funding and was left to what in hindsight looks like the least likely candidate, the Department of Transportation. This distinction at the federal level remains intact. The same federal agency in charge of keeping America's highways, airports, railways, and ports running also oversees all federal policy oriented toward pre-hospital medicine.

At the same time, the Department of Health and Human Services (HHS), assisted by the surgeon general, oversees much of the rest of the formal health-care system. HHS also oversees the Centers for Disease Control and the other aspects of the federal public-health system. Even the troubled Indian Health Service has been within what is now HHS since 1955, the year after Congress acted through the 1954 Transfer Act to separate indigenous health services from the Bureau of Indian Affairs (Bergman et al. 1999). The EMS system, therefore, remains separated from the near entirety of the federal apparatus for setting civilian health-care and public-health policy.

The EMS system is also managed separately from the rest of the public-safety apparatus. The United States Fire Administration, a division of the Federal

Emergency Management Agency, which itself falls under the U.S. Department of Homeland Security, oversees all federal policy for the nation's fire services. Reports by the U.S. Department of Transportation in 1966 and the Institute of Medicine (IOM) in 2007 both lamented the isolation the EMS system experienced from the rest of the public-health, public-safety, and health-care systems. The IOM characterized the current state of this relationship by noting that "local EMS systems are not well integrated with any of these groups and therefore receive inadequate support from each of them. As a result, EMS has a foot in many doors, but no clear home" (Institute of Medicine 2007, xx).

The lack of a distinct policy home has, therefore, meant that other groups have had to become the policy leaders for the nation's EMS agencies. In particular, it is leadership at the state level that most directly affects the operation of the EMS system today. Beginning in 1981 with the defunding of federal EMS policy initiatives, it would be states and sometimes regions within them who would assume the mantle of oversight for the growing patchwork of EMS agencies. Some states mirrored the federal government and placed EMS oversight within state-level departments of transportation while others placed EMS offices within their public-health apparatus. However, even in these states where policymakers positioned EMS as a part of the public-health system, the prevailing experience was one of isolation. Surveying the state of EMS in 2007, the IOM argued distressingly:

> EMS is widely viewed as an essential public service, but it has not been supported through effective federal and state leadership and sustainable funding strategies. Unlike other such services—electricity, highways, airports, and telephone service, for example—all of which were created and are actively maintained through major national infrastructure investments, access to timely and high-quality emergency and trauma care has largely been relegated to local and state initiatives. As a result, EMS care remains extremely uneven across the United States. (Institute of Medicine 2007, xx)

The patchwork nature of EMS care, first identified in the 1970s, therefore remains the reality in the United States. There are often at least four and sometimes five layers of oversight within states, including state EMS offices, regional EMS authorities, county and municipal governments, and hospitals (NHTSA 2013). Tribal authorities also oversee the provision of EMS care on reservations. Across many of these jurisdictions, EMS services are not always treated as an "essential service." As of 2021, just eleven states have legal provisions requiring municipalities to offer EMS services just as they do with fire and police services. While we often talk about the "EMS system," this remains a distinct aspiration for pre-hospital medicine in the United States. It is not one system, but many, and a legally optional one at that.

EMS Service Delivery Today

This unevenness is reinforced not just by the contradictions in how EMS is managed institutionally but also by the variation in EMS service delivery models. In many communities, like Chapman, a multi-jurisdictional approach to emergency medicine has been established. Most fire departments have some type of emergency medical services component, such as cross-training firefighters as emergency medical technicians or paramedics, and some police departments have incentivized their members to obtain EMS training, as well. These individuals are then dispatched to emergency medical calls ahead of ambulances and can provide stabilizing care until the transporting unit arrives. For these departments, EMS calls are now most of their work. One 2005 estimate found that 80 percent of fire department responses nationwide were for EMS incidents (Institute of Medicine 2007, 57).

Some areas are also served by "tiered response" systems where Advanced Life Support paramedic services are provided at a regional level to augment the local fire department and Basic Life Support transport resources (Nichol et al. 1996). In such tiered systems, there may be four or more agencies ultimately dispatched to a call: the local police department, the local fire department, a Basic Life Support ambulance providing transport, and a paramedic from the Advanced Life Support system.

For the transport portion of the EMS system, the actual providing of ambulance services as the public typically conceives them are effectively four models. Fire departments likely constitute a plurality of EMS systems (representative national numbers are notoriously difficult to come by). In many instances, this arrangement means fire departments offer both first-responder services and the EMS transports themselves. Fire-based EMS can be found both in small, rural volunteer departments and in large urban fire departments like those in New York City, Washington, D.C., St. Louis, and Los Angeles. Despite being most of these agencies' calls, EMS is often treated as a second-class citizen within these departments, with lower pay, smaller budgets, and a secondary focus on training (Institute of Medicine 2007, 56–58).

Another model for providing service are non-fire municipal services. These are public EMS agencies that are not formally part of the fire department. Instead, they offer EMS services on their own but often in conjunction with fire-based first responders who have received either mandatory or voluntary EMS training. Cities like Boston and New Orleans, for example, operate these

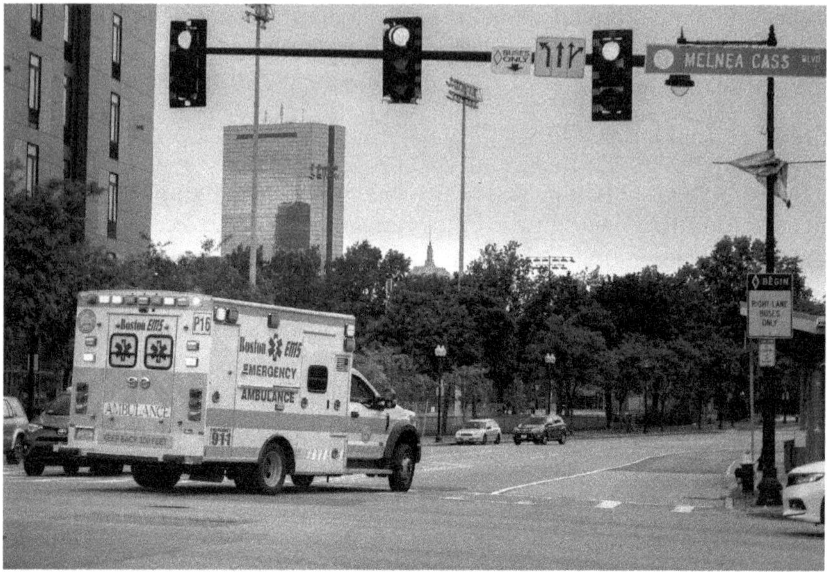

Figure 6. Boston EMS Ambulance (photo by Yassine Khalfalli)

public municipal EMS agencies (see Figure 6). They are often referred to as "third service" models, with the fire service and law enforcement being the other two first-responder services (Gresham 1994; Pozner et al. 2004), and likely account for less than 10 percent of systems (Institute of Medicine 2007, 56–58).

A third model is for hospital-based EMS systems. Some hospital systems, like New York's Presbyterian Hospital system, offer their own EMS transport services to surrounding communities. These likely account for less than 10 percent of systems nationwide (Institute of Medicine 2007, 56–58). In New York City, hospital-based systems take responsibility for responding to 9-1-1 calls in the neighborhoods immediately adjacent to their facilities. In other parts of the country, such as Southwestern Missouri, hospital-based systems cover much larger geographies.

A fourth and final dominant model for delivering EMS services is via a private company. This model is especially present in two contexts. In perhaps 35 percent of systems, private companies provide the 9-1-1 responses just as either a fire department, a non-fire municipal service, or a hospital-based system would handle them (Institute of Medicine 2007, 56–58). Private companies also play a significant role in communities that have one of the first three modalities for providing emergency responses. In those communities, health-care facilities, nursing homes, and other institutions contract with private companies to provide facility-specific emergency responses. Private EMS companies also provide nonemergency transports between hospitals and from hospitals to patients' homes, two services that fire departments and non-fire municipal services do not typically offer.

These models, therefore, coexist in several ways. Different service modalities may serve adjacent communities, and a community may have multiple private companies serving its nonemergency transport needs as well as providing emergency responses to local nursing homes and rehabilitation facilities. These private companies also provide "mutual aid," ensuring that emergency medical providers are available for responses during particularly busy periods or shift changes. There is also a considerable amount of regional variation in how these systems are structured. States like California are, for example, dominated by large, county-wide systems with a private company working with a single county-wide fire department.[2] EMS services elsewhere, in contrast, may be dominated by the local fire department and ambulance districts covering only a single town. Counties may therefore have dozens of fire departments and EMS agencies.

Finally, it is vital to recognize the role volunteers play in helping fire-based and third-service agencies operate. Volunteers make up a significant number of providers throughout the United States, though the exact number is not known. Many EMS agencies that once relied on volunteers have transitioned in two ways to declining numbers of volunteers. They have both begun to hire career personnel to supplement volunteers, particularly during the day, and to financially compensate volunteers for the number of calls or the number of hours they serve (Institute of Medicine 2007).

EMS Care Today

Providers at this study's field site, Private Ambulance, were fond of describing their care by noting that they could provide the same level of care that would be available in the first thirty minutes at a hospital's emergency department. Ray, a relatively new paramedic at Private Ambulance, described EMS work in the following way:

> My job, as a Paramedic, is to extend the capabilities of emergency room care to the scene for a patient who requires urgent, on-scene care. I have most of their capabilities that they can do in the first thirty minutes. . . . I can do [as well]. What I do not have is imaging, so I have to use my physical exam and the few tools that I have to make a differential diagnosis and treat the patient accordingly.

When compared to emergency medicine before the 1960s, this is a night-versus-day–like transformation. The words Ray uses to describe his work are highly clinical—"differential diagnosis," for example—and he is proud of the advanced set of clinical capabilities.

The expanding role of paramedics has had much to do with this capability. The EMS care delivered to patients occurs at two broad levels: Basic Life Support (BLS) and Advanced Life Support (ALS). Thomas, a paramedic instructor at Private Ambulance, describes the distinction between these two levels of training:

> If I was to describe it to a layperson . . . I usually describe the difference between an EMT and a Paramedic is that . . . Paramedics provide Basic Life Support just like EMTs do, but we can also administer medications, we can also start IVs. I tell the people that we can introduce breathing tubes in case someone, you know, needs that therapy . . . that we can do cardiac monitoring, that we can do EKGs and determine if somebody is having a heart attack, and people usually understand that stuff because they see it on TV. So that's usually how I define the difference between a Paramedic and an EMT, is that Paramedics can do more invasive or advanced skills.

In addition to differing based on clinical capacity, these two levels of providers differ significantly in terms of the educational requirements necessary to obtain certification. EMTs typically receive around two hundred hours of classroom training, while paramedics may receive anywhere from several hundred to several thousand hours depending on the state (Institute of Medicine 2007, 128–30). These educational requirements set EMTs and paramedics apart from other health-care providers, whose educational credentials typically involve a minimum of a bachelor's degree. EMS providers, therefore, have a reputation within health care as "taxi drivers" or "ambulance drivers," terms that carry a connotation of amateurism and belie the sophisticated clinical capacities of many paramedics (Whalley and Barley 1997).

One commonality, however, has been the increasing standardization of EMS training. The National Registry of Emergency Medical Technicians (NREMT) is a nonprofit agency with the responsibility for certifying most of America's EMS providers. As of December 2020, forty-six of the fifty states use NREMT as the basis for their credentialing process.[3] While states and localities still offer their training programs, the final exam process has been outsourced by oversight bodies to NREMT. This shift in certification testing has served to reduce the friction for providers who previously had to navigate complicated reciprocity systems if they wanted to move their EMS certification from one state to another. It also serves as a baseline, as state curricula must meet or exceed the NREMT's standards for the given level of training.

Structural Trends in the Provision of EMS Services

The trends described, including the development of the EMS system as both a balkanized, fragmented patchwork of services and the outsourcing of certification to a nonprofit entity, is not accidental. Indeed, the shift toward private EMS companies and nonprofit management (on the part of the National Register of EMTs) suggests that EMS services in the United States have a distinctly neoliberal flavor. EMS systems in a modern context emerged just as the privatization of the welfare state became a significant force in shaping civic services in America, and it is no accident that nearly 35 percent of the EMS systems today reflect this trend. The budgetary constraints placed on the public-service EMS systems, including both fire and non-fire municipal services, also reflect the retrenchment of the American state throughout the last forty years.

These broader economic trends have been mainly absent from social-science discussions of EMS work, with the lone, notable exception of Josh Seim's recent work (Seim 2017, 2020). There, Seim places capital as a significant force shaping management decisions alongside state bureaucracy. Like Seim's site, Private Ambulance itself is, as the pseudonym suggests, a private company. Unlike many private EMS agencies, it is a small company owned by a family rather than a regional or national entity with the backing of national or even transnational private equity firms (Ivory, Protess, and Bennett 2016). However, like Seim's own research site, Private Ambulance represents the unique ways in which capital influences EMS. It shapes municipal budgets, governs contracts, and implements policies seen as capital-friendly, including privatization and austerity. The character of EMS reflects the period in which it came of age, which was characterized by neoliberal economic policies that saw public services shrink. We do not see police services backed by private equity, nor do we see fire services similarly financed. Had the EMS system developed earlier, it is possible that it would look more like the nation's fire services, where privatization remains rare.

In terms of the National Registry, capital operates in the background. Since NREMT is a nonprofit, some of the financial pressures present in other spaces within pre-hospital emergency care are absent. However, the very fact that a nonprofit manages the certification and licensure of EMS providers around the United States is emblematic of the privatization of hitherto public resources under the banner of neoliberalism. The way EMS is structured therefore reflects the constellation not just of the demise of the general practitioner making home visits and the rise of pre-hospital medicine as a distinct discipline within medicine's division of labor, but also the profound structural changes that have shaped America's economy since the 1970s.

The Emergency Orientation within EMS

What ties all of this together—the various types of agencies, the different levels of care—is a united focus on providing pre-hospital medicine. Our popular imagination of this work focuses on emergencies: car accidents, heart attacks, strokes, traumatic injuries, and the like. For as long as the pre-hospital system has existed, these types of what providers call "calls" (which may have multiple patients) have been the "bread and butter" of EMS work. However, for just as long, there has been considerable tension between how we imagine EMS work and how providers experience it. To some degree, this is not unique (Ivory, Protess, and Bennett 2016).[4] The lived experience of many occupations differs from outside perceptions. However, the gulf between this reality and expectation in pre-hospital medicine feels like a yawning chasm.

"Real Emergencies"

Providers, like the general public, have a strong sense of their work and the ways in which it is often violated: "They tell you in school that 'you're there to take care of the sick people' and 'you're there to keep people alive until they can get to the hospital.'" This sentiment is the idealist version of EMS work, one in which EMS providers work to care for patients in their manifest function as purveyors of emergency services.

These patients and the calls they are a part of are what providers call "real emergencies" or "good calls." A shift with several "good calls" becomes one type of "good shift." When providers talked about "good patients" or "good calls," they talked about trauma patients and medical patients who required significant intervention. As this quote shows, it was easy for discussions of "good shifts," "good calls," and "good patients" to bleed together:

CP: How would you describe a good shift?

ED: The best shift that I've had here was like three months ago, right before I got my paramedic, and I had two really serious traumas in one shift. Which for [Chapman] is pretty rare, because there's not a whole lot of high speed roads . . . but I got two really good traumas. I had a really, really sick patient who was septic and needed a whole lot of

> interventions. I [also] had a really drastic heart attack that day that we were able to solve. And then a bunch of just a couple other, pretty interesting, I mean not like too serious, but hypoglycemic patients that actually needed interventions, not just a little juice and here you go, like unconscious.

This paramedic's descriptions of what types of patients constituted "good" calls provided a useful point of comparison to others' descriptions of "bullshit" work. There was a subtly implied hierarchy to this provider's views of "good" calls. "Really serious traumas" were at the top, along with a patient with a massive infection (sepsis). Below those patients were those who were "pretty interesting" but "not too serious," such as a patient with low blood sugar (hypoglycemia) who needed interventions. This paramedic also compared his diabetic patient to a hypothetical, less seriously ill patient with diabetes who only needed some juice to raise her blood sugar as opposed to a more medicalized intervention. Similarly, another medic compared a "real emergency," in which a patient crushed bones in his foot with a heavy object, with a prior patient "whose eyelash is in their eye and they want to go to [a top teaching hospital] and they want to see a specialist."

One distinguishing feature of provider descriptions of "real emergencies" was the frequency with which such calls required interventions. Ed's earlier quote invokes this connection between interventions and "good calls" explicitly. Identifying sepsis in a pre-hospital setting involves checking a range of vital signs including blood pressure, heart rate, and respiratory rate as well as assessing the patient for altered mental status and checking lactate levels using a small handheld meter. Treatment involves aggressive intravenous therapy with fluid boluses, which means paramedics must establish "IV access" quickly in these patients. Additional medications, such as norepinephrine, may also be provided to particularly sick patients.

Trauma patients and those experiencing diabetic emergencies (which more typically involve extremely low blood glucose or "blood sugar" levels than those that are too high) likewise require establishing intravenous access. Paramedics, in particular, have the ability to give patients fluids and medications in both cases. Moreover, trauma patients often require the management of bleeding, the stabilization of fractures, and treating internal injuries providers cannot as readily observe, such as broken extremities or profuse internal bleeding. The first call described in this chapter, involving arterial bleeding, is a quintessential example of the "good call" because of the degree of injury involved.

"Good calls" need not always be so gruesome and intervention heavy. Late one night, during an overnight shift I observed with Medic 7, we were dispatched to East Chapman for a patient who had fallen three stories off a fire escape. The perceived seriousness of the call meant a significant response, with several fire trucks and fire department paramedic units, police officers, and the crew I was observing. The firefighters packaged the patient in a tight gangway between the building she fell from and the structure next door. The firefighters then brought her to the ambulance. The crew I was with rapidly determined that, by some stroke of significant luck, she was not seriously injured. The medics did comparably little on this call because treatments were not clinically warranted, yet the dangerous mechanism (the significant fall) meant this was still a "good," exciting call for the providers.

"Bullshit Calls"

The comparisons just made, like contrasting the patient with a crush injury with the patient "whose eyelash is in their eye," tellingly reveals how "real emergencies" are defined relative to calls providers feel are not serious or are inappropriate.[5] These "bullshit" calls can unfold in several ways. Many providers shared a belief that the public did not know when and how to use EMS services appropriately and framed it as a critical challenge for their work. As Allison, a longtime paramedic, noted:

> I don't think people know when to use 9-1-1 for medical situations, or trauma situations. I've had people call because they were thirsty. I've had people call because they brushed their teeth and when they spit in the sink there was a little bit of blood. So in my mind, I think it's a poor use of the system.

These calls are frustrating to providers because they feel they are unwarranted. There is no reason, they believe, to call 9-1-1 in such an instance and request an ambulance. The issues, an eyelash in an eye, gingivitis, or thirst, would not be seen by the providers as being a "real emergency" because there is no apparent threat to the patient's life or health and because there is little providers could do to treat these issues.

The ability of providers to intervene clinically raises an important point about "real emergencies" and "bullshit calls." Just because a call is defined as "bullshit" does not necessarily mean a medical need is absent. Gingivitis can and should be treated by a dentist, for example, but its validity as a medical issue is not the same as its being what providers viewed as appropriate use of the pre-hospital medical-care system. Similarly, intoxication as we saw in the second vignette at the beginning of the chapter is an indicator of alcohol abuse or dependence. This is also a behavioral health issue, but one providers do not recognize as rising to the level of a "real emergency."

Providers often chalked these calls up to ignorance on the part of patients themselves. One provider put it diplomatically during an interview when he noted that "the public just doesn't know what I do for a living and what our capabilities are." Others were far more candid, suggesting that some patients lacked the intelligence to use the system correctly:

> It's more an education kind of thing. This is what you should call the ambulance for, this is what you shouldn't call the ambulance for. Because people don't know. But then there will always be people, you know, they go into Dunkin' Donuts and want filet mignon is how I think about it. But what can you do?

The implication this provider drew was that patients may never be able to figure out when to appropriately use services. Moreover, the idea of "what can you do?" belies a sense of hopelessness that is pervasive within EMS work. EMS providers have no ability to select their patients or control the call volume, and so are left to simply continue responding to calls as they come in regardless of how they perceive the validity of the patient's medical issue. Where a lack of knowledge was concerned, providers also placed some of their blame on the types of shows discussed in the introductory chapter:

> And when you see stuff like movies, or uh, TV shows and it's so freaken' dramatic or so dumb, then even if they have been told, it's supposedly telling them what real is, you watch those shows and they're ridiculous. They're the thing that gives people a false idea of what we do.

This false sense of what the EMS system is capable of and what it is for fed a broader misunderstanding, some providers believed, resulting in the misuse of the EMS system.

A second issue is born, providers believe, not out of ignorance but out of a desire to manipulate the system. For example, a provider told me that "there's a lot of abuse of the system for people calling because they stubbed their toe and if they take the ambulance they get seen in the ER quicker or Medicaid pays for it or whatever." During the pilot round of fieldwork in 2009, I observed a call where the patient was sitting in a folding chair out in front of her house when we arrived in response to her 9-1-1 call. She had a suitcase packed and looked as if she was waiting for some form of public transit. Providers immediately responded that this call must be inappropriate because she seemed prepared in a way that struck the medics as premeditated, and their assessment of the patient on the way to the hospital did not reveal what they perceived to be a valid reason for going to the emergency department.

Providers sometimes felt like they were being abused in situations like these by patients who were willing to let health insurance pay for an ambulance ride rather than having to pay for a cab ride out of their pocket:

> I feel like there is no perception of consequence of their call . . . both financial and both me and my end. They don't care about me or the hospital. People aren't being held accountable for the load that they are placing on the health-care system, financially, and as a result they call me because they don't have money for a cab.

Providers' perceptions of these circumstances often implied that patients were malingering or feigning symptoms. Providers imaged such an exaggeration or outright lie by patients to be a ploy to generate an ambulance response simply to avoid paying for a cab.

Sometimes perceived manipulation is more complicated. Private Ambulance does not do a significant amount of dialysis transfer work, which some private ambulance companies are heavily engaged in providing. Dialysis patients often need assistance getting to and from their appointments, and they frequently rely on ambulances for this purpose. During one afternoon with the crew of Medic 7, we transported a male patient to a dialysis appointment. During the ride, he revealed to the EMT who was riding in the patient compartment with him that he had explicitly scheduled the pickup to give himself time to go across the street and eat a submarine sandwich from the deli before his dialysis treatment began.

Perhaps there was a reason the patient needed to eat (such as maintaining his blood glucose levels during dialysis), and this was the best option for him. However, the EMT and his paramedic partner were irate after the transport. Their anger extended both to the patient and the broader system of interfacility transfers. While Private did not do many dialysis transfers, they did a significant number of transfers between hospitals in the greater Chapman area. Patients who would be brought to one hospital, sometimes by a Private Ambulance crew, would need to be taken to a different facility later for more specialized care. These transfers could be necessary for the patient because her condition was more severe than a local Chapman hospital could handle, or because she needed specialized care like inpatient mental-health treatment. One provider remarked:

> It's frustrating to take a psych patient in at noon and then . . . you're finally closing your eyes at like two in the morning and then they wake you up to go take that same patient down to some place that's like an hour away.

For providers, these types of calls were also seen as "inappropriate" or "bullshit" because they represented a systemic or structural abuse of what providers saw as a scarce and essential resource.

Consequences of "Inappropriate Use" of EMS Resources

The EMS providers who expressed strong opinions about what constituted a real emergency and what was an "inappropriate" or "bullshit" call also often held equally strong views about the potential consequences of these calls. The most commonly described consequence was the concern that "bullshit" calls meant the ambulances would be tied up and unavailable for "real emergencies":

> The only thing that bothers me is that they're taking our time away in a larger city, like, um, population to truck wise, they're taking our time away from, possibly, a sick person who needs an emergency intervention. So now we're transporting and a cardiac arrest comes in two blocks away [and we can't respond] because it started to rain and [a male patient who is homeless] didn't want to be outside.

The juxtaposition of the cardiac arrest and the patient who is living on the street was common among providers at Private Ambulance. For many providers, patients who suffered some form of housing instability were an essential category of "bullshit" calls who demanded what providers felt was an inordinate amount of their attention.

One of the most striking characterizations of this came from Tommy, a male paramedic:

> There have been times when five ambulances have been picking drunk patients up off the road and there has been no one available for real emergencies, and the time when that dead baby comes in and we can't go, or an ambulance that's farther away has to, because we're all picking up drunks.

Several providers shared this idea of the "dead baby" call. It was a hypothetical call, and none of Private's EMTs or paramedics could point to an example of this actually happening. One provider cautioned during an interview that the first-responder system was set up specifically to prevent this occurring in Chapman. Nonetheless, it occupied a significant space in providers' concerns about what *could* happen if "bullshit" calls became too frequent.

These fears, in turn, translated to the attitude with which providers sometimes approached patients during calls. Several providers felt caution about "rewarding misuse" of the EMS system and so actively changed their demeanor toward patients. One provider asked me rhetorically, "Why should I be as nice [to the homeless] when being nice rewards someone for abusing the system?" during an interview. Providers' management of their own emotions, their "emotional labor," sometimes boiled over into increased stress and frustration. One provider cautioned me that "it's very hard as a provider not to, when you witness abuse of the health-care system, not let it affect your demeanor and your affect toward patients."

Reacting harshly toward patients, particularly in public, could have its own set of negative consequences. For providers, while it may provide some immediate release of frustration, it could also lead both patients and bystanders to decrease their trust in specific providers or the broader system:

> When I walk up to that guy and go "hey, get in" . . . if the person that called saw that they'd probably think "that guy's totally smoked, what a burned out ambulance guy" but they don't know that that's probably the second time I've taken him today and the last time I took him he shit all over himself and the stretcher, so it's not good for anybody. It doesn't put a good image forward for EMS, and we're not actually helping [the patient].

Providers, therefore, find themselves at the center of a broader struggle over what the emergency health-care system, both pre-hospital and emergency department, is designed for. In attempting to police those boundaries themselves, they risk alienating patients. However, providers found it difficult to hold back in some instances, noting that the day-in and day-out toll of responding to calls they felt were inappropriate was grinding.

Advanced Marginality and "Bullshit" Calls

The types of calls providers would raise when discussing "bullshit" or "inappropriate" calls are important not just for helping define the scope of this work, but because of what they reveal about the larger orientation of EMS. Providers' discussions about "picking up drunk patients" or "homeless patients" invoke the extreme poverty many residents of Chapman lived in daily. Sometimes it was immediate. On a call in a public housing project one night, three drunk men were in the process of being arrested for assaulting each other with beer bottles. The police officers on-scene had requested the ambulance crew to clean up one of the men who had a laceration on the forehead. The dirty, sparsely furnished apartment smelled strongly of urine and stale beer. On other calls, particularly with those patients who were viewed by providers as street homeless, there may not have been so many immediate signs of poverty, especially when providers treated these patients on sidewalks in Chapman's generally upscale neighborhoods.

In other cases, the legacy of poverty was more complicated. A patient initially transported by Private Ambulance from a small but tidy apartment in a public housing project for a dental problem did not fill a prescription written by emergency department providers to treat an abscessed tooth. Instead, the infection festered, and another crew I was with returned later that month to find the same patient in septic shock. Accessing medication and following through on providers' instructions are part of the more complicated legacy of marginality and poverty for health outcomes.

These types of calls are the types providers at Private Ambulance would roundly dismiss. Yet, for paramedics in the United States, most calls do not rise to the level of "good" calls. The daily grind of the 80 or 90 percent of EMS calls that do not require Advanced Life Support is full of calls like these, where EMS providers confront the failures of the social safety net. Providers' acknowledgments that they are "there to keep people alive until they can get to the hospital" is rooted in a particular path dependency, where the development of EMS has continually reinforced the idea of "real emergencies." Addressing systematic failures in public housing and providing access to preventative health-care services and resources to mitigate poverty are not within the scope of EMS providers' views of their work. Moreover, they lack any real resources to help their patients who have these issues. Thus, these calls are dispiriting not only because they appear to be "abusive" or otherwise not the job of EMS, but also because there are no clinical interventions EMS providers can offer.

The Social Conditions of EMS Work

This tension between "real emergencies" and "bullshit" work, in a broader sense, captures the struggle over normative understandings of EMS work. When providers provide patient care, which I refer to as "interdependent work routines" in Figure 7, the patient care does not occur in a vacuum. Instead, it unfolds in dialogue with providers' understandings of what their jobs are and should be. The social construction of workplace norms and practices is therefore critical to how that work unfolds. The repeated emphasis on "emergencies" feeds an occupational culture that revolves around only the most serious calls. The notion of the "real emergency," as providers understand it, is tightly intertwined with the sickest patients.

Providers' view of "real emergencies" and their relationship with acuity rest in turn upon the development of the EMS system, in the 1960s and early 1970s, as not only a critical-care system but also a stand-in for general practitioners'

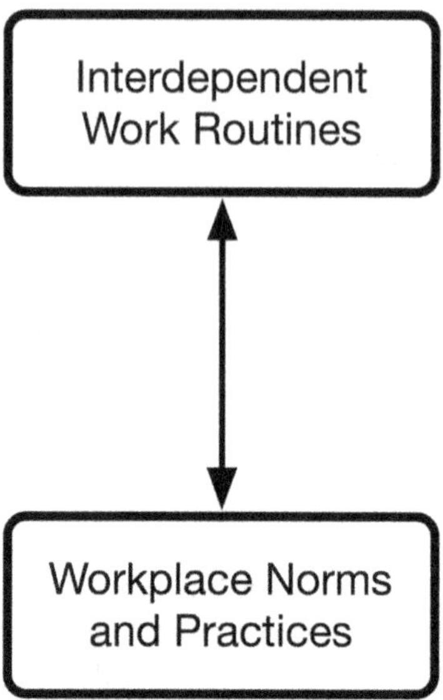

Figure 7. Evolving Theoretical Model—the Social Conditions of EMS Work (graph by author)

movement out of the business of house calls. The early social-science explorations of EMS work (Mannon 1992; Metz 1981) capture the idea of "street-level social work," a theme that has continued with more recent work (Seim 2020). The tension between the "good" calls, like cardiac arrests and trauma, with calls deemed not to be "real emergencies," has therefore been a central tension for providers since the earliest days of modern EMS work. It is not the product of recent trends in the organization or funding of EMS work but instead has always been an essential part of the experience. This experience is, therefore, fraught with tension. Providers articulate a sense of discord between how they imagine EMS work and what the reality of the job entails.

These social conditions contribute to the fundamental "structural marginality" of EMS as an institution. It is not an explicit part of either the first-responder or medical communities, having developed separately from these institutions that have existed for centuries longer than modern EMS. Though it shares hallmarks of both institutions, in some cases strong affinity with other first responders, it is also marginalized from both by low pay and more austere work conditions. Moreover, the EMS system is often not a fully integrated element of either the more comprehensive first response system or the health-care system (Institute of Medicine 2007).

Several additional factors contribute to this marginality. The degree of balkanization within the EMS system, with thousands of different agencies composed of volunteers, per diem staff, and career staff across multiple different organizational types (for-profit, third-service), makes treating the EMS system as a singular entity virtually impossible. Private Ambulance, as a for-profit company serving Chapman alongside a public fire department, is emblematic of this to a degree. They are not a major, national corporation backed by venture capital and publicly traded like some EMS companies. They do have a close working relationship with the fire department. It is, therefore, essential to acknowledge that balkanization does not necessarily mean that the quality of care delivered is challenged. Instead, on a systemic level, the orientation of EMS work has been defined by fragmentation rather than a systematic organization. Providers sit in the midst of this fragmentation, straddling boundaries among a variety of institutions they must navigate and negotiate repeatedly during work shifts.

2
The Ambulance Drivers Are Here!

"I've also had people that will say 'how 'bout you just take me to the hospital' or 'I called because I needed a taxi, let's go!'" (Allison)

An Early Morning Interfacility Transport

It is early in the morning, and the crew members of Medic 7 were sitting outside a small grocery store on the south side of Chapman named "Downtown Variety." It was just shy of "oh-six-forty-five," or 6:45 A.M., and both providers were waiting sleepily for the store to open so they could purchase breakfast sandwiches and lottery tickets. The store did not open until "oh-seven-hundred," and so Medic 7's crew had little to do but wait. Janelle, the more experienced of the two medics staffing Medic 7 that morning, sat with an iPad on her lap. In contrast, Tim, the junior medic, opened the newspaper he bought at a drugstore around the corner from Private Ambulance's headquarters before we drove downtown. At 06:45 hours, the radio, which had been generally quiet, jumped to life. It was the dispatcher, requesting Medic 7 respond to the Mather Hospital for an "interfacility transfer" (an "IFT" in the seemingly endless dictionary of abbreviations used by EMS providers).

The IFT in this case was for a patient in need of cardiac catheterization. Placing small, flexible tubes in the arteries around the heart is a common intervention for patients who have just had a myocardial infarction (a heart attack) or have partially blocked arteries around the heart resulting from coronary artery disease. The Mather Hospital lacked a cardiac "cath lab," shorthand providers use to describe the units where cardiac catheterization takes place, and so the patient needed to be transferred. That morning, the Muir Hospital had a spot for the patient. "The Muir," as providers call it, was located on Chapman's north side. Charlie opened the tablet computer as they drove toward the Mather and began writing the skeleton elements of his narrative in the run report software, explaining that he could get all the essential elements of a transfer outlined before they ever made patient contact.

Janelle parked the truck by the ambulance entrance off to the side of the Chapman's emergency department. The two providers took the ambulance's cot and piled their cardiac monitor and Advanced Life Support equipment onto it. Once it was loaded, they rolled the ambulance cot into the hospital and headed for a bank of elevators. The patient was staying on an upper floor of the hospital. They got off at the patient's floor, and, as they entered the unit, a nurse looked up from her place at the nurse's station and remarked, "Oh, the transporters are here!" Perturbed, Janelle shot back, "Oh, the transporters? We're the paramedics." The nurse responded defensively, saying she just meant that "transporting" is what Medic 7 was doing. Charlie attempted some levity, saying sarcastically, "At least you didn't say that we're just ambulance drivers. When anyone says that, I just nod and walk away." The nurse was now visibly upset and walked away without saying anything.

The transfer itself went on without issue. A second nurse came up to the nurses' station, gave the paperwork to Janelle and Tim, and provided a quick update on the patient. While Janelle spoke with the nurse, Charlie called medical control to get orders to maintain the medications being delivered by an intravenous pump that a nurse had already affixed to the patient's bed. Since those medications were not standard, the two paramedics needed permission from a medical control physician to administer them. Medical control physicians are always available to EMS agencies for these types of requests, and providers use dedicated phone lines to reach them. The paramedics at Private kept the medical control numbers stored in their cell phones so they could quickly obtain orders if needed. Once they got their orders from medical control and the report from the nurse, they worked together to "package" the patient. This involved transferring him from the hospital bed to the cot while they kept the tangle of cardiac monitor wires ("leads") and the IV line organized. At the other end of their drive, there were more reports to be given to the nurse working in the Muir Hospital's cardiac catheterization lab.

Locating "IFTs"

Interfacility transfers are more routine at some EMS agencies than others. Some agencies do not take on transfer work, focusing instead on solely responding to emergency calls dispatched through the 9-1-1 system. A complete focus on 9-1-1 is especially common for fire-based and third-service–type agencies. Other agencies, particularly private companies, dedicate themselves mostly or even exclusively to IFTs, whose regularity offers a base of revenue for ambulance companies. Private sits in between these two extremes. While 9-1-1 work is the focus of the agency, they do provide IFT services to the two major medical centers in Chapman, transporting patients between the hospitals or from these hospitals to another destination, like a rehab center, their home, or a hospital in another city.

Providers at Private Ambulance distinguished among four types of interfacility transfers:

1. "BLS transfers," which typically transport patients home from the hospital or to rehab facilities,
2. "psych transfers," which involve transporting patients from emergency departments to psychiatric facilities,
3. "ALS transfers," which involve transporting patients between hospitals when maintaining medication delivery or cardiac monitoring is required,
4. and "vent transfers," which require at least one additional crew member because the patient is dependent on a ventilator to breathe for them

Most providers at Private expressed some disdain for transfer work. ITs are predictable, often dull, and frequently time-consuming because of the distances that must sometimes be covered. Even ALS transfers, which require some additional sets of skills, were not immune from this disdain. Vent transfers, which would seem to be interesting to the lay observer because they required the most technical skills, were subject to strong dislike. They took upward of two hours and often required the primary ambulance crew to return to Private's headquarters in North Chapman to pick up the ventilator unit. Even after they obtained the ventilator, every step of the vent transfers observed seemed to take a longer amount of time than providers expected it should.

None of these types of transfers fit the stereotypical mold of critical-care work providers themselves and the public hold of EMS work. Long, boring, and often with very little in the way of clinical work, interfacility transfers embody a particular perspective on EMS work providers disdain: the "ambulance driver."

The Symbolic Ambulance Driver

A long-standing focus of sociology has been the "division of labor," a term describing the ways status and power play out in hierarchies within a single workplace or a society more generally.[1] Central to the concept of the division of labor is that occupational roles in society often have significant symbolic meaning. This symbolism connects to the amount of control that workers in a given role have over their jobs, the prestige these jobs themselves convey, and the monetary rewards associated with the work they undertake.

Medicine is but one of the classic examples of modern divisions of labor. The tightly stratified hierarchy of health-care professions begins at the bottom with technicians in a hospital who conduct routine, mundane tasks. Then there are nurses, physicians' assistants, and finally physicians themselves. Each "rung" of this hierarchy includes increased compensation, responsibility, and autonomy in how individuals can control the pace and direction of their work. Within these occupational categories are smaller divisions and subdivisions, such as the distinction between licensed practical nurses, registered nurses, and advanced practice nurses. Similarly, there are gradations within the ranks of physicians between interns, residents, fellows, and attendings.

When the nurse invokes the idea of "transporters" to Janelle and Tim, or when others call EMS providers "ambulance drivers," it serves as a symbolic reminder of their low position in medicine's division of labor. Pierre Bourdieu's notion of symbolic power is an excellent tool for understanding the negative connotations of these terms and why they resonate so powerfully with EMS providers (Bourdieu 1979, 1984). Power, in Bourdieu's eyes, "is of the order of belief, credit and discredit, perception and appreciation, knowledge and recognition—name, renown, prestige, honour, glory, authority, everything which constitutes symbolic power as recognized power" (Bourdieu 1984, 251). Critically, this form of power is typically viewed in Bourdieu's work and by others as tacit and unconscious. In other words, individuals do not regularly think about how we deploy symbolic power in our own lives or how others deploy power against us. Much as the fish may not be conscious of water, symbolic power is an omnipresent yet subliminal tool for exerting social domination.

In this case, the terms "transporters" and "ambulance drivers" are a potent reminder of the highly structured division of labor within modern medicine. They were offensive to Janelle and Charlie precisely because they highlight a common misconception of EMS work, framing it not as the site of acute care described in Chapter 1 but rather as a sort of medical taxi service. Thomas, a paramedic with several years of experience, articulated this tension:

> A lot of people are very sensitive to the term "ambulance driver," you know? Yes, we do drive the ambulance, but we do other things in the back as well. I like to tell people that we can provide the same amount of care that the emergency room will provide for about the first fifteen

> to twenty minutes, unless you're really, really sick and you need the operating room.

The paramedics hear "transporters" as not reflecting their skills, training, and experience, but rather highlighting how they differ from their colleagues in other health-care occupations. Their work is defined by a practical interpretation of one facet of EMS care, transporting patients, without any recognition of the other facets of their work. Other health-care providers may, for example, argue that the "real" work of health care happens at the hospital, without recognizing the large share of patients that EMS providers treat without ever transporting them.

While the maligned emergency medical technician or paramedic may be well aware of these stereotypes, the nurse in the exchange presented earlier seemed oblivious to how calling the providers "transporters" could be seen as offensive. The nurse's ignorance fits with Bourdieu's notion of symbolic power as being unconscious. The nurse in the earlier vignette uses language highlighting differences in the division of labor without thinking or purposely trying to be divisive. Nevertheless, the phrases are divisive and injurious and are not universally applied. Providers were able to identify these inconsistent applications of injurious terms:

> We're not ambulance drivers. We do do that [drive ambulances] but we do other things as well. I'm not calling the physician's assistant a doctor's helper, or I'm not calling a nurse a doctor's go-getter. We're not ambulance drivers. They don't understand the connotation that has or even [that] the mindset is kind of offensive.

In this way, there is not just symbolic power in the division of labor but symbolic violence as well. Symbolic violence refers to the deployment of language to reinforce the marginality and powerlessness of a lower status group by a higher status group. Ask EMTs and paramedics what they think of the term "ambulance driver," and they will be quick to tell you they dislike it.

During another transfer I observed, hospital staff told the EMS providers to utilize a freight elevator rather than a more conveniently located elevator that was also open to patients' use. The paramedic I was with was aghast at what she saw as a deeply personal affront. The request to use the freight elevators came from a nurse, as had the conflict originating over the use of the term "transporters." Tensions between nurses and paramedics at Private Ambulance were not an everyday occurrence, particularly at the hospitals where providers spent most of their time. However, these friction points are revealing for what they illustrate about the medical division of labor.

Viewed another way, the frustration providers shared with transfer work can be tied directly to broader frustration with being identified as "ambulance drivers." When asked during both shift observations and interviews, providers would describe transfers as frustrating. Some even saw transfer work as a threat to both the workforce as a whole and their skills. Providers might leave Private Ambulance if they were doing too much transfer work. Since transfers did not involve many of their sophisticated skills, they took away from valuable opportunities to practice them on 9-1-1 calls.

However, taking a step back, it is clear that at least some transfers do involve sophisticated clinical skills. The transfer described earlier was typical of many of the Advanced Life Support transfers observed. During the IFT, providers had to use at least some of their technical skills with intravenous access, cardiac monitoring, and medication administration. What all transfers have in common, however, is the notion that the ambulance itself is just a means to an end—a way to get the patient from place to place. Transfer work, therefore, is the embodiment of the identity of "ambulance driver" in a way 9-1-1 responses and other forms of EMS work do not entail. The term "ambulance driver" therefore locates EMS work as "dirty work" in the eyes of others not just because it involves patients who may be dirty, but also because it is symbolically dirty work in the eyes of other health-care providers. It is the blue-collar work that "sanitizes" patients for treatment in the hospital.

Discretion in EMS Work

This notion of an "ambulance" driver gives away the mistaken impression that EMS providers fulfill a medical taxi service. While transfer work may approximate this function, emergency calls involve a significant amount of decision-making on the part of providers. Rather than framing EMS work as "technician work" where decision-making is somewhat absent,[2] a more appropriate framework for developing an understanding of EMS work is Lipksy's notion of street-level bureaucrats (Lipsky 1980). This idea originated during the 1970s during a period in which neoliberalism came to the fore and austerity confronted many American public services (Evans and Harris 2004; Lipsky 1980). Lipsky used the idea of street-level bureaucrats to understand how individual works made decisions and navigated larger structures as they executed the fundamental tasks associated with their work.

While EMS providers at Private Ambulance are not public employees and therefore, in the strictest sense, do not fit into Lipsky's focus on civil servants, they are all "frontline workers" who serve as gatekeepers to services and execute government policies.[3] Whether they are employed by public or private agencies, the ability of providers to act based on their training and decision-making process within the confines of a broader regulatory structure represents the hallmark of "street-level bureaucracy." Discretion in Lipsky's work is a source of conflict, particularly with management (Lipsky 1980). It is an acknowledgment that, for street-level bureaucrats, there are gray areas between what Davis calls the "effective limits on [a bureaucrat's] power" (Davis 1969). Researchers have widely explored the nature and limits of discretion for these occupations (Evans and Harris 2004), framing them not just as a source of potential conflict with supervisors but also as a site where inequalities may emerge.[4]

Acknowledging discretion is an essential departure from the "technician" view of EMS work (Whalley and Barley 1997), which frames providers as the enactors of policy in a tightly regulated structure without significant agency. For EMS providers, discretion varies in two crucial ways. The first involves the level of training providers have. As I have noted previously, emergency medical technicians (EMTs) have a more limited set of skills they can practice and a correspondingly more limited set of interventions they can offer. Paramedics, on the other hand, have a far more comprehensive set of skills. Discretion, therefore, exists on a spectrum between these two levels of care.

The other axis of discretion exists for paramedics, in particular, based on what they have "standing orders" for and what they need permission from medical control to do. The vignette at the beginning of this chapter captured the medical control process, where providers were unable to maintain a particular prescription medication during the transfer, given their regular protocols. At most other points during my fieldwork with Private Ambulance, providers were able to act within their scope of care to provide interventions, medications, and treatment to patients without requesting permissions from the medical control system.

Discretion is present not just in clinical care but also in terms of patient disposition. Decisions to transport a patient to an emergency department, which emergency department to go to, or whether the patient can leave without care (or even against the advice of EMS providers) all represent additional spaces EMS providers ultimately have control over. As with clinical care itself, there may be guidelines Private Ambulance supervisors expect providers to follow. For example, trauma patients are immediately transported by Private Ambulance to Benton General Hospital, Benton Medical Center, or Benton Jewish Hospital. All of these exist in the larger neighboring city and have more significant trauma services than the capabilities at the Mather or Muir hospitals. It is left to providers to make the decision about which facility is best, particularly in cases where patients do not have a preference in terms of where treatment occurs.

Axes of Control in EMS Work

While EMS providers do have discretion over many facets of the clinical care they provide, this discretion does not occur in a vacuum. However, it is exercised by providers in a space where there are multiple and sometimes competing institutional actors who also help shape the labor process of EMS providers. Figure 8 summarizes the web of relationships providers must regularly manage during both individual calls and more generally during shifts.

The most immediate relationship most providers have to confront is their relationships with each other. Once they have completed training, all providers work in pairs with what they call a "partner." These pairs are intentionally structured based on each provider's experience level. The least experienced EMTs will be paired by management with other EMTs. Once EMTs at Private Ambulance gain experience, they have the option to begin working with paramedics. Likewise, new paramedics will work with more experienced paramedics. A medic who has obtained the requisite number of hours can begin to work on MB trucks with another EMT. The control management exerts, along with the oversight EMS dispatchers provide, are the two other relationships providers must manage within EMS agencies themselves.

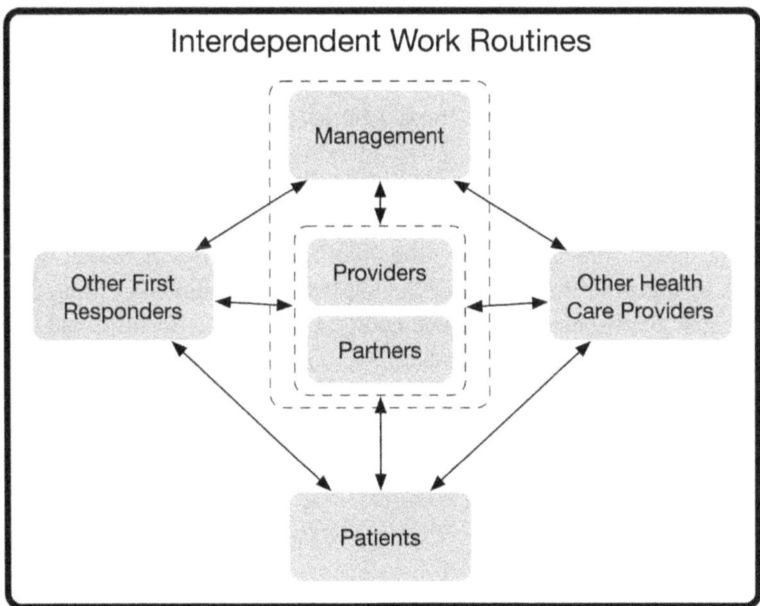

Figure 8. Evolving Theoretical Model—Interdependent Work Routines in EMS Work (graph by author)

Outside of EMS agencies, the next most immediate relationship for EMS providers is with patients, with whom providers must work during what is rarely a "good" day for the individuals who require EMS care. EMS providers work with two other external constituencies to ensure each patient receives the appropriate care. The first occurs mostly at emergency scenes themselves, where providers join with other first responders—namely, police officers and firefighters—to offer pre-hospital medical care to their patients. If the crew determines additional care is needed, they will transport the patient to an emergency department where they will interact with the final constituency: other health-care providers. They also work with physicians remotely via the medical control system and during the interfacility transfers described previously.

Each element of interaction summarized in Figure 8, from partners, management, and dispatchers to other first responders, health-care providers, and patients themselves, is regulated both internally within EMS agencies and often externally by other bodies, as well. So, while providers have control over facets of their work and can even make determinations about whether a patient requires additional care at an emergency department, they are not entirely free to carry out their work. The number of actors with whom they must interface and the bodies of regulations they work within mean that EMS work, then, is defined not just by discretion but rather by constrained discretion.

What is critically important about the degree of constrained discretion in EMS work is that these spaces of discretion are both contested and evolving. Such an environment evokes the classic idea of "negotiated order," which describes the shared, sometimes tacit agreements among participants in a social organization (Strauss 1985, 1988, 2008). The order is understood as "negotiated" because it is always in flux; participants frequently reevaluate and restructure the rules constituting the order (Hall 1987). Negotiation is, therefore, a response to inadequate or incomplete norms and rules in an institution. Such an absence of guidance could be because of institutional failure. However, negotiation may also be particularly necessary where additional flexibility is required, such as in street-level bureaucracies. Such negotiated orders may occur on a small scale between individuals or on a larger scale between organizations or groups within organizations (Maines 1977). However, the degree to which negotiated orders operate varies (Hall and Spencer-Hall 1982).

Street-Level Negotiation at Private Ambulance

Negotiation and discretion are everyday activities that are part and parcel of the experience of providing pre-hospital health care at Private Ambulance.[5]

Moreover, they are necessary components of jobs that are difficult to routinize because the scenarios providers confront from one call and shift to the next are so varied.

Negotiation in Practice

Negotiation is particularly important for providers during calls because they find themselves interacting with a wide array of people throughout a typical call. Take this example, from an evening call Matthew and Nora, two paramedics, responded to at a university in Chapman. Like many larger cities, Chapman's economy transitioned over the twentieth century from a primarily industrial base into one where the "knowledge economy" is ascendant. Former factories now housed lab and start-up space, and the footprint of "meds and eds" in the city had grown significantly. College students were, therefore, a significant portion of the call base for providers.

The specific call the Private Ambulance dispatchers assigned to Matthew and Nora was for an ill student in a fraternity house. On the fifth floor of the fraternity house, they found fire department paramedics treating the patient, who was unsure about going to the hospital despite suffering an allergic reaction. Matthew entered the cramped dorm room bathroom to help the other paramedics while Nora remained in the hallway with the university police officers and several student bystanders. Matthew found that, unlike some of their other university patients, the young man was not intoxicated.

Two of the female bystanders approached Nora with questions about how the 9-1-1 system worked. As Nora and the officers addressed their inquiries, Matthew was busy working to convince the patient that it was in his best interest to receive medical treatment at a hospital. The patient, who was frightened and confused, relented after a few minutes of speaking with Matthew. With Matthew's help, the firefighters on-scene assisted the patient down the five flights of stairs and into the waiting ambulance. The Chapman firefighters were present as part of the broader relationship with Private Ambulance, where firefighters responded to more serious calls, provided initial BLS and sometimes ALS care, and then helped move the patient to the ambulance. Likewise, police officers (be they Chapman police, an officer from one of the universities, or transit police officers) were also present at a large proportion of Private's calls. However, they were typically less involved in patient care than the firefighters were.

Nora climbed into the rear of the ambulance and began obtaining the patient's vital signs while Matthew got into the driver's seat. The trip was an uneventful but expedited one. Throughout the roughly eight-minute trip to the hospital, Nora continued to monitor the patient's blood pressure and heart rate. She also asked follow-up questions, trying to obtain an understanding of what transpired before the patient became ill. Once they arrived at the ED, Nora and Matthew worked together to pull the cot from the ambulance and wheel the patient through the hospital's sliding glass doors.

Inside the hospital, they were greeted by a nurse who questioned Nora and the patient about the patient's symptoms. The nurse repeatedly asked Nora whether the patient had been drinking, which Nora denied and tried to steer the conversation back to the patient's symptoms. The nurse did not appear to listen at first and insisted several times on placing the patient in the waiting room. The frame of college students as intoxicated, particularly during the evening shift, is a powerful one, and this nurse appeared unwilling to let go of it. However, after several minutes of back and forth with Nora, the nurse relented. Matthew, who had been watching the scene while cleaning the cot with anti-bacterial wipes, expressed his frustration. "This is an emergency room, people are going to come here when they're sick," he said, wondering aloud why hospital staff sometimes got mad about admitting patients to the ED who were not critically injured or sick.

While Matthew finished cleaning the ambulance's equipment, Nora worked with the hospital staff to register the patient in the hospital's computer system. She then returned to the ambulance, and, as they made the drive from the hospital to Private Ambulance's headquarters, she worked to complete the call's digital paperwork, which the providers call a "run report." These documents contain details about the call, such as location, as well as information about the providers' clinical assessment of the patient and notes about the care they provided. The provider who rides with the patient in the back of the ambulance to the hospital is typically the one who fills out this paperwork, since this provider has the most interaction with the patient. As we pulled into the headquarters, Nora "synced" the "run report" wirelessly from the ambulance to Private's electronic run report servers, and with that submission, this call was complete.

Working with Partners

As the vignette shows, EMS workers regularly negotiate with their partners and other first responders at emergency scenes. The pairings of partners I observed were the result of both an active effort to pair specific individuals by management and the product of swaps and call-outs that inevitably changed the pairings that at least some partners experienced each week. Each pair of partners was responsible for staffing a single ambulance based on the pair's clinical experience and level of training. Thus, on any given call, partners could have different roles; when and how these roles were assumed were products of negotiation. For some calls, there was a formal, regulated aspect to the division of labor, since critical patients were required by state protocols to be treated by paramedics.

On some calls, however, partners determined who would lead patient care based on individual strengths. One paramedic, Samantha, described such an arrangement:

> Working consistently with a partner, whether it's the same day each week or multiple days in a week, you really get a feel for what their strong points are and what yours are, and you can play off each other. I've worked with a partner for about six months, and he's very good tactically. He's very good at extrication, he's very good at splinting and I'm very good at talking to patients. So regardless of who was responsible for patient care and who was driving, we would just approach it. We didn't have to talk to each other about it. We just went in and I would get the information from the patient, and he would deal tactically with the patient.

Private Ambulance is relatively small for an EMS company, and many providers worked with regular partners, at least for particular days and shifts. Working with new partners can be complicated because there are numerous preferences providers hold related to providing clinical care. Many partners, especially when they both had the same level of training (i.e., both were paramedics, or both were EMTs), would swap calls. Sometimes more senior medics would let the more junior partner do most of the clinical care unless they had a particularly sick or injured patient. Matthew fell into this camp as one of the most experienced medics at Private Ambulance and one of the few who was present during both periods of fieldwork.

During many calls, the distinction between one partner as the clinician and one partner as the driver was blurred. As in the earlier vignette, one partner may do an initial assessment on-scene and then hand off clinical care to the other, or both may initially work together before deciding which partner would finish the call in the back of the ambulance while the other drove. As Samantha noted, partners would often have different strengths, and pairs who had experience working with each other were able to play to those strengths.

For Samantha, negotiation occurred not only based on clinical strengths but also along gender lines, as well:

> It's interesting to go to a call and have an Engine company of three guys, a Squad of two guys, a Rescue company of four guys, a police officer who is a guy, and your partner who is a guy and the patient is the women who is bleeding vaginally because she's having complications in her second trimester, and they're all like "Samantha"? What would they do if I wasn't here?

Decisions made by providers about who was responsible for patient care were made, therefore, along several informal axes in addition to state protocol requirements and clinical strengths. A provider's gender, comfort in speaking with specific populations of patients, and/or simply whose turn it was to provide patient care were all determining factors.

Like other first-responder occupations, it is men who make up the predominant share of EMS providers. Approximately two-thirds of paid EMS providers are men, and Private Ambulance is no exception. The majority of the providers I worked with during all phases of data collection were men. The personnel from Chapman's fire and police departments who responded to calls with Private Ambulance were also overwhelmingly male. Samantha's story about being the only female provider on an EMS call was not unusual.

Among Private Ambulance's providers, there were regular signs that this was a masculinized workplace.[6] Some of the paramedics would get together to ride motorcycles at very high rates of speed on area highways during their days off. Another paramedic had the nickname "ball bagger," a reference to testicles. During one shift, I sat with a group of providers from several crews as they discussed an iPhone application used for rating the "happy endings" (i.e., sexual acts) available at different massage parlors, much to the discomfort of the one female medic present. Dispatchers would refer to ambulance crews where the providers were both women as "broad squads" to me and their colleagues.

This type of language and discussion, sociologists argue, creates an environment that potentially places female providers at a disadvantage. While I did not witness overt sexual harassment of providers by colleagues, there is at least some evidence to suggest it is common (Bigham et al. 2014; Boyle et al. 2007; Koritsas, Boyle, and Coles 2009). For EMTs and medics, there is not a way to walk away or obtain truly private space during shifts. Providers eat, sleep, and work together in close quarters, and the frequent downtime discussed in Chapter 5 leaves them with less-structured time. Their work is frequently out of the view of supervisors or peers, and so can be physically and socially isolating. Understanding gender dynamics in EMS work is, therefore, not just a question of how providers arrange the division of labor for themselves, but also an entry point for understanding how EMS work can become toxic for providers.

Working with Other First Responders

In addition to negotiating with partners, providers often found themselves negotiating with other first responders. In Chapman, the fire department responded to most of the EMS requests placed by callers through the city's 9-1-1 system. The unique nature of each call and the combination of responders made formal arrangements between EMS providers and others challenging. Therefore, informal negotiation was repeatedly required. On some calls, the firefighters who had already begun treatment continued while the Private Ambulance paramedics acted in a supporting role. As in the vignette, firefighters sometimes assisted in "packaging" and "extricating" the patient from the scene into the ambulance. Extricating the patient most often involved helping move them to the stretcher and, often, downstairs and out to the idling ambulance. Firefighters would also help move equipment, such as the bags and the cardiac monitor, for providers. All of this was determined on a case-by-case basis and sometimes occurred in an unspoken manner. Personnel would see a need and act on it without being asked.

More intricate scenes, however, sometimes demanded greater coordination. One afternoon while I was riding with two paramedics, Max and Thomas, dispatchers assigned them to respond to a fall at a construction area. They were among the first units to respond along with one of the local Chapman fire department companies. Chapman police officers were already on-location, hurriedly gesturing Max and Thomas to park and guiding us to a temporary stairwell on the exterior of the still unenclosed structure. We walked up five flights of stairs and then across metal forms laid down in preparation for concrete floors to be eventually poured by construction crews.

When we arrived at the patient, we found firefighters beginning to move him onto a "backboard," a plastic board sometimes used for spinal immobilization after falls. Max and Thomas immediately got to work with the firefighters, hooking the patient up to a cardiac monitor and establishing IV access. The providers expressed concern about the height the worker had fallen from, two stories further up on the steel beams. As they worked, additional fire companies arrived, including paramedics from two additional fire companies and a ladder company, which positioned itself next to the structure as we worked on the patient.

Once the patient had been packaged on the backboard and was ready to be extricated, the firefighters coordinated the next moves. A fire officer had arrived on the fifth floor and asked a firefighter on the ground to move the ambulance to a better loading position. Other firefighters moved the patient in a Stokes basket to the ladder truck's basket. As we walked down another temporary stairwell, the ladder truck's members lowered him in the truck's basket. They then facilitated moving the patient to the ambulance. This scene was among the most complex I observed, one where over a dozen firefighters worked with Max and Thomas to move the patient from where he had fallen to the ambulance, several floors below.

Relationships with police on-scene were different. In many cases, police officers did not respond to EMS calls with Private Ambulance. If they did respond, the officers were not typically engaged in patient care as firefighters were, even if the police officers were first on the scene. As with the example of the fallen construction worker, they often stood by, letting EMS providers and firefighters work on the patient. Officers would direct traffic, as they did at this scene, or help usher bystanders around the providers as they worked.

Alternatively, if dispatchers were unclear about the nature of the 9-1-1 call, "they'll usually send the police with us." They would, on occasion, help carry equipment back to the ambulance or fire trucks, but their role mostly appeared to be present in support in case they were needed. As James, another paramedic, described:

> The police are very good about protecting us, protecting our safety. If there's any question about someone being violent toward us or we're put in a bad situation, the police in this city swarm like killer bees. You get a very secure feeling being on the streets and knowing they're looking out for you. That's pretty good.

The relationship between EMS providers and police, in particular, spoke to the unpredictable nature of EMS work. Dispatch information about particular calls could be sparse in Chapman, and providers reported during interviews that they would sometimes be unsure of what they would find when they arrived on-scene. Police presence at calls provided reassurance for providers who might be worried about violence on-scenes. Officers also assisted in finding patients, mainly when they were able to arrive on-scene first. This was particularly helpful in confusing neighborhoods or apartment buildings.

Management of EMS Work

The second group that EMS providers found themselves negotiating with was Private Ambulance's management, who remained present in the background of the vignette. The company's management was multilayered, extending from the immediate road supervisors to several senior paramedics who oversaw the daily operations and quality-improvement activities. Immediate supervisors were, according to company policy, purposefully placed on the road in an ambulance with a partner. Private Ambulance, unlike many EMS services, intentionally did not give supervisors different uniforms or marks denoting their elevated rank. As one supervisor noted, "You would never know that I was a supervisor unless you asked, and I told you." Placing supervisors in such a position was seen as beneficial, according to the same supervisor, because:

> The supervisors aren't riding around in a truck, making sure your tie is on. They're working, so they get the intricacies of the place. They have

> the same issues that you do. They have the same arguments with the nurse that you have, so they get it. They have a great working knowledge of what goes on, so it's easy to identify with the field providers.

These supervisors worked with providers daily to ensure that shifts ran smoothly, but largely in subtle ways. If providers needed to be switched between ambulances or a vent transfer came in, supervisors often helped coordinate these moves.

Upper-level managers, on the other hand, took responsibility for ensuring that the providers of Private Ambulance provided excellent patient care. Doing so in a diffuse and fluid work environment could be challenging. EMS supervisors at Private Ambulance did not have the luxury other managers may have had. Employees could be spread out over a wide geographic area and not be concentrated in a single location like many other service workers would be. Private Ambulance, therefore, relied on several pieces of technology to provide virtual, if not physical, oversight of EMS work. These efforts, which all occurred in the background of the vignette, included tracking ambulances with Global Positioning Systems (GPS), which assisted supervisors in allocating resources and shortening response times to calls.[7]

Management also monitored using cameras located in the cabs of the ambulances. These cameras would record audio and video from the cab in the event of a collision, hard braking, or quick turning. The video systems could also be used by the operations staff to discipline providers for their driving habits, giving management a way to oversee a massive, dangerous part of EMS work without being physically present. Leaving Benton General Hospital one afternoon, Noelle triggered the camera by braking too hard. She was texting and loudly cursing when she realized the camera was recording her. Managers had already warned Noelle about texting while driving, and she feared the latest recording could be cause for termination.

Videos sometimes attained "cult" status within Private Ambulance, being passed around and viewed by many providers as a source of entertainment. During the first fieldwork phase in 2009, providers reminisced about a video captured during a disaster response Private Ambulance had participated in several years beforehand. The ambulance crew in question was driving across train tracks at an at-grade crossing. The storm had damaged the crossing's lights and barriers, and the crew reacted with extreme horror when they realized they narrowly avoided being struck by a train.

These "cult" videos do not just provide entertainment when providers pass them around amongst themselves. Instead, they serve to normalize surveillance in the workplace and reify it not as a part of the digital panopticon many mobile workers find themselves in but rather as a source of entertainment.

However, they allow management to peer in on providers' behavior without being present, and the use of automatic push alerts means managers can quickly be made aware of possible deviations from the driving standards Private Ambulance uses.

The same is true for the monitoring of patient care, which is subject to similar surveillance by management. As in the vignette, all providers entered their "run reports" on tablet computers and then delivered their electronic call records wirelessly to Private Ambulance's quality-assurance supervisor, who read each call to determine the appropriateness of the care given. Providers expressed a range of emotions about this practice, with a minority of providers feeling "micro-managed" at times while others, often younger and less experienced providers, expressed appreciation for the guidance given.

Many of the providers reported attempting to head off any potential negative repercussions by finding the supervisor before he had had a chance to read the call. These defensive acts by the providers appeared to serve two purposes. First and foremost, the providers were able to ensure that any care deviating from Private Ambulance's expectations could be explained in person, and therefore may have been less likely to result in a prolonged confrontation with management. One provider, who was not a supervisor, noted:

> There are other dynamics on a call that don't get documented that need to come out when people are asked about the call. Because, if you're just looking at the numbers, you're not going to see that there were three flights of stairs to get down, and that's why the capnography was off. The patient wasn't able to be bagged in that situation because it wasn't feasible.

Providers relied on their ability to tell their side of a call's story as a means to prevent or mitigate any criticism, constructive or otherwise, that management may give once they review the call. Second, providers would use the time with the supervisor to get insight into how they could handle unique or uncommon calls in different ways. Some of the providers spoke of the processes of seeing the supervisor as an educational experience. Given the supervisor's advanced training and experience, providers appreciated being able to talk about different ways to handle similar situations. In both cases, the electronic "run reports" allowed management into each patient-care experience, giving them insight into the care delivered and the actions of their EMS providers.

Management of EMS work, therefore, shares some commonalities with service work, where cameras, recording devices, and digital quality-assurance tools are increasingly the norm (Levy 2015). From management's standpoint, these tools allow them to manage a mobile and spatially disparate workforce.

For providers, however, the systems become mostly unavoidable. Orr's essential ethnography (Orr 2016) discusses the practices of copier-repair technicians, whose workday activities happened primarily outside of the gaze of management. Fast-forward twenty years, and the avoidability of road supervisors is a thing of the past (see also Rolland and Monterio 2002).

Negotiating the Role of EMS with Patients and Bystanders

Negotiation with patients and bystanders often reflected EMS providers' beliefs that the public had little understanding of what EMS providers do. Jason, a paramedic, told me he felt that "the public just doesn't know what I do for a living and what our capabilities are." This ignorance meant providers often spent time on calls describing their role and why they were doing interventions instead of quickly transporting a patient to the hospital. The bystanders at the call described in the vignette spent several minutes questioning Nora and the police officers on-scene about how the 9-1-1 response system worked.

While Nora was not providing direct patient care at that moment, other providers reported patients and bystanders who were more intrusive. Seth, a paramedic supervisor, argued:

> I think once family members get educated on what the paramedics are doing, we're not just sitting there taking a blood pressure and a heart rate and a respiratory rate, they're treating you. And once you've explained that to family members, I've seen family members come to terms with that, understand that, and accept it and I've also seen the side of family members just not caring at all, saying, "You're not a doctor just go to the hospital and that's how it's going to be." And sometimes that can make situations a little dangerous when you have agitated family members.

The notion that EMS providers should just "go to the hospital" parallels the idea of the "medical taxi" described earlier. It reflects what providers feel is a broad misunderstanding about their role among members of the public, who seem to have a much stronger sense of what firefighters and police officers do.

EMS providers, therefore, rely on negotiation with patients and family members to be allowed to provide the needed care or to convince them that being transported to the emergency department was in their best interest. Tom, another paramedic, described this:

> I've also had people that will say, "How 'bout you just take me to the hospital" or "I called because I needed a taxi, let's go!" Well, I would

> be totally fine with that if you weren't complaining of ten out of ten chest pain and you're diaphoretic and pale.

Many providers were frustrated by these patients because they were well equipped to treat such acute cases. However, some patients did not understand this and often believed the ambulance was there simply to ensure they got to the hospital safely.

Equally painful could be convincing patients who were injured not to risk further injury. On a call with Jason, a patient insisted on using the bathroom even though he had fallen and moving could have risked further injury to the patient. Jason, his partner, and the firefighters on-scene tried to prevent the patient from moving around, but the negotiations with the patient were futile. This situation prompted Jason's remark about how the public did not understand his job and the role of the EMS system.

Patients also do not always call 9-1-1 with a decision made about whether they want to go to an emergency department and, if so, which ED they would like to go to for care. The patient in the vignette seemed unsure about what was the best decision for him, and it took some convincing from the firefighters and Private Ambulance providers on-scene to get the patient to go to the hospital for an evaluation. Another paramedic, Sam, noted that some patients were not sure about going to the hospital because they believed the EMS providers could treat them in their homes. He told me, "A lot of people will call and think that we can show up and prescribe them something as if we're doing a house call and you have to explain to them, obviously, that we don't do that." This idea harkens back to the days of the general practitioner who could make house calls, which largely predates the modern EMS system.

Other patients, Nora noted, requested that the providers give them a diagnosis while still in the patient's home. Simulating an exchange with a patient, she stated:

> I've had people tell me, "Well, you tell me if I need to go to the hospital." Legally I can't do that. I will always advise you to go to the hospital. I am not a doctor and I can't tell you one-hundred percent one way or the other if you need to be emergently seen or if you can go by your own means. We're always going to advise that you come with us and get evaluated.

Working with patients to understand their options, and in some cases to convince patients to seek treatment or accept treatment from EMS providers, was a frequent and sometimes frustrating element of their work.

Providers' inability to offer a diagnosis and the requirement to always leave emergency department transportation on the table as an option for patients is another result of the peculiar legal structure of EMS work. Providers are required to transport patients to emergency departments if the patient requests it, and they cannot refuse transportation even if the providers themselves are sure it is not clinically warranted. At the same time, they are also legally not allowed to tell patients they do not need to go in a definite sense, because they cannot offer a formal diagnosis. Providers develop rhetoric for communicating options to patients but are left to negotiate the outcome of each call with patients who are free to disregard their advice.

Working with Other Health-Care Providers

The final group of individuals providers regularly interact with are the staff in emergency departments, especially the nurses who help assign patients to beds and take initial reports. These nurses are called "triage nurses," and providers interact with at least one every time they transport a patient to the hospital. As with patients who failed to understand the role of EMS providers, EMTs and paramedics sometimes interacted with triage nurses and medical professionals who failed to understand the role the EMS providers played in patient care. With the patient Nora and Matthew brought to the ED several hours after his allergic reaction, Nora had to negotiate with a triage nurse who was operating from preconceived notions about the patient.

Samantha believed that "the seasoned emergency room staff definitely understand EMS's role. Newer emergency room staffs will learn it . . . within a six-month period." However, she cautioned:

> I think that some of the emergency facilities that we wouldn't take traumas to, or we wouldn't take seriously sick people to, don't have the same understanding because they don't get the seriously sick people, so they don't see EMS's role.

Providers did not believe all of Chapman's (and the neighboring cities') emergency departments were equal in their abilities. Samantha's cautionary statement about ED staff exposure to EMS, therefore, highlights the perceived gulf between ED staff who see EMS work with critical patients regularly and those who do not. Every provider interviewed expressed strong preferences for individual hospitals over others. Providers primarily based these preferences on how they felt the medical staff treated them when they went to those facilities with patients. If transfers of care required extensive negotiation or if providers felt disrespected by the staff, they seemed likely to dislike going to the facility as a whole.

Other providers reported similar difficulties in negotiating their place within the medical hierarchy. At other facilities, often where the providers stated they had secure professional networks with the staff, providers reported more positive experiences with tasks like transferring care. Staff would be attentive and appear to take the providers' clinical observations seriously. At the facilities where they transported patients frequently, such as the Mather Hospital, providers regularly spent downtime in the ED joking with staff and even reported spending time outside of work with some of the providers in the hospital.

At other hospitals, especially those where Private's crews transported much less frequently, the ED staff would sometimes appear distant and at times even seemed to ignore providers. This could be true for new providers at places like the Mather Hospital, where there was an expectation that they had to prove themselves to ED staff. One new paramedic worried that after "the first five words out of your mouth, if it doesn't start off well, the triage staff will just tone you out." Another emphasized the need to "paint a picture" for every physician so they had as many relevant details as possible. Regardless of how providers felt hospital staff treated them, these interactions were critical for their patients, and providers tried to communicate as much information as possible.

The Interplay between Workplace Practices and Interdependent Work Routines

EMS providers engage daily with more individuals, and in more diverse ways, than many service work settings sociologists have examined in the past. The emerging model of EMS work, modified to capture this expansion (see Figure 9), attempts to capture the multiplicity of different power structures and alliances shaping EMS work. It also identifies how these axes of power develop in relation to the wider norms and practices of EMS work. Like other service workers (Leidner 1993), there have been efforts to routinize these interactions through protocols. These protocols, however, cannot plan for the uniqueness of each patient. Interpersonal negotiation, therefore, becomes a tool for organizing and providing patient care in settings where routinization is impractical. It is not just that EMS providers have discretion in the way patients' care is administered to them. In EMS settings, the sheer number of parties involved requires continual assessment and reassessment of how to use their discretion most effectively. Providers must decide which of the pair will provide treatment and what other first responders are or are not needed, and they must work with other health-care providers to ensure that patient care is transferred from providers to hospital staff appropriately.

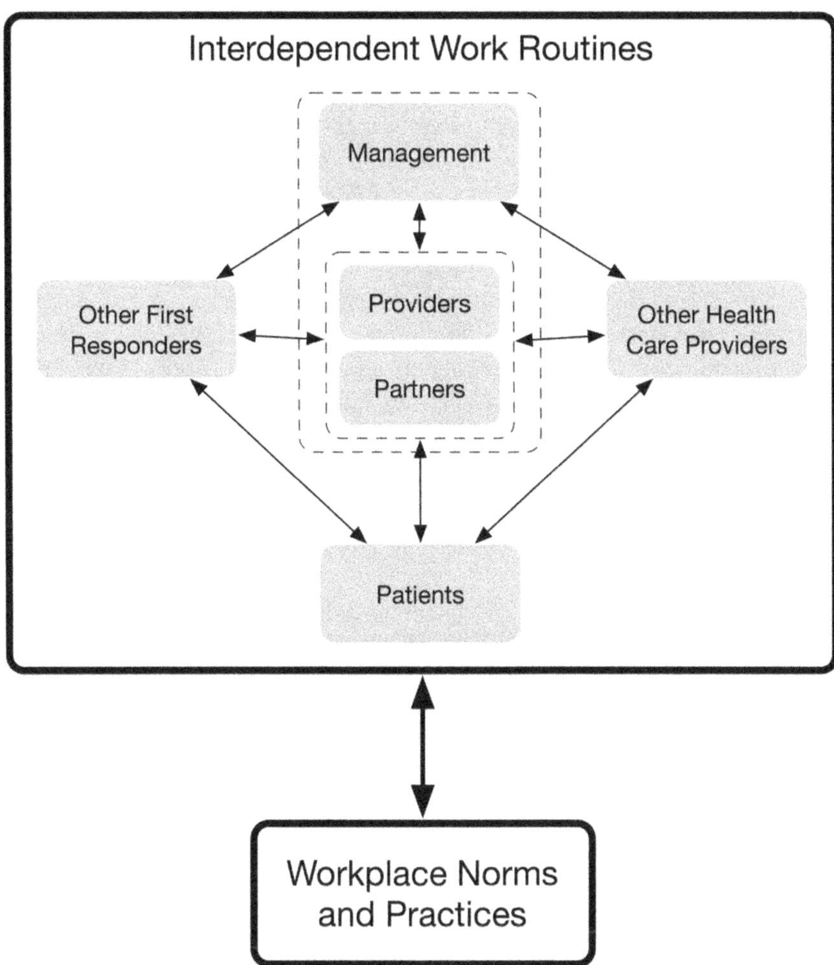

Figure 9. Evolving Theoretical Model—Integrating Interdependent Work Routines and Workplace Norms (graph by author)

Discretion, however, can also be misleading. Those unfamiliar with the EMS system, including patients, bystanders, and even other health-care providers, may misunderstand the level of discretion providers have. Patients assume they can be diagnosed by EMS providers or simply be given a ride to a medical facility. Hospital staffs assume providers can serve as gatekeepers, limiting their exposure to undesirable patients as in the earlier vignette. In both cases, navigating the terrain of discretion happens through continual negotiation. In the case of EMS providers at Private Ambulance, providers exercise discretion through continual negotiation.[8] Importantly, providers in this case are also negotiating the boundaries of their very existence, not only with other health-care providers in terms of professional boundaries (Abbott 2014; Freidson 1988) but also with patients themselves. Negotiation, therefore, serves not only to allow providers to do their jobs but to justify their occupational existence.

Some of these negotiations rest upon the familiar terrain of gender dynamics. Others have noted the often hypermasculine culture of EMS agencies and first-responder work more generally (Boyle 2002; Chetkovich 1997). Such internal forces also shape the terrain of negotiation and discretion if, as Samantha noted, providers assume that certain types of work will be done by female providers on-scene. These observed gender dynamics are a critical point that gets to the heart of one weakness with the triangular-service work models. Not only do they implicitly assume an equilateral relationship between customers, management, and employees, but they also assume homogeneous effects within each of those categories. The internal negotiation identified here shows the essential disparities and uneven power dynamics even within those categories.

There is a more substantial, and perhaps even more vital, critique to make with these data. The sheer number of different constituent groups present in our data provide a useful empirical example of the limits of a triangular model for service-work interactions. The different groups identified may be present to varying degrees on calls or, in some cases, may not be present. Attempts to theoretically model relationships between EMS providers and others on-scene may, therefore, come up short because of the variety of possible permutations of bystanders, patients, first responders, health-care providers, and the ever-present eye of management keeping watch over the virtual shop floor.

This "electronic panopticon" (Bain and Taylor 2000) is, along with the gradual expansion of clinical interventions (Institute of Medicine 2007), the most substantial change within EMS since the beginning of the twenty-first century. Today, technology has become an essential mediator in this relationship by allowing EMS managers to oversee EMS work without being present. By using GPS technology, management can track the movements of ambulances, which allows Private Ambulance to decrease response times to emergency calls and gives managers oversight of the activities of their providers. Such a bird's-eye view is akin to a virtual window overlooking the shop floor. Cameras and electronic "run reports" allow managers to zoom in on specific interactions of importance, including safe driving and the delivery of medical care. Individuals' driving and medical care can be tracked over time and across hundreds of data points. These technological innovations mean EMS management is not present physically, much as they are absent in Orr's study of copier-repair workers (Orr 2016). However, the virtual overview of the shop floor means they are effectively always present, which is a departure from previous studies of mobile service workers.

This chapter and Chapter 1 paint a particular picture of EMS work, one that differs substantially from media representations and our population's imagination. The EMS system is a marginal entity within the American healthcare system. Such marginality is visible not just in the system's history and contemporary organization, but in the daily interactions providers have with each other and the institutions they work closely with to provide patient care. It is a system, like a thoroughbred, engineered for a very particular set of circumstances. Yet the reality of EMS work is much different. "Real emergencies," as providers term them, do indeed happen. However, the term "ambulance driver" epitomizes much of the work EMS providers engage in regularly. This pejorative captures the positionality of EMS in the wider division of labor in medicine. The term "ambulance driver" also captures the sub- or non-acute nature of the patients EMS systems regularly care for, a topic we will return to in Chapter 5.

Conclusion

Like law enforcement and fire services, the Emergency Medical Services (EMS) system in the United States has its roots early in the country's history. However, unlike these two companion first-responder institutions, the EMS system became professionalized far later. It was not until the 1960s that policy changes at the federal level allowed for America to develop and institute a formal training curriculum for what we now recognize as emergency medical technicians. Policymakers, providers themselves, and other health-care providers understand the system as a part of the critical-care system. It is there, we are told, for car accidents, acute injuries, heart attacks, strokes, and the like.

This view is paradoxical, given that many of the same policymakers and health-care providers also frame EMS providers themselves as relative amateurs compared to nurses and physicians. While EMTs continue to receive relatively limited levels of training, paramedics receive extensive training that often outstrips the skill set nurses in emergency departments receive. The framing of EMS personnel as "ambulance drivers" ignores the clinical sophistication of these providers and unsurprisingly is a source of much frustration for them.

While it minimizes their role, the idea of the "ambulance driver" as the clinical equivalent of a taxi driver captures the institutional marginality of EMS work perfectly. This is underscored by their role in interfacility transports (IFTs), which are an area largely ignored in other EMS research. While others have focused on emergency calls, IFTs provide a crucial glimpse into how the "ambulance driver" is socially constructed. Moreover, this is an identity that providers must constantly manage, negotiating with others around them as a daily part of the job as they justify their presence, their skills, and their role in health care.

In terms of defining the relational aspect of marginality, the "ambulance driver" concept and the role of IFTs both serve to highlight the different status of EMS providers relative to other health-care providers and first responders. Consequently, the EMS system is not a fully fledged member of either the health-care system or the first-responder world. While it may be central to the delivery of some critical-care services and pre-hospital transportation, we can see how this centrality is simultaneously subsumed by marginalization from both the health-care system as a whole and other first-responder fields. Both low wages and low occupational prestige accompany this outsider status. The working conditions, particularly for career EMS professionals (as opposed to volunteers), that providers experience are also challenging. The occupational marginality that complicates the EMS system's institutional position is the subject of Part II.

PART II
EMS as Marginal Work

Like all professions, working in Emergency Medical Services requires the adoption of a particular vernacular. Ambulances are "trucks," "rigs," or "buses." "Load and go" or "scoop and shoot" serves as shorthand for a patient whose illness or injury is so significant as to require immediate transport from the scene. Ambulance shifts themselves at Private Ambulance also have nicknames. An "eight" is an eight-hour shift, a "twelve" is a twelve-hour shift, and a "twenty-four" is a shift that lasts for a full twenty-four hours. At Private, twenty-fours are the mainstay of the Advanced Life Support shifts, with each ambulance staffed by either a paramedic and an emergency medical technician (an "MB" truck) or two paramedics.

Providers experience a lot over twenty-four hours. The "twenty-fours" at Private Ambulance are staggered, beginning at either "oh-six-hundred" or "oh-seven-hundred" hours (i.e., six or seven in the morning) and ending at the same time the next day. Staggered shifts are an effective way to ensure that ambulances are always available in the field for calls. This approach to scheduling is particularly crucial in Chapman because of the location of Private Ambulance's headquarters at the northern end of the city. Ambulances stationed ("posted," in Private's vernacular) in Midtown Chapman, therefore, have to drive north in rush-hour traffic each morning for shift change. Staggering their shift changes means that there is typically at least one ALS ambulance located in the neighborhoods around Midtown to respond to an early call.

In Chapters 1 and 2, which constituted Part I, I argued that the Emergency Medical Services system exists apart from the rest of the health-care system. This institutional marginality defines the system itself, how interactions with other health-care providers and first responders unfold, and how the public see EMS providers. EMS work, however, is also itself marginal. It is impossible to understand EMS work without reckoning both with its temporal aspects (the pace, the timing of events, the long hours) and its spatial aspects (where work occurs, how travel unfolds). Long hours spent in ambulances define the experience of the "twenty-four." Providers at many EMS agencies spend these hours not in a station but instead in the ambulance itself. This time in the "truck" is essential to understanding how the marginality of the work itself comes to define EMS work. Here, EMS providers experience challenging work conditions unlike the control of a traditional hospital emergency department.

Part II makes an analytical distinction between two overall categories of Emergency Medical Services work: emergency calls and downtime. Emergency calls are responses to requests for medical assistance. Emergency calls, or what providers refer to as "calls" or "jobs," are the central focus of their workday. Since they are unscheduled in the sense that providers do not know from one minute to the next if they will be sent to a call, there are periods between calls when providers wait for dispatch to their next call. These periods are termed downtime and can encompass a variety of activities, including paperwork, searching for meals, using the bathroom, driving to a location to provide "coverage" for a neighborhood of the city, and sleeping. It is critical to understand that downtime does not necessarily mean it is break time for providers. Many downtime events, for example, involve paperwork or running work-related errands as requested by Private Ambulance's dispatchers. Both phenomena are, therefore, integral to the overall experience of a shift for providers.

3
The Twenty-Four
The Rhythm of EMS Shifts

"Moments of craziness followed by hours of downtime." (Kyle)

Shift Work

Like with other first responders and health-care occupations, life at Private Ambulance revolves around shifts. Private Ambulance's supervisors schedule providers for standard shifts that are eight, twelve, or twenty-four hours long, though there are other increments used for scheduling, some shorter and some longer. The "twenty-four," as providers call it, is the standard shift for the ambulances that have at least one paramedic on-board. The Basic Life Support ambulances tend to work shorter shifts during the day. "Twenty-fours" at Private Ambulance begin at either "oh-six-hundred" or "oh-seven-hundred" hours (six or seven in the morning; everything in the EMS world unfolds on a twenty-four-hour clock).

Within the fire service, firefighters sometimes refer to these long "twenty-fours" as "tours," a wonderfully descriptive turn of phrase for describing shifts. Calling them "tours" evokes the notion of them as a linked series of events that take first responders throughout (and sometimes outside) their district. The idea of seeing EMS work as a series of related events is essential for understanding the grind that shifts represent. Focusing on downtime or patient interactions as isolated events belies the cumulative way these moments contribute to something greater. The cumulative nature of shifts is crucial, considering the typical number of hours worked during an American workday is just eight hours. Therefore, our typical concept of time spent at work is only a third of what a paramedic or EMT working a "twenty-four" experiences during a workday.

Shift 99

This shift was a "twenty-four" where I was present for over sixteen hours. It highlights both the spatial and temporal aspects of EMS work that are the primary focus of this chapter.[1] For most of the shift, Medic 7 was staffed by Janelle and Charlie. Janelle was scheduled for the entirety of the "twenty-four," while Charlie was scheduled to be relieved after twelve hours.

Downtime: Rig Checks and Breakfast (45 Minutes)

It was a few minutes before "oh-six-hundred hours" (or six in the morning) when the dispatcher buzzed me in at the front doors of Private's headquarters. When I reached the windowless dispatch office, he checked a list on a clipboard and let me know I would be riding with Charlie and Janelle that day. Charlie walked up from Private's cavernous garage just as we were discussing my assignment. He turned, waved me back, and I followed him around, past the operations offices and the two bunkrooms, and down into the garage itself. Charlie began going through the ambulance, checking each bag and cabinet to ensure they contained the appropriate supplies. Charlie was younger than many of the other paramedics and seemed to pay fastidious attention to these details in a way the more seasoned paramedics did not.

As he did this, he began talking to several other providers about a "man down" call he had on his previous shift. Like other notable calls, the story of this particular patient at the nearby Bullhead Transit station had already been making the rounds since it had occurred. Charlie relayed to the other paramedics that he thought it would be what he called "the usual morning drunk" but it turned out to be a minor who was quite sick. The providers spent time discussing the clinical particulars of the call, with Charlie happy to have someone to kill time with as we waited for Janelle to arrive.

Janelle breezed in, several minutes after the official start of our shift, hair still wet from her morning shower. Unlike Charlie, she had significant experience as a paramedic and was considered the more senior of the two providers. Charlie had not received clearance from management to work alone yet, meaning he was not able to be paired, for example, with an EMT instead of a more senior paramedic. When Janelle got downstairs, they debated who would drive, with both providers angling to be the person not driving that morning. Janelle ultimately made an executive decision that she would drive, and we headed downtown, stopping at the CVS in Bullhead that was down the street from Private's headquarters. We all went inside, with Janelle purchasing some toiletries she was out of while Charlie and I bought drinks for the morning. After flipping through several options, Charlie also bought a *New York Times* to read in the truck.

Back in the ambulance, we drove downtown without any specific instructions from the dispatcher. Different dispatchers had different attitudes about where ambulances post, Janelle told me through the passageway between the cab and the chair where I was sitting in the patient compartment. The dispatcher that morning was not posting trucks but was working on what Janelle called the "spread yourselves out" idea. The University Plaza area of Chapman, at the northern end of Midtown, was a regular spot for spending downtime. If we saw one or two ambulances already there, the idea of "spread yourselves out" was to find an area either farther up or downtown to post on our own.

At this hour, both the Old Quarter (where University Plaza was) and Midtown were mostly empty except for commuters heading to work. Charlie and Janelle switched to discussing the relative merits of the burger and burrito takeout restaurants in the Old Quarter as we headed south toward "Downtown Variety," where Janelle had decided she wanted to get breakfast. The store was mostly unremarkable, with its stocks of cigarettes, sodas, chips, lottery tickets, and local newspapers all for sale inside. Downtown Variety was, however, legendary for the breakfast sandwiches served at its deli counter. It was these sandwiches that had drawn Medic 7's crew to the sleepy neighborhood at the beginning of their shift. Downtown Variety did not open until "oh-seven-hundred," and so Medic 7's crew sat outside, waiting for them to open.

Call 1: ALS Interfacility Transport (49 Minutes)

As I noted at the beginning of Chapter 2, breakfast was delayed by a call involving an interfacility transfer. On the way to the Mather Hospital to pick up the patient, Janelle honked the ambulance's horn at a Chapman firefighter headed to work and gave him a wave.

Downtime: Breakfast and a Nap (1 Hour, 7 Minutes)

After leaving the Muir Hospital at the conclusion of the first call, Janelle decided to try to get breakfast sandwiches again. During our drive back to Downtown Variety after the call, the subject of dispatchers again came up, with Charlie criticizing dispatchers as largely powerless and emphasizing his belief that posting ambulances was about "exerting what little control they have" over providers' work routines. He followed up with a John F. Kennedy–inspired voice, adapting the famous line from Kennedy's 1961 inaugural to "ask not what your dispatcher can do for you, but what you can do for your dispatcher." Both the Old Quarter and Midtown were busier at this point in the morning, with tourists mingling with commuters and tour buses packing some of the streets near the heart of the Old Quarter.

The call came in after we had been sitting for over twenty minutes and lasted another fifty, so by the time we got back to Midtown Variety, it was well over an hour after Janelle had intended to eat breakfast. We each ordered a sandwich, and Janelle bought coffee from the cook. The deli itself sat behind a high counter at the rear of the store, where a simple sandwich menu hung over the rear wall. The menu's display evoked an earlier era. It was a Coca-Cola–brand menu board containing menu offerings manually arranged out of small black plastic letters with the prices in red next to each item. During early mornings, the store smelled of cooking eggs and breakfast meats heaped onto deliciously greasy sandwiches.

We paid for our sandwiches at a register in the front of the store. The cashier was flanked by lottery tickets and cigarette cartons, and both Charlie and Janelle bought lottery tickets. As we waited for our food, they talked about what they would do if they won the Powerball drawing, which was worth hundreds of millions of dollars. Back in the ambulance, Janelle drove us around the corner. We ate in silence, Janelle using her iPad and Charlie reading the *New York Times*, and then the three of us fell asleep in our chairs.

Call 2: Report of Seizures on a Metro Train (1 Hour, 1 Minute)

After resting for about forty-five minutes, Charlie and Janelle were jolted by the dispatcher's voice. We were being sent outside of Chapman to treat a patient who was reportedly having seizures. Janelle drove quickly—the call is a significant distance away, and she weaved in and out of traffic and through intersections as quickly as she could. We met the neighboring community's fire department and their Basic Life Support ambulance crew at a train station where the patient's train had stopped. The patient had not had seizures and was already "packaged" and ready for transport in the fire department's ambulance.

In the back of the ambulance, Janelle and Charlie quickly made a plan: Charlie would gain IV access while Janelle drew up a dose of Zofran, a medication to treat nausea. The call did not go as planned nearly from the outset. At one point, Charlie openly disagreed with Janelle in front of both the patient and the firefighters about the plan. Janelle had planned to drive their ambulance behind the BLS ambulance to the hospital. However, Charlie's dissent caused her to ask if he was comfortable with providing care. When he demurred, one of the firefighters offered to drive so they could both treat the patient.

In the hospital garage, Charlie and Janelle debriefed the call. Janelle verbally reprimanded him for the way he disagreed, telling Charlie, "Some of the guys here would bite your head off for saying that," but assuring him he did not "have to worry about me because I'm cool." Charlie had also pulled the patient's IV out during the transport while setting up an IV drip that Janelle had thought was unnecessary. He was visibly frustrated when Janelle walked away, and we drove in silence back to Chapman from the hospital, with Charlie working on his run report while Janelle drove. Charlie looked up at one point to make fun of a call for a "man down." "Maybe he just likes lying on the sidewalk," Charlie mused, implying he was not seriously ill.

Downtime: Restocking (49 Minutes)

Back at the Mather Hospital, Janelle restocked the IV supplies while Charlie and I used the restroom. Janelle and I met up outside, and we talked about the previous call. She told me she felt bad for Charlie, she had been there before, and it could be intimidating working in front of firefighters whom you did not know. We spent time sitting in the ambulance, with Janelle sharing "war stories" about calls she had been a part of. After twenty minutes, one dispatcher called Medic 7 over the air and requested they post to provide "downtown" coverage. Charlie came out of the hospital, and we drove around the corner to a convenience store, parking in its lot. Charlie kept working on his run report while Janelle smoked a cigarette behind the ambulance.

Call 3: Public Assist (8 Minutes)

We were only there for a couple of minutes, however, when the dispatcher sent us to a "public assist." We were tasked with checking in on an individual who missed an appointment with her mental-health-care provider that morning. The call was nearby, and we were soon on-scene with both the Chapman Police Department and Chapman Fire Department's Truck 2. Charlie and Janelle carried their equipment up to the house but were quickly told by the CPD sergeant on-scene that the patient was all right—she had overslept—and we were not needed. We packed our gear back up, passed several officers standing idly in front of the house, and prepared to drive back to the convenience store.

Downtime: Driving (6 Minutes)

We drove back in silence to the store. Janelle parked the ambulance and we all sat for a moment.

Call 4: ALS Inferfacility Transfer (1 Hour, 40 Minutes)

The dispatcher almost immediately sent the crew on another call. It was a medical interfacility transfer to a facility several cities away. Janelle attempted to get Medic 7 out of the call, offering to take another nearby one for a "man down." However, the dispatcher declined, selecting an ambulance farther away because Medic 7 was heading in the opposite direction. Janelle dismissed this as "silly," but Charlie began to rant, criticizing the dispatcher at length while he began filling out the paperwork for the interfaculty transfer.

The call was long, and we were out of Chapman for well over an hour while we drove to the suburban hospital and then returned to the city. It was not a particularly exciting call for the crew. Charlie spent much of the first part of the long drive describing the patient's medical history and the labs listed in the patient's chart. For a time, Janelle found herself stuck in a construction-related traffic jam on an interstate. We made it to the hospital once traffic opened up beyond the constriction created by the construction work and transferred the patient to a hospital bed on an upper floor after reporting to a nurse at the entrance.

Downtime: Lunch (49 Minutes)

On our drive back into town, Charlie and Janelle talked about coworkers for a few minutes before beginning to decide on their lunch plan. We stopped at a chain Mexican-style restaurant. Janelle told me she loved the food there but ate it so frequently. She also said she was not sure if she wanted it now or for dinner. Charlie and I walked inside and ordered a burrito, and we used the bathroom while Janelle stayed in the truck, using her phone. After we got back into the ambulance, Janelle decided she wanted something from one of the markets in the Old Quarter. We drove south and parked in the fire lane out front of a small grocery store. Janelle ran in while we ate our burritos quickly in case another call came in. A burrito left sitting in the ambulance during the call would end up soggy and perhaps inedible. She came back with a salad and managed no more than a few bites before the dispatcher came on the air again for Medic 7. They were sending us on yet another call.

Call 5: Abdominal Pain (25 Minutes)

The call was for abdominal pain in a nearby apartment building. Charlie asked if I had been there before and mentioned that it was a public housing complex that Private's crews responded to frequently. We took the elevator to the patient's floor and spoke with the firefighters who were already on-scene. The patient, who was having complications from diabetes, was sitting in a folding camping chair in the dark. There were trash and empty beer cans strewn about the sparsely furnished apartment, and a mattress lay directly on the floor in a corner. The firefighters helped transfer the patient to the cot Charlie and Janelle brought with them in the elevator. Charlie tried to talk to the patient about managing his diabetes during the ride to the hospital. Once we arrived there, Charlie told me a bit more about the patient, whom he had treated several times before both for diabetes and complications related to alcohol abuse. The frequent contact Charlie has had with this patient, and others, meant he knew a wealth of information about their medical history.

Downtime: War Stories (1 Hour, 16 Minutes)

After transferring care to the emergency department from the prior call, we sat on the rear bumper of the ambulance in the ambulance bay and talked with each other and, later, with another crew. It was shady in the ambulance bay because there was an awning covering it, protecting us from the bright afternoon sun. Ambulances have unusually wide bumpers (relative to passenger vehicles) to facilitate climbing in and out of the rear door of the ambulance. Private Ambulance's bumpers were metal and provided plenty of space to sit and lean with your back up against the rear of the ambulance.

At first, a former Private Ambulance member now working at the Mather Hospital joined us. The emergency medicine world is a small one. Throughout Chapman, there were current and former members of Private Ambulance who worked at the area hospitals, local fire departments, and other EMS companies. The Mather Hospital was no exception, and this former member spent his break catching up with Charlie and Janelle. They compared what it was like working on an ambulance—long, sometimes unpredictable hours—with what it was like working in the hospital, where shifts were shorter in length. They also described how hospital work has more predictability than EMS work because staff were assigned to a set number of patients and transferred care to a colleague at the end of each shift. Their conversation segued into a discussion of why the former member decided to leave Private Ambulance.

Once the former member's break was over, he went back inside, and Charlie and Janelle switched to telling "war stories." These included stories about calls they had been on, hospitals they have transported to, and what EMS work was like for them.[2] They spent time talking about time-consuming psychiatric transfers. Since in-patient beds were few, patients often had to be driven considerable distances from the hospital they first presented at to a facility where an in-patient bed was available. Janelle talked about one overnight transfer she did during a blizzard to a facility located about an hour away. When they returned, they realized they had forgotten some essential paperwork and had to do a second drive out to the facility and back. Janelle also tells us about times she had damaged ambulances, including a front tire she flattened. Her partner was so tired that despite hitting a curb, he did not wake up until Janelle had realized the tire was flat.

They also talked about nurses. They both preferred the staff who work at the Mather Hospital relative to the other major medical center in Chapman, the Muir Hospital. At the Muir, Charlie said, the nurses could be "crabby." If he took a patient in who was hurt, in Charlie's words, "bleeding everywhere and covered in shit," the nurses at the Muir would look at them and say, "Why the fuck did you bring him here?" Janelle concurred, grumbling that "we like the nurses at the Mather Hospital better."

Janelle got up after a while and moved into the cab of the ambulance out of view while Charlie continued to talk to me about tattoo designs he was interested in. After a few minutes, another Private Ambulance truck pulled in behind us. We heard them dispatched for a scheduled transfer of a patient earlier in the afternoon. One of the EMTs hopped out of the truck and asked if we heard a police officer had been shot in a neighboring city. We had not; an officer being shot was "fucked up," Charlie says. The EMTs went inside, and Charlie was left sitting on the bench, visibly upset. He talked about the recent shooting in the city and the shooting of some firefighters in Webster, New York, the previous Christmas. "It really makes you think," he said. "I understand firefighters being killed in a collapse or in a cold storage warehouse, but [these shootings] just don't make any sense. People say 'oh he had a bad childhood,' but it doesn't matter." Charlie trailed off, seemingly lost in his thoughts. He shook his head, and his radio crackled to life.

Downtime: Coffee and a Cigarette (10 Minutes)

Our conversation about gun violence was interrupted by the dispatcher, who directed us to "come out" from the hospital and cover downtown. Janelle drove, blaring classic rock through the ambulance's radio, and pulled into a Dunkin'

Donuts on her way downtown. Instead of continuing farther, we ended up parking there. Janelle got a coffee and smoked another cigarette, and Charlie slumped down in the passenger seat as he played on his smartphone in silence. We were at the Dunkin' Donuts for a few minutes, just enough time for Janelle to get most of the way through her cigarette, when the dispatcher came back on the air with our next call.

Call 6: Pediatric Trauma (35 Minutes)

The call the dispatcher sent Medic 7 on was at one of the university campuses within Chapman for a traumatic injury to a pediatric patient. Given the nature of the reported injury, the fire department responded along with Medic 7 to the scene and helped move the patient from the location of the call out to the ambulance.[3] This call took us out of Chapman again to the regional children's hospital, whose emergency department was quiet. They quickly accepted the patient without keeping Medic 7's crew waiting. Janelle had "teched" the call, and Charlie drove back into the city where we were yet again requested to post downtown.

Downtime: Downtown Coverage (27 Minutes)

Charlie picked a new spot, not far from Downtown's central plaza, and got out of the truck to make a phone call while Janelle worked on her paperwork from the pediatric trauma. Charlie told me this was one of his "secret" posting spots because there were no residential parking restrictions, and they were close to the busiest parts of downtown Chapman.

Call 7: Medical Alarm Activated (8 Minutes)

Medic 7 was dispatched for the report of a "man down." The dispatcher provided an update after a minute or two, letting the crew know the call was for an activated medical alarm. The dispatcher also clarified that the patient may not be at the exact address given to the crew initially. Instead, the patient was possibly somewhere in the area around the given address. To help Medic 7 locate the patient, the dispatcher also provided them with a physical description of the patient from the medical alarm company.

Janelle used a map book to determine what the cross streets were for this address and directed Charlie to the reported scene. When we arrived, the street was mostly empty, and Janelle commented that no one looked to be in distress. Janelle called the dispatcher on the radio to let him know we were "out in the area" and looking for the patient. She had Charlie drive two blocks north, turn the ambulance around, and then drive a few blocks back south on the same street. Charlie slowed at one point, checking to see if a person we were passing matched the description of the patient. He did not, and we checked a public parking lot nearby for anyone matching the description before calling back in service.

Downtime: More Downtown Coverage (1 Hour, 25 Minutes)

The dispatcher requested we continue to provide downtown coverage, and Charlie decided he wanted to head back to where we were before. When we parked, Charlie got out of the ambulance and came around to the passenger side. I opened the side door and sat on the step that takes you up into the patient compartment. Janelle was on the phone inside the ambulance, and when she hung up, she got out and lit another cigarette. We talked about smoking, and Janelle says it was "like clockwork [for her] between calls. Have a smoke. I don't even want to, but it is a habit." As with a sizable portion of Private's employees, she was a regular user of tobacco products, she says, telling me that many of the guys who worked at Private did not smoke but "dipped" (used chewing tobacco) instead.

While we talked, we heard the Chapman Fire Department, which had already had several structure fires today, dispatched for the report of "smoke in the area" nearby where we were posting. This latest fire report led the providers to talk about Janelle's boyfriend, a firefighter, and the risks in firefighting work. They also talked about beer and vacations, since Janelle was heading to a neighboring state this coming weekend for some time with her boyfriend. After chatting for a while, Janelle decided to go inside a nearby shop to look around, and Charlie started to talk to me about going out to bars in downtown Chapman. The bars were frequented by what Charlie described as "that pastel shirt and jeans crowd wearing what they wear to work." He contrasted this with his preferred outfit, a T-shirt and shorts, and then described a couple of the bars where he felt comfortable in the area.

We were interrupted by a phone call for Charlie, and Janelle came back out from the shop. We talked about the differences between working with a strictly "medic-basic" (or "MB") system, where paramedics were always paired with an EMT and have less backup, and a system like Chapman where there are other paramedics available on neighboring ambulances as well as with the fire department. Janelle commented about how great it was to have that level of support before getting into the ambulance to use her iPad. Charlie had just finished his call, so we talked about the woman he was on the phone with and his relationship with her. Charlie decided it is about time to start to head back to Private, since his shift would end at nineteen-hundred hours. With rush hour traffic, getting back would take quite a bit of time.

Downtime: Changing Partners (57 Minutes)

We started driving, and Charlie talked about how happy he was, having moved recently to the area and started working at Private. He and Janelle had ample time to talk in the heavy traffic, and Charlie went back over the details of his relationship with the woman he spoke to on the phone. As we slowly made our way north, another Private Ambulance crew ambulance responded to a call for "the psych," and Charlie commented out loud "for a crazy person." When he spoke, Charlie drew out both syllables of "crazy" for additional emphasis so that it sounded like "craaaa-zzzzee." Charlie added he was glad it was not assigned to us since he had "gotta get back, it's almost 7 o'clock."

We were getting close to the Old Quarter now, and the two paramedics started to talk about where they should park if the dispatcher still had not called us to return to base by the time we got into the Old Quarter itself. They talked over a couple of different options, including a gas station halfway between the Old Quarter and Private's headquarters Charlie suggested. Janelle disagreed, saying the gas station employees might be "all butt hurt if we do that" (sit there) and instead suggested a different option. Before we got there, though, the dispatcher requested we return for the partner swap, and Charlie continued driving north to Private's headquarters.

After we parked outside, Charlie went into the men's locker room to change, and Janelle headed upstairs to the dispatch center, where she spent about twenty minutes chatting with the dispatcher. They spoke mostly about their families, and then both Janelle and I went to the bathroom. After our break, we met Adam in the crew room at the top of the stairs down to the garage, and Janelle introduced me to him. The new crew of Medic 7 walked back down into the garage and out the main door into the alley where Janelle and Charlie had left the ambulance. As we walked out the main door, Janelle commented to me about another paramedic whom Adam was talking to. "He's crazy," she told me, "They're all crazy here. You have to be crazy to do this [work]." With this reflection on life at Private Ambulance, she climbed into the ambulance with Adam close behind, and we began driving back downtown once again.

Call 8: Psychiatric Problem (31 Minutes)

Just a few minutes into our drive, the dispatcher Janelle spoke with at Private's base came on the air to send Medic 7 to a psych call at a nursing home. We arrived at the facility to find a patient sitting in a wheelchair inside the front entrance. There were two staff members nearby, but neither of them had a complete understanding of why the patient needed hospitalization. The only information they had, which they kept repeating, was that the patient's nurse requested it. The nurse, however, was nowhere in sight, and neither Adam nor Janelle made an effort to find her. Adam started with patient care, such as it is with "psych patients." He spoke with her about how she was feeling, while Janelle got the cot out of the ambulance. In the back of the ambulance, Adam sat and quietly chatted with the patient. At the same time, we rode down to Chapman City Hospital, which housed the city's only psychiatric emergency department (what providers called the "psych ED").

At the hospital, Adam and Janelle wheeled the patient back to the psych ED. Janelle helped the patient into a bed in a sparsely furnished observation room. Thick glass separated the room from the nurses' station, allowing the staff to monitor patients from a central station. Adam and I walked through the room and talked to both staff members who were present, a younger nurse who was in charge and an older nurse who appeared very new. The older but newer nurse seemed excitable and moved quickly around the station, ready to jump into treating the patient. The senior nurse tried to calm her down, and Adam shared what little info he had on the patient. They seemed a little annoyed that he did not have more details.

We went into the registration room to get the patient registered, a process that took a while. Adam made a comment under his breath and then looked at me and said, "It's like pulling teeth in here." Once we were outside of the ED, I asked him how often he felt it was a challenging process. He said, "All of the time. I mean, [the nurses] have to have worked somewhere else. You have to have taken a report from a [paramedic]. I only know what I'm told. I can't figure out what's wrong. That's your job." Adam sounded exasperated as he said this and then turned toward the ambulance.

Dinner (1 Hour, 45 Minutes)

We got back into the ambulance, and Janelle again tuned the radio to classic rock. She decided she wanted Middle Eastern food for dinner and asked if I was okay with that choice; Adam had already eaten dinner. When we parked near the restaurant, Adam stayed behind working on his run report from the previous call. We went inside, and Janelle told me how much she liked the restaurant. A group of young Arab men staffed the counter, and their menu offered a range of Mediterranean and North African food choices. We waited for our food by a side counter stocked with napkins, utensils, and condiments.

Once our orders came up, I followed Janelle out to sit in the square, not far from the ambulance. Adam had wanted a soda, which Janelle bought and brought over to the ambulance before she joined me at a table.

As we ate, Janelle talked to me about homelessness in Chapman. She used the Private Ambulance code "37-Delta" for them. I asked her if she knew where the code came from, and we discussed how providers used the term. Janelle told me some more "war stories," this time about several bad homeless calls she had responded to along the river during the winter. She described calls during lousy winter weather where the medics would find severe frostbite on their patients. Janelle said she could not imagine living on the street. She also told me she thought that the homeless were different there than in neighboring cities. Janelle adds that they are "rougher" in Chapman.

Eventually, Adam joined us after buying some pastries from the Middle Eastern restaurant, and the conversation switched to talking about vacations and travel. The discussion about travel carried over into the ambulance as we drove north toward the Old Quarter. After a while, the conversation wandered back toward the previous call, and Janelle mentioned she hated doing geriatric psych calls: "It's just so sad. When I first started, I took this little old man in that we had to restrain because he was so violent." Janelle paused, and then repeated herself, "It's so sad."

As she drove into the Old Quarter, Janelle mentioned we might not be able to park in our usual spot. She tells us the city traffic department "meter maid" had been kicking Private Ambulance crews out of a strip of roadway providers have regularly used in the past for posting. Located off the main square, this strip consisted of a fire lane in front of some retail shops near a small grocery store. The grocery store was open twenty-four hours a day and offered restrooms, making it a favorite for providers. As we pulled in, Janelle complained that "it's busy," putting an emphasis on busy. She groused about the college students filling the square on a busy, temperate late summer evening. "UGH," she yelled. We then sat for about twenty minutes with little discussion in the ambulance.

Call 9: Psychiatric Problem and IV Drug Use (24 Minutes)

The radio broke the silence, with our dispatcher on the air with another call for us. It was another reported "psych call" nearby, and we soon met two Chapman Police Department units on-scene. The patient was sitting on the front stoop of a storefront church. The street was very dark, with a few nearby streetlights providing only some dim lighting. According to a bystander, the patient had asked him to call 9-1-1 because he was sick. The patient was whimpering and told Janelle he was in a significant amount of pain. Janelle asked him about any recent substance use, and she and the patient discussed issues related to both intravenous drug use and chronic infectious diseases as well as infected sores. The patient asked to go to the Mather Hospital, so Janelle walked him back to the ambulance while Adam got into the cab. They did not make an effort to take the cot out for the patient. Instead, they had him climb into the ambulance on his own.

During the quick ride to the Mather, Janelle asked him to tell his story several times over. She seemed to be looking for (and later tells me is confident she found) inconsistencies. Janelle focused in on slight changes in his recent medical history, the medications he reported taking, and the reasons the patient gave for recent hospitalizations. He told Medic 7's providers about using harm reduction services, and Janelle nodded. At the hospital, they used the cot to wheel him in and help him to a bed in an emergency department room. Adam and I went back outside with the cot while Janelle went to register the patient, and Adam looked at me and sarcastically deadpanned "another life saved" as he slid the cleaned cot back into the ambulance.

Ice Cream and Waiting to 60 (44 Minutes)

Still at the hospital, Adam slept in the front of the truck while Janelle worked on the run report in the driver's seat. After fifteen minutes of napping, Adam decided he wanted frozen yogurt and so drove us uptown slightly from the hospital to a local ice cream and frozen yogurt shop, located along Main Street in a low, one-story building. The street was quiet, and there was some momentary confusion regarding whether the shop was still open. Janelle decided she would "hold back" that night, telling me she liked her frozen yogurt but was not in the mood for it that night.

When Adam got back in with his dessert, he drove the ambulance down the street to a traffic island in the middle of a park near the Old Quarter. As he drove, Janelle asked him if he thought her previous patient, whom she called "my guy," "was a seeker?" Adam responded, "I dunno?" Janelle continued, "He didn't have a fever or nothing," and Adam then concurred, agreeing that "he looked like a junkie." Janelle doubled down on the point of his IV drug use—"He admitted to it, definitely a junkie." She also felt suspicious about the patient's request to go to the Mather Hospital when, according to their records, he usually presented for care at another safety-net hospital in a nearby city. If he was a drug seeker, she surmised, the other hospital would have records of this behavior and that could be why he did not request to go there tonight.

At the park, Adam and Janelle settled in to wait for the dispatcher to call them back for the evening. Private's providers referred to this condition as "waiting to 60" (or return to Private's base) for the night. During overnights, dispatchers station (or "post") two ambulances at the Mather Hospital where there is a bunkroom. They also station an additional ambulance at Private's base where there are couches and bunkrooms available for sleeping. Dispatchers and providers both refer to this ambulance as the "base truck," and Medic 7 was the base truck that evening. Since the base sits away from the significant population centers in the city, the base truck has a reputation for being a bit quieter than the other units stationed at the City Hospital, and Adam and Janelle were anxious to get back and get to sleep. While they waited Janelle smoked another cigarette, and Adam called his wife to say goodnight.

60ing (18 Minutes)

When Janelle finished with her cigarette, she got back in the ambulance, and the dispatcher called soon after. They gave Medic 7 permission to return to quarters. As we drove back north through the city, Janelle decided to fill up the ambulance at a gas station just south of the ambulance base where Private had a corporate account. Adam got out of the ambulance and filled up the tank. While we sat, the dispatcher came back on the air and requested Medic 7, our ambulance, expedite our return to pick up the portable ventilator. After this, Medic 7 would be taking an interfacility transfer from the Mather Hospital to a hospital with a specialized intensive care unit. The patient was on a ventilator, and this would be what providers called a "vent transfer."

Ventilator transfers were the subject of a significant amount of derision among providers. Providers felt that the calls took a long time, in part because getting the paperwork in order for a complicated case was extensive. Moving the patient from the hospital's ventilator to the portable one and then back to the new hospital's ventilator also took a significant amount of time and work. They also required additional providers because, in the event of a failure, there needed to be at least two providers in the back of the ambulance to perform CPR. Crews, therefore, had to return to headquarters each time to pick up the ventilator and often a third crew member; sometimes a second ambulance would be taken out of service to staff the transfer. We drove back to Private Ambulance, and Adam bounded inside to pick up the ventilator while I packed my bag and wished them both luck with the transfer. I watched from my car as Medic 7 pulled out of the parking lot into the night, headed south back toward the Mather Hospital.

Rhythm in Shift Work

Each shift I observed at Private Ambulance unfolded similarly to "Shift 99," and yet each was exceptionally different. This incongruous experience reveals a central paradox of EMS work—it is at once very predictable and yet, at the same time, not predictable. When asked to describe their jobs, EMS providers at Private Ambulance often focused on how each day was different. Many enjoyed the fact that they did not know what each new call or shift would bring in terms of patients and challenges.

However, there were also readily distinguishable patterns between shifts. Each felt as though it had a rhythm. None were exceptionally busy, going from call to call to call without any break. While some shifts featured more calls and others less, each shift featured repeated periods of downtime or driving, like regular commas in a run-on sentence. Like "Shift 99," the temporal rhythm of each shift, therefore, felt like a continuous oscillation between boredom and excitement where it was difficult to predict what each new event would bring. Providers like Charlie ate quickly, as we did with lunch, not knowing if their meal would be interrupted. Providers were never particularly frustrated when this happened, acknowledging that these interruptions were just part of the job. They did, however, frequent restaurants where they could get takeout and quickly leave if they needed to. Providers treated opportunities to sleep in much the same way as eating. Adam and Janelle were excited to get back and get to sleep toward the end of their shift precisely because they did not know how long it would last.

One way of understanding how demanding shifts can be is through providers' discussions of the "flow" or "pace" of shifts. During the semi-structured interviews, providers identified the pace of a shift (though not always using the word "pace") as one significant factor affecting whether they believed a shift was "good" or "bad":

> CP: What's a good shift?
>
> SAM: A good shift? There's the, you know, the white rhino of an EMS shift is probably busy all day, so you know it makes [the] day go by. You're occupied. You're not really bored sitting around whatever and then sleeping at night. Getting a good amount of sleep. You know, getting a call or two, but that's about it. That's a pitch perfect EMS shift. Pretty rare.

Sam continued, describing that it was also possible to be too busy during the day. He described a state of business so frantic he felt like the shifts were "brain-numbing":

> SAM: [the busiest] shift I ever worked would be an example of that. We did a 24 on a Friday [and] I did twenty-seven calls in a "twenty-four." Twenty-three of them were ALS, so it's like full work up. Twenty-five of them were transports, and then we got held three hours after the shift for [a] 4 alarm fire standby. That can be brain-numbing.

Both quotes focus on the idea of pace. A fast-paced shift, with too many calls, does not allow for rest or proper sleep. A shift that feels too slow, on the other hand, can introduce boredom into the workday.

The question of pace and sleep is especially critical for providers who work on twenty-four-hour shifts. Downtime is therefore not "wasted" time but rather plays an important role in offering a mental and physical break for many providers. A period of rest is even more essential when work periods stretch to twenty-four hours or longer, as in the example Sam gave, when they were held three hours after their shift while they stood by at a large structure fire. Without these breaks for both sleep and mental rest, providers reported feeling like they were sometimes pushed nearly to their "breaking point":

> DWIGHT: . . . most of the time you feel like you're getting your nuts kicked in for 24 hours. [It's] busy during the day, sometimes you don't have enough time to think between calls. You're just constantly moving . . . but it feels like right before you reach your breaking point there's a lull and then you kind of just chill out . . .

These tensions, in particular the notion of the "breaking point" or a "brain-numbing" shift, speak both to the lack of control providers have over their work routines and the more general challenges shifts present to workers, whether they are EMS providers, firefighters, police officers, nurses, or workers on an assembly line.

Unlike assembly-line work, however, patient care is involved. "Shift 99" is typical of the shifts I observed. Few of the shifts featured only very ill patients. Patients who had significant injuries or illnesses, those patients with "real emergencies," were few and far between. The mix of patients described in "Shift 99" was typical of the shifts I observed. Vent transfers are emblematic of much of what is awkward about this pace of the calls themselves. They are unpredictable, the patients are sick, but they are also generally stable. These could be tedious, time-consuming calls where the prospect of things going wrong in a hurry was never far off. They required a significant amount of driving because the hospitals to which vented patients needed transport were all outside of Chapman's city limits. A vent transfer at the end of the shift could mean staying for hours over the official end of a provider's shift because of the timing involved. Typically, vent transfers were like most of the other calls: time-consuming and ultimately not about using many of the advanced skills the paramedics, in particular, had acquired.

Temporal Context and the Emerging Model of EMS Work

The importance of rhythm in shift work for providers is that the pace of shifts and the way they unfold impact everything else about the shift. How much of a break they have between calls, if they can get a meal, or whether the meal is interrupted are all consequences of this temporal context. The pace itself is what we will refer to as the "temporal context" of work (see Figure 10).[4] The temporal context affects providers' interdependent work routines, affecting who they see, when, and for how long. Busy shifts may mean they get little time to interact with other crews, as opposed to slow shifts where they may have ample time to sit on the rear bumper of their ambulance and people watch.

Shifts also blend for providers. Providers experience a "loop," where the rhythm of one shift feeds into other shifts as well. They arrive at Private Ambulance, check their truck over to make sure it is ready, post, go to a call or two, post again, and so on. This loop happens day in and day out for them. Some days are busier than others, but there is a sense of repetition with EMS shifts. Therefore, working in EMS can feel like being stuck in a constant loop of downtime, responding to calls, trying to sleep or nap, and responding to more calls. This loop suggests that marginality is not just structural and occupational, but temporal as well.

Time is something that EMS providers cannot control, and yet the pace of shifts is an essential part of the broader norms and practices of EMS work. Critical calls require a "fast" pace, driving quickly to the call, moving deliberately on-scene, and transporting patients with expediency. This pace comports with how providers and the general public view EMS work. The temporal context also impacts the social workplace practices through the occupational tricks of the trade providers develop. This includes knowledge about how to order meals that are easy to eat in an ambulance or that will sit well if a meal is interrupted by a call. Taking advantage of public restrooms or those in hospital emergency departments because you do not know when you will get a break again is another example of the way the unknowns inherent in EMS work's pace structure the work itself.

The ways in which provider time is shaped by outside institutions fits with the concept of a "web of time" (Clawson and Gerstel 2014). This idea of a web is meant to underscore the different institutional forces that shape workers' abil-

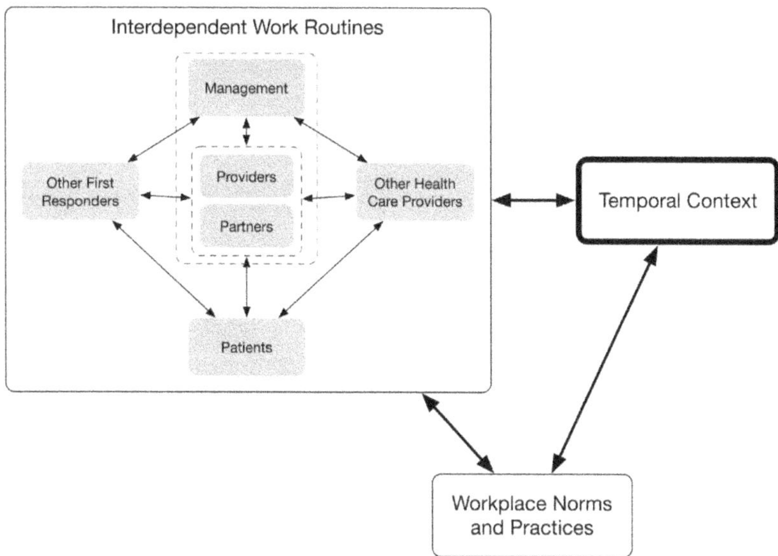

Figure 10. Evolving Theoretical Model—Integrating Temporal Context (graph by author)

ity to schedule their work as well as their own time and that of their families. For EMS providers, their "web of time" is shaped by a variety of institutions. Within Private Ambulance, supervisors are in charge of scheduling, while dispatchers dictate when providers are assigned to different calls. The speed at which those calls unfold is dependent on their interactions with patients as well as with other first responders. This rhythm is also dependent on how busy hospitals are and how quickly nurses and hospital staff can direct their patients to a room. Even their movements around Chapman are structured by forces like time of day, which impacts how much traffic they must contend with. Each of these factors contributes both to the rhythm of their shifts and to the larger "web of time" that influences EMS work.

Many of these activities are also examples of "downtime," which as we can see from "Shift 99" is a constant presence in EMS work. Part of the pace of shifts is the inevitable breaks, even during those shifts providers feel are "brain-numbing" because they are going from call to call. These breaks are crucial for providers to catch their breath, get a bite to eat, and get some sleep. Downtime is therefore a temporal phenomenon, but it is also one affected significantly by *where* it takes place. These temporal and spatial elements of downtime are the subject of Chapter 4.

4
Hurry Up and Wait
Passing Time and Avoiding Conflict

"It's flipping through my phone. Facebook. Taking naps, eating, if we have a chance." (Liam)

Naps and Lunch

Early in the morning on one of the first crisp fall days in Chapman, I was riding with Emily and Marianna, two of Private Ambulance's EMTs. We had just finished a call, and Emily had parked outside of Eaton Plaza in the Old Quarter. The women told me they could not park in the Plaza anymore, and so Emily had picked a spot a few blocks away. Once she parked, she took out her tablet computer and started reading while Marianna spent time on her iPhone.

After a few minutes, Marianna fell asleep. After she had been asleep for a while, Medic 5 pulled up next to us, blocking traffic. The medics started to take pictures of Marianna sleeping, and Emily motioned for them to be quiet. However, Marianna woke up, laughing as she gave Medic 5's crew the middle finger and a hard time for hassling her. A car pulled up behind Medic 5, which forced the crew to drive on, since there was no parking. A short time later, Marianna was asleep again, and B10 pulled up alongside us. Its crew began to take photos of her as well. Emily gestured for them to stop, and like Medic 5, they had to pull away when a car pulled up.

Marianna fell asleep again, and a spot opened up behind us. A Chapman police officer occupied it briefly, and then Medic 5, who had been circling the neighborhood, grabbed it when the officer left. They sat for a few minutes until their dispatcher assigned them a job.

Likewise, B10 had been circling the neighborhood, as well, and parked behind us once Medic 5 went to their call. One of the EMTs came up to our ambulance to visit. Marianna, who was now awake, and Emily talked to him for a while. They discussed new electronic music releases, and Marianna plugged the EMT's phone from B10 into our ambulance's stereo so we could listen to music together. The other EMT from B10 joined us but spent most of his time on his phone a few feet away from the ambulance. The EMTs spoke for a few minutes as they listened to music, and then Emily and Marianna decided they wanted coffee.

They drove to the other side of the Old Quarter and parked in front of the same market we visited in Chapter 3 for lunch. They used the bathroom and bought coffee at the Starbucks adjacent to the grocery store. With our food, we drove back down to where we had parked before. B10 was still there, and we talked to the EMTs again, making small talk until Emily and Marianna decided they wanted lunch. Emily had food with her, and we headed to the Mather Hospital to use the microwave in the ED break room. However, we did not make it far before we were interrupted for a call.

Downtime in EMS Work

The unpredictable and uncontrollable nature of EMS work, the subject of Chapter 3, is a critical attribute that shapes individual shifts as well as the more general temporal quality of EMS work.[1] One aspect of this temporal climate is that the amount of time between calls, which I describe as "downtime," is both unpredictable and uncontrollable. Emily and Marianna had no idea how busy they would be when they began their shift, how much time they would have to relax, or whom they would get to socialize with between calls.

Nevertheless, downtime is also reliable. During "Shift 99," a total of ten hours and forty minutes, or about two-thirds of the shift, was spent on downtime activities. This ratio matches the general trend with downtime, which accounted for 64 percent of the total number of shift hours observed. While providers do not know how much time they will have from shift to shift, they can reliably assume they will have some time on each shift that is considered downtime.

Another critical feature to emerge from Chapter 3 is that downtime (and calls, though we will return to this in Part III) happens *somewhere*. Providers may, therefore, see large swaths of geographic territory during their shifts, and so time spent at work for EMS providers is also time spent *in place*. The spatial nature of EMS work adds significant complexity and potential conflict to the shifts EMS providers work. All work, of course, takes place somewhere, but often within the confines of a single site like an office building or a factory. What is essential about EMS work, along with the work of other first responders, is the way it unfolds in a myriad of locations during a single work period. Downtime happens at a coffee shop near the Mather Hospital, at the hospital itself, at Downtown Variety, or at one of a variety of other locations in Chapman where providers go when they are not responding to calls.

Providers' decisions about where to spend downtime illustrate another facet of the complex relationships between time, the social features of work, and interdependent work routines. To this point, these features of EMS work have been described mainly in terms of how our evolving model of EMS work applies to emergency care. The same forces shape downtime, and this chapter explores downtime in greater detail. However, this chapter also adds a second dimension of complexity, highlighting how the core axes of work time are themselves also shaped by *where* they occur. This emphasis on place has been acknowledged by social scientists unevenly despite the "spatial turn" a variety of disciplines have experienced.[2] For sociologists of work, in particular, there is limited exploration of space and place for how these relate to the broader interests of urbanists for work occurring in cities.[3] For EMS providers, in particular, tensions emerge over whether they have a "right" to the city itself, especially when it comes to where downtime takes place during their shift.

Experiencing Downtime

In Chapter 3, I noted how EMS work is one occupation that fits into the idea of a "web of time" (Clawson and Gerstel 2014). In Chapter 3's context, the "web of time" helps to underscore how the temporal rhythm is shaped not just by one organization but by an array of organizations around EMS work. The myriad of linkages and connections that shape EMS work broadly also affect specific facets of shifts, like downtime. Downtime, as I have already described it, is the time between emergency calls. It is not scheduled and not necessarily leisure time, but despite its unpredictability, it is a regular feature of EMS shifts.

Downtime Activities

This tension between "work time" and "downtime" is visible in the range of activities providers engage in during downtime. Broadly, these activities are one of three types: (1) purely personal, such as running errands; (2) activities that help providers through their long shifts, such as eating and sleeping; and (3) purely work-focused, such as running errands for dispatchers or completing paperwork. Each of these appears in Chapter 3's thick description of

"Shift 99," which began with personal errands Janelle, one of the two paramedics, had to run. Our first stop of the morning was a drugstore located in a strip mall nearby. Janelle went into the back to purchase some toiletries while Charlie and I bought coconut waters and Charlie bought a copy of the *New York Times*. This particular downtime event also illustrated the fuzzy boundaries between the three categories just noted. In essence, it was purely personal in the context of Janelle's errands but also involved purchasing drinks and a *New York Times*, which are perhaps better described as self-care.

Activities that help providers through long shifts, such as sleeping, eating, and staying entertained, constitute a significant element of downtime. During "Shift 99," there were trips between calls to get breakfast, lunch, and dinner at a variety of takeout restaurants or neighborhood grocery stores. Providers occasionally brought food from home, but more often than not, as in "Shift 99," meals were picked up on the go when there was time during shifts. Typically, providers would select a restaurant together, though there were instances when providers each had different ideas about meals, and they spent time going to each of those restaurants. There is a downside to splitting restaurants for providers, though, because downtime length is not predictable, and there is no guarantee both providers would be able to eat. The negotiation over where to eat and, more broadly, how to spend downtime illustrates the social context within which downtime occurs. Providers work off a set of shared norms that govern priorities during downtime and emphasize the need to be accommodating to partners.

"Shift 99" also illustrates the flexibility providers have with downtime. If providers have errands to run, such as picking up toiletries from a convenience store, they often can complete them between calls. Providers also can sleep if they would like, which is another essential element of managing the length of shifts. At several points during "Shift 99," including after breakfast, one or more of the providers napped in the ambulance. During the interview phase of data collection, a provider noted how sleep is imperative, especially on long shifts such as "twenty-fours." During downtime, this paramedic would "usually get some sleep in there, maybe take a nap if I can. If I'm going to be on a twenty-four, then I definitely try to get a nap in." The unpredictability of EMS work makes napping particularly crucial because there are no guarantees that the overnight segments of shifts will be quiet and restful.

The third element of self-care that was ubiquitous during shifts was the use of personal electronic devices, typically smartphones and tablet computers. Providers would connect these devices to the internet through the wireless hotspots installed in the cab of each ambulance. Every provider I rode with or interviewed had a smartphone, and 40 percent of those interviewed also reported having an iPad or Kindle they used at work. During "Shift 99," Janelle had an iPad with her that she routinely used during downtime activities. Providers use these devices for a range of activities, including accessing Netflix-style streaming services, reading, using the internet, checking Facebook, texting with friends, and playing games. When pulling into a downtime location, checking smartphones was often the first thing providers would do once they were parked. Some providers also used their smartphones to stream music through the ambulance's stereo system while we drove or sat at a post.

Finally, downtime during shifts consisted of the third group of purely work-focused activities. These periods allowed providers to run errands for Private Ambulance itself. Company-oriented tasks included picking up billing information ("face-sheets") from area hospitals, fueling ambulances, taking ambulances in need of maintenance or annual inspections to the mechanic, or delivering chocolates to area emergency departments during the holidays. These are all necessary tasks for the company itself that providers support during their time between calls. Providers also use downtime to complete "jobs," the patient-care reports they write up for each patient they make contact with on calls. They complete these reports using "Toughbook"-type tablet computers, which transmit data via the wireless hotspot in each ambulance.

Temporal Marginality and Downtime

Beyond providing providers with a chance for self-care, there is another purpose to downtime. EMS providers have relatively little control over their work environment, a phenomenon I describe in Chapter 3 as temporal marginality. They cannot control the pace with which they see patients or where those patient contacts take place and may not have the time to step out for a lunch break or a nap before returning to the grind. They receive their directions via dispatchers who control much of the daily workflow EMS providers are subject to during shifts, thus Charlie's dry paraphrase of John F. Kennedy: "Ask not what your dispatcher can do for you." These are important points because they underscore the lack of autonomy providers experience during their workday.

Downtime becomes a temporal space over which providers have a significant degree of control. If they want to people watch, nap, or eat, those are all options that are available to them until the next request comes in from their dispatcher. Thus, the dining decisions made during "Shift 99" for breakfast, lunch, and dinner were all choices providers made based on their mood and what types of food they were interested in when they had a free moment to eat. Downtime is not just a mental and physical break but a chance to exert control upon a work environment over which providers often have little control.

This lack of control itself shapes what downtime looks like for providers. Providers reported not being able to feel like they could fully relax. Meal selection occurs with mindfulness about whether the food would be edible should a call come in and disrupt their consumption. Even sleep comes with caution, as providers turn the volume up on their radios so they do not miss a call. They sleep in their uniforms, with work boots stashed nearby at the ready in case they have to be quickly put on to respond to a call. Downtime, then, is not a complete rest, but rather one full of anticipatory caution:

> SETH: . . . the thing about it . . . it's like, all right, you're anticipating, you're just like [in] constant anticipation . . . like I better get this done because I'm not going to have a chance to do it because we're busy, and anticipating the next call. . . .

Anticipatory readiness is a particular challenge for providers with downtime because, while rest is both welcome and necessary, it is never complete. Providers were careful not to wander too far from the ambulance, sometimes joking that if they decided to get food or go to the bathroom a call would come in.

Good shifts were not just those with the right mix of patients, but those with a rhythm to them during which providers were busy but also got rest and sleep. Bad shifts were either too busy or not busy enough. Not busy enough could be a challenge for providers, who, for practical reasons, could not stray far from their ambulances. During the second observational period, iPads and smartphones were far more common than they were during the initial round of observations in 2009. These digital devices, as well as Kindles, were regularly used as entertainment. Providers would use the hotspot in their ambulance to watch films or TV shows on streaming services like Netflix or stream videos from YouTube. Wi-Fi also enabled a variety of other activities, like using social media platforms such as Facebook or reading a news website. Other providers would bring print books, and nearly everyone carried a backpack or bag with personal items they would stow in the cab of the ambulance.

Unlike other social-science accounts of boredom, which focus on a genuine lack of activities and opportunities for individuals to engage in, providers were not "bored to death" (O'Neill 2017). Instead, boredom operated in a gray area where providers felt like the pace of their shift was defying expectations of a "good" shift but did not lack activities to fill that boredom. Occasionally boredom was welcome. Providers enjoyed the slow pace of Sunday shifts, for example. They would sometimes gather at diners for breakfast, taking advantage of the typically slow pace of calls to sit down for a meal as a group. At other points, providers would arrive at work exhausted from a prior shift, a late night with their partner, or a hangover. Boredom then was an opportunity to recover. At other times, providers were restless, left wanting something to do. Downtime is, therefore, something to be *managed*.

Interdependent Work Routines and Downtime

Managing downtime, of course, also means managing relationships with partners.[4] More often than not, partners would negotiate over food choices, trying to find a restaurant that would suit both of their tastes, for example. Staging decisions were similar. Providers would discuss where they wanted to park when they were assigned to a post in a particular neighborhood or ask their partner if they were all right with running a couple of errands. These errands covered a range of activities, from shopping at a camping store to going to a local mall to pick up toiletries. One evening, a supervisor even stopped to pick up a six-pack of beer for an after-work drink.

Providers would also try to meet up with other ambulances, something often difficult to accomplish because of posting assignments and the different pace of calls various crews experienced on a given shift. Interacting with other ambulance crews was challenging because of the difficulty of finding places where multiple ambulances could park. Space and the lack of interaction inherent in mobile workplaces like EMS therefore present a challenge for developing occupational communities.[5] Providers were able to bridge these gaps in time and space during the workday and therefore develop virtual occupational communities by using ubiquitous smartphones they carried (as I noted earlier, every participating provider had one). When interactions were not feasible, either because of call volume or dispatcher requests to post in specific locations, providers relied on smartphones to stay in touch with each other during shifts.

Smartphones, especially during the second period of observation, filled a variety of needs for providers. The first was that texting between providers allowed them to facilitate meeting up with other ambulance crews during shifts.

> CP: How do you kind of all end up congregating?
>
> SETH: So we either do preplanning, so we'll preplan like, oh, you want to do this later? And I'm like, oh yeah, let's try. Or we get group text messages going and go to [an ice cream shop] and get coffee and whatever, just kind of see where everyone is.

These group text messages allowed providers to make plans even if they did not cross paths physically with each other. Another provider described a similar process for arranging meetups with friends, adding that there was an additional advantage to meeting up with other crews during a shift:

> CP: How often do you do that, the texting other crews?
>
> RACHEL: Pretty frequently. Especially if it's like I'm closer to some people than others. But if someone's on [i.e., working], I'll be like "hey where are you posted" and if it's kind of a slow day, we'll like meet up, you know, down wherever they're posting and just kind of hang out. Get out of the truck for a bit, socialize with someone else. Because I mean you spend twenty-four hours with the same person, you want to sometimes get out and socialize with someone else.

Meeting up, therefore, was also a relief valve for managing relationships with coworkers. Providers spent long periods with only one other person in the cramped ambulance cab, and meeting up with others allowed them to expand their social network during shifts.

Texting and using other applications with messaging capabilities were not just means to an end (in terms of arranging meetups) but ends in themselves. It allowed providers to maintain off-duty relationships with each other and stay in touch during workweeks that could stretch to sixty hours or more:

> JOHN: Most of the time, like probably 70 or 80 percent of the time it's non-work stuff or just [about] hanging out doing stuff. I mean I'm pretty good friends with a lot of people here so usually hang outside of work, too. I would say, more than not stuff we did, stuff we want to do. Plan stuff.

Interactions that could happen in person in many workplaces, such as arranging plans to spend time together outside of work, were more easily facilitated via text messages during shifts. Not all providers were at work each day, and, even if each of the providers in question was at work, the pace of the shift may make planning in person difficult.

The second purpose was that texting also allowed providers to share information informally that was relevant to their jobs. This information was sometimes not related to patient care but was helpful to know during a shift. For example, several providers concocted a "selfie" game involving several public bathrooms in the city of Chapman. They would send around pictures of themselves in these bathrooms, and then the others would guess where the bathroom was:

> Sam laughs because he has just received a picture from Harrison of him in a pink bathroom. Sam doesn't know where he is, but Olivia and Drew tell him that they think Harrison is in a particular ice cream and coffee shop's bathroom. Sam shows them several other photos, including a picture of Sam in [the deli we are parked out front of]. Olivia had been talking about how she needed to go to the bathroom,

> but after seeing Sam's photo (and asking him where the bathroom is) she decides not to use it: "That's disgusting" [she says]. Sam agrees that it's not a great bathroom and points out the "communal soap bar" as evidence.

This game, carried out via messages sent between smartphones, was an attempt both to pass the time and to inject humor into shifts. The game also served to share knowledge about the quality of bathrooms around the city. Not only could providers who played the game create a virtual communal experience during shifts, but they were able to expand their knowledge of public restrooms they could use or avoid later.

Providers would also informally share knowledge about patients with each other. Since calls were all dispatched on the same radio channel, providers hear dispatchers send their colleagues on "jobs" and use their smartphones to provide them updates on potential patients:

> CHARLIE: . . . sometimes if we went to an address, maybe we just give them like an unofficial heads-up like listen I was there earlier. They're, maybe they refused or the guy is going to be tough, doesn't want to go, but he really needs to go. If it's something pertinent like that, we can kind of head someone off on the pass. If we know who's on that truck going to that address.

Providers, then, used text messaging in informal ways to provide background on patients they recognized and try to facilitate a smoother experience for their coworkers who were treating a known patient. Messaging, therefore, allowed providers to stay in contact, plan meetups, share jokes or funny photos, and share information about patients to try to help their coworkers through a call.

Spatial Context and Downtime

For EMS providers, their ability to engage in downtime activities is governed not only by the shared norms and the temporal marginality of work but also by its spatial context. EMS downtime, then, is impacted by where it occurs within the city, with specific activities concentrated in particular neighborhoods. This spatial context is an essential quality of EMS work and one that has been largely ignored by social scientists interested in work and its meaning in our lives.[6]

The Spatial Concentration of Downtime

Chapman's neighborhoods can also serve to enable or constrain downtime. For instance, Sirgi's is one of many restaurants in the Old Quarter. Importantly,

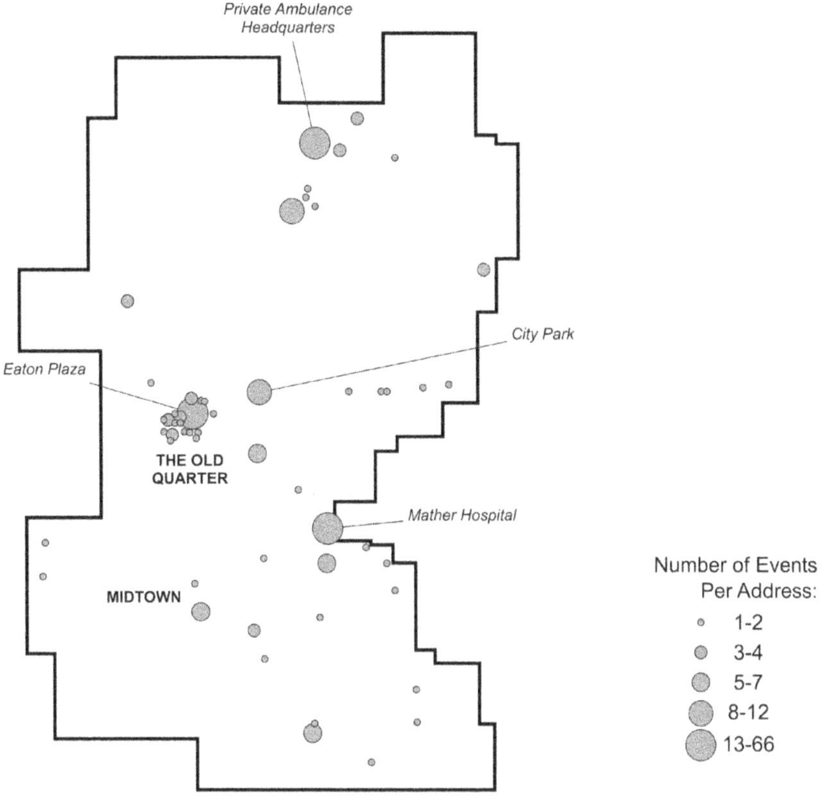

Figure 11. Private Ambulance Crews' Downtime Locations (graph by author)

this density includes many restaurants fitting the "fast-food" category, since a neighborhood with a high density of fine dining establishments would do little for time-constrained EMS providers. A broader analysis of dining by providers, particularly events where at least one provider visited a convenience store or restaurant to purchase food, illustrates visible clustering of these events in the Old Quarter (see Figure 11). Beyond the institutional imperative of remaining "centralized," this clustering may reflect providers' preferences for dining:

> [The dispatcher] calls us, asking us to stage in [Midtown]. Harrison and Micah start to talk about what they want for dinner. Both providers express frustrations about being posted there. They go through their [Midtown] food options, which are already limited, according to them, but even more so since we [were] already at [Shwarma Cafe] today. They talk about going to [a burger chain] and mention that

> pizza is an option, but they don't like [the pizzeria's] pizza all that much. Both providers agree that they'd rather go to [Uptown Plaza] and eat at [Sirgi's pizzeria]. Micah calls [the Dispatcher] on his cell phone and asks if they can go grab dinner in [the Old Quarter] first. [The Dispatcher] agrees, and we get into the ambulance.

The need to stay centralized does not wholly determine dining patterns. Instead, the Old Quarter is a neighborhood where providers believe their options are not constrained like they believe they are in Midtown. During the shift observations, providers patronized several coffee shops, two different local grocers, two pizzerias, and several burger joints in the Old Quarter. In Midtown, for comparison, providers limited their dining to a single cafe located near the Midtown fire station. Negotiating with dispatchers for the ability to eat meals in the neighborhood of choice becomes one additional element of emotional labor for providers.

Dining is not the only downtime activity with its spatial logic. A number of the categories identified through qualitative analysis as downtime activities show varying degrees of concentration (see Table 3). Some activities occurred at only a few addresses. Others occurred at many of the downtime addresses. Providers' errands, whether for personal purposes or at the behest of a dispatcher, also show concentration in several areas, particularly in North Chapman, the Old Quarter, and the Tory Plaza area of Chapman. The clustering in North Chapman reflects several services that Private Ambulance works with regularly to keep its vehicles running smoothly and a gas station where Private Ambulance maintains a corporate account. Other activities, such as bathroom use and sleeping, show tighter patterns of concentration. Bathroom use, which was not a trivial activity when providers spent hours in an ambulance at a time, was also highly concentrated on a small number of locations. Providers' use of restrooms was limited to just seven addresses out of the total fifty-

Table 3. Spatial Concentration of Downtime Activities by Address

Activity	Number of Addresses	% of Downtime Locations
Bathroom	7	11.86%
Dining	36	61.02%
Errands	20	33.90%
Paperwork	16	27.12%
Sleep	8	13.56%
Socializing	14	23.73%

Note: Data drawn from the main period of field observations during 2013. Valid addresses are those within the city of Chapman.

nine downtime addresses. Of these seven addresses, providers only used three more than once. Sleeping, similarly, was limited to eight addresses but only occurred with regularity at four.

Focal Points

For Private Ambulance providers, there were specific areas of Chapman with particular importance for how downtime was spent and structured. These areas, which I refer to here as "focal points," since they served as hubs for downtime activity, facilitated and enabled certain types of downtime activities.[7] These focal points underscore the importance of specific locations for providers. In other words, not all downtime locations in Chapman were created equal. An analysis of the frequency and type of downtime events by location reveals four addresses that together accounted for two-thirds of downtime activities. These focal points were the site of a large proportion of each activity for providers, particularly for the use of bathrooms, for sleeping, and for socializing. Thus, while the overall distributions of particular downtime phenomena varied spatially in different ways, these focal points served as magnets enabling many of these activities in a single place (see Figure 11, where focal points are individually labeled).

A closer examination of socializing occurring at these locations also illustrates the broader context and importance of these locations (see Table 4). These four locations accounted for 80 percent of all the socializing crews did with each other and other medical providers during their shifts. These focal points shared several common features. They offered parking for multiple ambulances and, Private Ambulance's headquarters aside, were centrally located within the city of Chapman. They fulfilled the functional requirement of providing coverage to the city while at the same time allowing providers to socialize with each other, since multiple crews could occupy the same post.

In North Chapman, the main focal point was Private Ambulance's headquarters itself (24 percent of all downtime events; 73 percent of North Chapman downtime events). Though providers did not typically return to the headquarters during their shifts, they started and ended their shifts there. This meant providers would often cross paths at shift change both with coworkers who were on duty during the same time period and others who worked before or after a particular shift:

> SETH: . . . you see everyone [who works at Private Ambulance] every day, you know what I mean? The shift going off, that's probably an eighth of our workforce every time, every morning that leaves. And then a new crew comes in, so you're just constantly seeing people.

Table 4. Focal Points' Share of Downtime Activities

Activity	Private Ambulance	Eaton Plaza	City Park	Mather Hospital	Total
Bathroom	13.04%	17.39%	0.00%	52.17%	82.60%
Dining	5.71%	25.71%	0.00%	0.00%	25.00%
Errands	0.00%	3.92%	0.00%	8.57%	39.99%
Paperwork	4.65%	25.58%	2.32%	34.88%	67.43%
Sleep	16.13%	22.58%	16.13%	32.26%	87.10%
Socializing	40.98%	11.48%	3.28%	26.23%	81.97%

Note: Data drawn from the main period of field observations during 2013.

Passing each other at Private's headquarters could be the only time providers on the same shift cross paths if a shift is particularly busy. Additionally, there was always an ALS ambulance crew based there on the overnight. There was therefore ample opportunity to interact face-to-face with colleagues, dispatchers, and EMS supervisors here.[8]

There were also regular training opportunities providers were expected to attend, such as monthly training known as "rounds." These events gave providers both the continuing medical education their certifications required and an opportunity to catch up with coworkers. At one such "rounds" I attended during the EMS shift observation phase of data collection, providers ate breakfast together and joked with each other about calls from the previous week. The medics I sat with spent a considerable amount of time making fun of both the presentation itself and the physicians who were in attendance. These events were shared experiences where providers were able to develop a sense of community with each other.

The Mather Hospital, which was the primary safety-net hospital for the city of Chapman as well as a location where Private Ambulance maintained a bunkroom, was the main focal point. In addition to the bunkroom, providers would congregate at the nurses' station in the emergency department. Spending downtime there would allow them to socialize with the hospital staff and in the ambulance bay outside of the ED. Providers also congregated in the ambulance bay described at the beginning of the Introduction. The bay was, in actuality, a driveway with space for six or more ambulances to be stacked up one behind the other.

Though providers were not encouraged to spend time here during the day, they frequently transported patients here. Nearly a third of the calls observed where providers transported a patient had Mather Hospital as the destination, a rate twice that of the next-most-common medical center. Thus, after they had completed providing patient care, providers had an opportunity to interact with their colleagues and take their time cleaning their equipment before heading back out on the road. Such interaction was present on many shifts, including "Shift 99," where the crew sat outside the ambulance and chatted with other ambulance crews as they arrived to drop patients off or take patients away.

In addition to Private's headquarters and the Mather, there were two other focal points in the Old Quarter. One was an observed focal point; providers reported the other as a focal point during the interviews. Eaton Plaza, which I discuss in greater depth in the next section, was one of the most common downtime locations during the first two-thirds of the shifts I observed. During this period, Eaton Plaza accounted for 57 percent of all downtime in the Old Quarter. However, it became untenable for ambulances to post there, and its share of overall downtime dropped precipitously during the last third of the shifts observed. Its centrality as a focal point shifted to several locations, including the "City Park" post that Janelle and her partner used at the end of "Shift 99."

Socializing at these focal points could take on various forms. One weekend afternoon at the Mather, five of us sat in the back of one paramedic ambulance parked in the ambulance bay. Providers chewed tobacco, spitting into doubled-up pairs of nitrile exam gloves and filling them with the dark sludge left over from the wads of tobacco in their mouths. As they dipped, they talked about both work-related topics like patients they thought were humorous and a range of non-work-related things.

During the interviews, one provider described similar impromptu gatherings in the back of an ambulance to watch movies:

> HARRISON: . . . you know at night when it's slow, sometimes we'll all, if it's slow enough where we can all meet up, sometimes someone who has one will just put on a movie on Netflix and sit in the back of the truck and watch it.

At other points during the shift observations, particularly at Eaton Plaza, providers would congregate around one ambulance, standing outside the cab and talking about their shifts or topics unrelated to work. Socializing like this required focal points because these were the areas where it was most comfortable for the ambulances to congregate.

These interactions, like those at Private Ambulance's headquarters, gave providers a sense of community despite a work environment whose transience made regular interaction more challenging than in many other workplaces. This sense of community was important for providers because it provided connections that could be lost during busy shifts when providers are merely "passing in the night" between calls rather than seeing each other for any length of time. It also provided a means for developing "occupational communities,"[9] which embody the shared meanings and practices of EMS providers. Socializing provided a concrete means for sharing the knowledge, norms, and culture that constituted the world of EMS work.

Public and Private Focal Points

The four focal points described previously can be divided into "public" and "private" locations.[10] The two focal points in the Old Quarter, "Eaton Plaza" and "City Park," can both be described as "public" places where the providers and their ambulances occupied public spaces in plain view of passersby, residents, and local businesses. The other two focal points, Private Ambulance's headquarters and the Mather Hospital, are both "private" places. Private Ambulance's headquarters were, for the most part, obscured from public view. They were set back off a side street and easy to miss without specific directions. The ambulance bay at the Mather Hospital was physically partitioned from Chapman Street by a high concrete wall. Similarly, the bunkroom within the hospital was set back in the corner of the emergency department and was physically separated from the patient-care spaces within the ED.

Spending downtime in public-facing focal points opened providers up to interruption. During the field observations, the crew I was riding with spent part of a particularly dull afternoon in Eaton Plaza. During one ten-minute period, they were repeatedly interrupted:

> About five minutes after arriving at [Eaton Plaza], a woman walks up to the ambulance and asks directions to an area restaurant. Jason gives her directions (Preston did not know where the restaurant was), but the woman still seems confused. After she leaves, Preston asks Jason about where the restaurant is, and Jason gives him a description of the building.
>
> After another five minutes, a man walks up to the ambulance and reports that someone who appears drunk is at the foot of the stairs going down in the [Old Quarter] transit station from [Eaton Plaza]. He asks who he is supposed to tell about this, and Jason responds, "Us." Preston tells me that they [individuals who are homeless or use substances] like to hang out down there because it gets slightly less foot traffic than up "here" [in Eaton Square]. He says, though, that the [Regional Transit] police are through there "every five minutes" and that if there is a problem, they will call. I ask if the walk-ups to the ambulance occur frequently. Jason says that they do, and Preston adds that it is not every day but regularly. He also adds that "I've never had it not be for a homeless person."

These were two very different types of interruptions, but they are interruptions that are far less likely to happen when providers post in "backstage" locations. Providers, therefore, had to maintain a certain level of availability and professionalism in those "frontstage" areas, since they were a public presence, readily identifiable from a block or more away. In both cases, providers served as a sort of public clearinghouse. They were able to point a pedestrian toward a restaurant of interest in one case and accept (though not act on) an individual's concerns about a homeless person in another.

Spending time in public locations did not just mean interruptions. When parked in a "frontstage" space such as "Eaton Plaza" or "City Park," providers would climb into the back of the ambulance where they would not be readily visible to passersby. At "backstage" or not-public locations, providers had more flexibility to sleep in ambulance cabs or the bunkrooms at both the Mather Hospital and Private's headquarters. As long as they were not called out of the Mather to post, they were free to sleep in more relaxed ways than in a "frontstage" area of the city.

Conflicts over Space in Chapman

Providers' posting in residential neighborhoods did not just affect their behavior. When providers occupied parking spaces or loading zones with their ambulances, they shaped the behavior of those around them. Their posting decisions opened themselves up to conflict with both other public servants and members of the communities in which they posted. Despite their public role in responding to emergencies, providers found that Chapman's residents did not universally welcome them when they were not on a call.[11]

Contested Locales

One distinction between the "frontstage" focal points and the "backstage" focal points is the "backstage" areas frequented by providers keep them from conflict with residents and business owners. In comparison, both "frontstage" focal points generated controversy during the study period. Providers' use of any "frontstage" space, focal point, or otherwise was determined in part by the availability of parking. Providers were sensitive to parking spots and the amount of time they spent in a given location. Considering parking was particularly important to providers when they utilized private parking lots for downtime, such as at convenience stores in Uptown or Tory Plaza. Both locations had parking lots providers would use, though they would be careful not to occupy more than one spot or not to monopolize a space for an extended period.

On the street, there were other rules providers followed to determine whether a spot was "fair game":

> Charlotte: We don't park in handicapped spots. But as far as streets, I mean as long as we are really adhering to like one-ways, you don't want to be going the wrong way down a one-way or something like that. We try to avoid bus stops. Like all the bus stops along [Main Street] and [in University Plaza], they don't want us parking there, which is understandable. There's really, most of it's fair game. Loading zones, if we're in the truck, are pretty fair game, too, because we can just move if someone comes.

Loading zones and other areas designated by the city as "no parking" zones were commonly used by providers when posting on the street as opposed to in a parking lot. Providers occasionally discussed conflicts with a "meter reader" from the city of Chapman who would ticket ambulances if providers had parked them in loading zones. At first, these seemed to be isolated events, albeit events that were surprising to hear about, given the deference usually given to first responders. However, after Eaton Plaza emerged as a point of conflict between Private Ambulance and neighboring businesses, these small-scale struggles over turf took on a different meaning.

The Eaton Plaza Conflict

For the first two-thirds of the shifts I observed, providers would frequently park their ambulances in an area known as Eaton Plaza (see Figure 11). Eaton Plaza was a predominantly commercial area located in the Old Quarter. There were numerous stores in several different commercial strips, including two chain coffee shops, a third local coffee shop, a pizzeria, and a chain Mexican fast-food restaurant. There were also various retailers, both local and chain, carrying a variety of types of clothing, footwear, jewelry, and sporting goods. Providers would park their ambulances along a stretch of Eaton Plaza marked as a loading zone. This stretch could accommodate two or three ambulances at any one time and offered easy access to the stores and restaurants in the Plaza.

Most importantly, it offered quick access to a small grocery collectively referred to by a nickname—"the Market." Within the Market were a salad bar, a hot bar, sushi, a deli counter offering sandwiches made to order, and a restroom for customers. During the two-thirds of the shifts I observed during this period, we visited the market eleven times (approximately once per shift) to buy drinks, snacks, and sandwiches and to use the bathroom. Eaton Plaza and the Market were a frequent presence during this first period of observations, with 21 percent of the downtime events during these shifts occurring in Eaton Plaza (see Table 4). Eaton Plaza, in short, was the primary "frontstage" focal point for providers.

However, in the fall, a change occurred. Though Eaton Plaza had offered a significant degree of convenience because of the availability of dining establishments, shopping, and the Market's bathrooms, it had also been the site of a running conflict between Private Ambulance, the city's traffic department, and a particular business in Eaton Plaza. Parking enforcement officers had occasionally forced ambulances to move:

> After idling for about a half an hour, a [Chapman] Traffic Enforcement officer asked the ambulance to move up to the front of the loading zone (when B6 first got into [Eaton Plaza], there were cars in part of the loading zone; once they left the ambulance was left in the middle and Liam had not moved it). Preston commented that "she kicked us out of here yesterday."

While providers had occasionally reported run-ins with parking enforcement officers at other locations, they had indicated that this was a growing problem. Providers blamed a local business owner for it:

> Dispatch directs us to "head into the [Plaza]" [to post]. When we get into [Eaton Plaza], Pam wants to park [in the loading zone], but Charlie says that he doesn't want to get yelled at by either the jewelry store people or the Chapman Parking attendants. Pam responds, "Fuck that woman and her jewelry store, go in and ask her if she has anything tasteful."

Unlike other business owners, who did not vocally protest Private Ambulance using curb space or even their private parking lots, the providers reported being subject to repeated harassment in Eaton Plaza. Not only did parking enforcement officers step up ticketing of Private's ambulances, but the store owners began photographing ambulances parked in loading zones and calling Private Ambulance's headquarters to complain. Eventually, providers believed, their calls became so frequent that Private Ambulance's management decided to ban their crews from parking in Eaton Plaza.

After management handed down the ban against crews spending time in Eaton Plaza, the amount of time spent there dropped dramatically (see Table 5). While a significant amount of downtime was spent there over the first two-thirds of the shifts I observed, I only returned there once after the ban. Visits to the Market declined as well, with crews I was with patronizing it only twice during the remaining seven shifts. This drop-off meant that providers were pushed out of one of the primary locations of the Old Quarter and into more peripheral areas, which often lacked the amenities of Eaton Plaza. One provider described his strategy,

Table 5. Downtime Events by Neighborhood and Focal Point, before and after the Eaton Plaza Ban

	Pre-Eaton Plaza Ban		Post-Eaton Plaza Ban	
Neighborhood	Frequency	Percent	Frequency	Percent
North Chapman				
Private Ambulance	47	25.5%	19	20.7%
All other addresses	13	7.1%	12	13.1%
Subtotal	60	32.6%	31	33.7%
The Old Quarter				
Eaton Plaza	38	20.7%	1	1.1%
Eaton Plaza, Adjacent	3	1.6%	5	5.4%
City Park	5	2.7%	7	7.6%
All other addresses	21	11.4%	12	13.%
Subtotal	67	36.4%	25	27.2%
Tory Plaza				
Mather Hospital	26	14.1%	20	21.7%
All other addresses	5	2.7%	4	4.3%
Subtotal	31	16.8%	24	26.1%
All other Neighborhoods	26	14.2%	12	13.0%
Total	184	100%	92	100%

Note: Data drawn from the main period of field observations during 2013. Eaton Plaza "adjacent" events were within a block of the original posting site.

saying "There are other places, [we can] move up [Eaton Street] toward West [Chapman] or just find different spots until someone else complains." A particular area that saw an increase in traffic was along a city park on the northern end of the Old Quarter. This post saw a jump in traffic after Private Ambulance stopped parking in Eaton Plaza. It constituted 7 percent of all downtime in the Old Quarter area before the change and 28 percent of all downtime in the area after.

Providers expressed a range of opinions about this change. Some providers were ambivalent about it, with one going as far as to say he understood the business owners' concerns because "you can't, can't blame them, I wouldn't want a diesel truck running in front of my business all day." Other providers were more critical of the owners. Idling ambulances, one of the rumored complaints the business owners had made about Private Ambulance, served a function for providers. One provider described their working conditions in the following way:

> PAM: It's kind of discouraging because we're not doing anything malicious. Like I get when people like leave their trucks on and stuff like that, but it stinks because everyone gets air-conditioning and heat in their office,

> you know what I mean? Like, this is my office. Like, I'm sorry you guys don't like the emissions that I'm producing, but I'm not a truck that's delivering like a little keychain to your house from Amazon. I'm here with a ton of equipment that's plugged in. And it's like sixteen degrees outside, or it's eighty-four degrees outside, and it's a big box, a big metal box like out in the sun. So it's definitely disheartening that people literally don't know what we do and what the capacity we do it.

Pam went on to describe the "people" she was referring to as the jewelry store owners. Her point about the ambulance as their office during all kinds of weather is particularly crucial for understanding providers' mindsets regarding downtime. The ambulance served not just as their office but as their home. Some providers, therefore, viewed the conflict over Eaton Square as if the ban had been tantamount to an eviction.

While providers were generally critical of the owners themselves, they also focused more generally on how the change had affected their shifts. Ben described the change as "difficult":

> BEN: It's been difficult. Things seem more disjointed. Like I used to be able to go there and talk with crews a lot because that's where everybody would usually be if they were in [University Plaza]. And now it's like, unless you communicate directly with another truck, like by texting [them] or whatever, it's pretty much like if you run into them you run into them.

Eaton Plaza's role as an informal meeting place with other crews was among the most significant effects the ban on parking there had. No other locale in the city of Chapman had the same constellation of parking and amenities.

> HARRISON: I mean, sometimes it wasn't even like you were working because you could park there, get out of the truck, sit on the bench, have a coffee, watch some guy on stilts do tricks for an hour and a half. And if you needed to go to the bathroom, it's right there. Everything was right there. Now we're kind of like kicked out of there, and it's not a struggle, but it's inconvenient to try to have to find food and a bathroom and all this other stuff that I think people don't really take into consideration when you're working twenty-four hours inside of a van.

One of the common themes providers raised was the division they felt between themselves and people who worked in an office. They highlighted the aspects of their job that kept them on the streets, working long hours in their ambulances without a base to return to for downtime. Providers felt that residents and business owners in Chapman did not fundamentally understand what first-responder work was like for them.

The Social Construction of Place

While the specifics of the conflict over Eaton Plaza are unique to that space, it is essential to see the eviction of Private Ambulance's crews in a broader context. Providers had reported a much longer running conflict with parking enforcement officers before Eaton Plaza emerged as a contested space. When they moved to City Park, conflict followed them. After a few months of increased traffic there, residents began to complain to Private Ambulance about traffic and the idling diesel engines.

These conflicts are, at their most basic, about whether it was appropriate for ambulances to use and occupy these areas of the city. From the perspective of EMS providers, their priorities for using space differed from those of residents and business owners. They emphasized staying warm or cool, which necessitated idling the ambulance's engine while parked. They also prioritized staying in a central location with numerous amenities for an extended period. In both cases, outside parties had a different conceptualization of what was appropriate in "Eaton Plaza" and "City Park" and were vocal in protesting what they saw as misuse. EMS providers' presence did not fit in, according to the providers themselves, with other actors' conceptualizations of "Eaton Plaza" as a prime, high-rent shopping area or "City Park" as a quiet residential corner of the neighborhood.

In other parts of the city, providers' use of public, "frontstage" spaces did not draw the same ire. We can account for the difference by understanding not just differences between public and private space but variation in public spaces themselves. Prime public spaces are those mainstream society uses and values. Marginal spaces, on the other hand, do not have the same use-value. Sociological studies of homelessness, for example, document the pushing of individuals who live on the street out of prime space and into marginal spaces.

In much the same regard, the movement of EMS providers out of Eaton Plaza and later out of City Park represents pressure on Private Ambulance by residents to avoid prime spaces. Providers were attracted to these primary locations, notably Eaton Plaza, because of the unparalleled combination of amenities and ample, if not strictly legal, parking. Moreover, these locations were primary spaces because they allowed providers to stay "centralized" and, during the day, to follow a dispatcher's typical insistence that providers avoid posting at the Mather Hospital for extended periods. Providers were therefore squeezed in several directions toward "City Park," only to have a similar conflict over this space emerge a few months later.

The inevitability of these conflicts for EMS providers is perhaps unique among first responders. For police, the weight of their authority may keep citizens from vocally opposing their presence in particular neighborhoods. Firefighters, in comparison, have physical stations to return to between calls. In many urban EMS systems, EMS providers are not afforded the moral authority of law enforcement officers. They also lack the physical infrastructure fire departments have invested so heavily in out of necessity. All these occupations, however, are "blue-collar" in nature. In Chapman, the neighborhoods in and around the Old Quarter are decidedly not "blue-collar," with multi-million-dollar homes, private schools, boutique shops and restaurants, and exclusive hotels.

Providers recognized these differences and regularly raised them when discussing the neighborhood. They are part of the layers through which providers see urban space. Importantly, however, this view from the ambulance cab is not just about identifying prime and marginal spaces, but about seeing these as conflicted spaces. The Eaton Plaza conflict reinforces this idea that urban space is to be competed over. Providers are not only victims in this competition. Instead, they also play a role in policing others' use of space, particularly individuals who lack stable housing. As we consider the unique prism through which EMS providers view the city, understanding space as a source of social conflict is an essential consideration.

Spatial Context and Downtime

Chapters 1, 2, and 3 have each added a layer of complexity to our model of EMS work. With this chapter's turn toward a spatial understanding of EMS work, our model must continue to evolve (see Figure 12). The essential ways in which EMS work, in particular downtime, is *located* in Chapman means we must take seriously the effects of space on every aspect of EMS work we have discussed so far. For providers, time and space are intricately related. Driving consumes large parts of shifts. Providers must snatch opportunities to sleep and eat when they are available because they have no idea how much longer their downtime will last. Place, therefore, shapes the norms and practice of downtime, since both food and sleeping options are dictated by where downtime occurs. Since providers must make decisions about this together, these same factors shape the interdependent nature of working with a partner.

With this in mind, Figure 12 adds a large box around our existing model to emphasize how all these activities are also *spatial* ones. At first blush, perhaps, it may seem that spatiality is a novelty of EMS work or other mobile occupations. However, I want to suggest that this need not be the case. For service work, even when it is rooted in a fixed place, *where* that place is can shape the

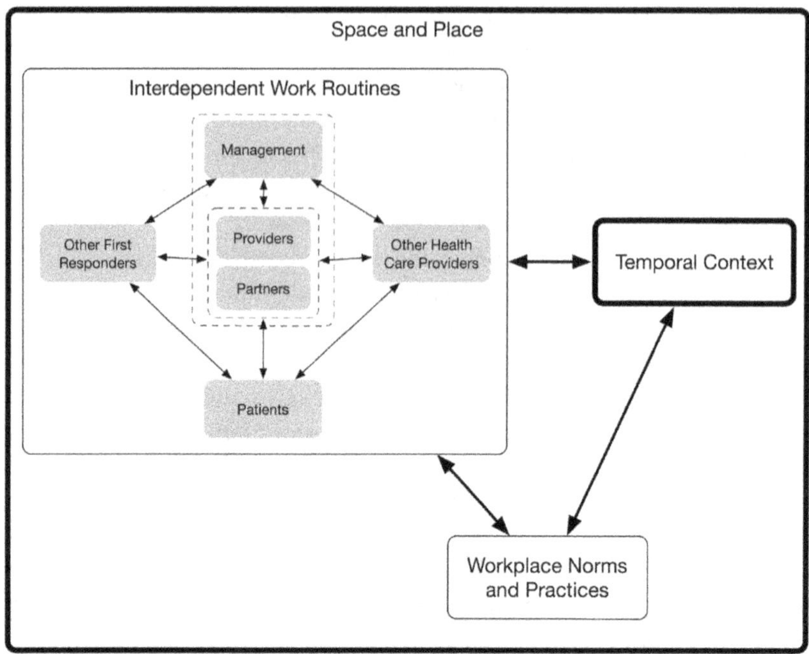

Figure 12. Evolving Theoretical Model—Integrating Space and Place (graph by author)

work itself dramatically. Think of work in a fast-food restaurant, for example, which may have different features or clientele depending on its neighborhood. Likewise, professional workers may find that the specific locations of offices dictate opportunities for how they spend leisure time and lunches and their ability to access other amenities.

However, space is present in EMS work in ways that, even though all work occurs somewhere, makes mobile work a notable departure from other types of jobs. Every moment of EMS work is an experience with the location where it takes place. This experience can be physical, such as having to navigate different topographies, experiencing different weather conditions when treating patients injured outdoors, or even imbibing the sounds and smells of urban life. There is no isolation from the outside world here, which office workers may experience only when they walk past a front lobby or a guard at an entrance to a building. For EMS providers, space shapes every facet of the day, from the moment EMS providers leave Private's headquarters to the moment they return at the end of their shift. As conflicts over space show, providers' access to space is contingent on the broader social construction of the spaces within which they work.

Conclusion

Whereas Part I focused on institutional marginality, Part II is about occupational marginality. EMS work is hard on providers in part because it is both unpredictable and uncontrollable. Each shift has a pace, but providers have no way of knowing what that pace will be, how many patients they will see, and if they will be able to end work on time. Downtime is one area where providers have some control over their work, but it is an area of tension. First, dispatchers sometimes choose to exert influence on where providers post, and so providers do not have complete control of their options for downtime. Second, downtime can be tedious. Providers have no way of knowing how long it can last or when it will be over. And yet downtime also provides needed mental breaks, sleep, and chances to eat during shifts that can stretch twenty-four hours or longer.

These tensions, between downtime as a needed break in an otherwise chaotic day and downtime as a site of boredom, are part of the paradox of EMS work. Like military occupations, there is a sense of "hurry up and wait" among EMS providers that creates a condition of anticipatory readiness. This mindset makes it harder to sleep or relax when you may have to change gears quickly and respond to a call. Anticipatory readiness is the fundamental paradox that shapes downtime in EMS work. EMS work is marginal work because there is no ability to clock out, take a fifteen-minute break, or reliably stop and go to the bathroom without the potential for interruption and a quick exit from the back of a grocery store to respond to a call.

Where downtime occurs is also critically important for providers. Accessing grocery stores, restaurants, and event bathrooms are contingent on those amenities being available in the neighborhoods where dispatchers station EMS crews. EMS work is therefore marginal not only because providers do not know when breaks will come, but also because they do not know where they will be able to spend them. This lack of control makes the conflicts over downtime focal points in Chapman even more frustrating for providers. Residents and business owners may not always welcome providers' idling ambulances. Private Ambulance's EMTs and paramedics find themselves facing yet another form of marginality, with particular neighborhoods demarcated as "off-limits" for them. This territorial conflict prefigures the ways in which providers socially construct others' acceptable use of public space, something we turn to in Part III.

PART III
EMS in the Marginal City

It was mid-afternoon, part of the way through a shift, when Private Ambulance's dispatcher sent Medic 5 to a call for an unconscious patient. We arrived on-scene before the fire department medic unit or police officers who were also responding. A building maintenance worker was waiting for us in front of the patient's apartment, which was squalid. Someone had piled the furniture on the side of the room. A picture frame lay smashed and broken on the floor, and a bike was blocking our path. In a bathroom near where we found the patient, there was an overflowing cat litter box. The bedroom, where the patient lay unresponsive, was full of empty beer, liquor, and vanilla extract bottles. Andy bent down at the patient's side and made a fist in his gloved hand. With his knuckles, he rubbed vigorously on the patient's sternum, the bone in the middle of the chest that connects each side of the rib cage. The patient responded to the sternum rub but did not fully wake.

Chapter 1 presented the notions providers hold of "bullshit" and "real emergencies." It seems reasonable to ask whether an unconscious patient, having consumed too much vanilla extract for its alcoholic properties, falls into the category of "bullshit" or "real emergency." Despite the possible complications of unconsciousness and chronic alcoholism that manifests itself with individuals drinking from small bottles of vanilla extract, providers at Private Ambulance described these calls invariably as "bullshit." For the EMTs and paramedics at Private Ambulance, if they spent two-thirds of their time fighting boredom during downtime, most of their time on calls is spent on "grunt work." This involves responding to "bullshit" calls that providers see as falling outside their responsibility.

Chapter 5 introduces "grunt work," while Chapter 6 connects it to how providers construct notions of stigmatized neighborhoods. These chapters rely on unique spatial data that help to capture providers' connections between the patients they see and *where* those patients are found. Together, these chapters capture the final facet of marginality that defines the EMS system. Not only is it marginalized from other health-care and first-responder institutions, but a significant number of its patients are themselves marginalized from the health-care system and instead turn to ambulances for care.

5
The Daily Grind of Grunt Work

"Shitty vodka. We see mouthwash too sometimes, or like vanilla extract. Stuff people have to buy when they get kicked out of the liquor stores for the day. And other than that it's just beer, but mostly hard liquor." (Oliver)

"37-Delta Fresh"

It was past midnight, and Randy was sitting awake in the dispatch area. Randy's partner, Laura, was asleep in one of the bedrooms in the middle of the night. Laura and I awoke to Randy and the dispatcher rousing us for a call, an assault in a high-rise apartment complex. When we arrived on-scene several minutes later, we found the parking lot full of police cars whose light bars lit up the surrounding buildings with red and blue flashes. Randy got out of the ambulance and told me there were many "frequent fliers" in this building because it had a lot of residents who received Section 8 vouchers for housing. A Chapman Police Department sergeant was waiting for us and took us up to the apartment in the elevator.

The apartment itself was dark, barely furnished, and disgustingly dirty. There were empty bottles, broken glass, and pools of blood all over the floor. The apartment smelled strongly of both alcohol and urine. Three men were sitting under a dim light in what would be the living area of the apartment. Two were handcuffed and sitting on the dirty sofa. One of the men repeatedly tried to get up, despite being handcuffed and having an officer standing over him. A third was sitting in a chair, bleeding from the head after having been struck with a glass bottle. Laura worked to bandage the patient's head while

Randy, with the help of the officer holding a flashlight, looked at the two other men in the apartment. Once Laura had finished bandaging the primary patient's head, Randy and Laura led him to the elevator and out to the ambulance, where they buckled him into the cot.

The smell of urine and alcohol followed the patient into the ambulance. After having dropped the patient off in the emergency department exam room assigned to him by the triage nurse, Randy looked at me as we cleaned the cot at the hospital. The patient, he dryly noted, smelled "37-Delta fresh," a reference to the pungent mix of alcohol and urine. The term "37-Delta" was one of several labels, including "drunks," that providers used to discuss patients they believed to be intoxicated with alcohol. Randy mused aloud, wondering if he smelled so bad after a night of drinking. Laura responded, telling me it takes something special to build up that smell and that Randy might not be able to reproduce it. Randy agreed and continued musing about the possibility of bottling the fragrance.

"You 37-Delta Motherfucker": Labeling Alcohol Calls

Long before ambulances existed in the United States, Americans were imbibing at eye-popping rates. Some of the founding fathers were daily consumers of alcohol, and Americans drank whiskey and beer at rates far higher than we do as a nation today. Early in the nineteenth century, activists began to rail against the consumption of alcohol. Early propaganda from the temperance movement captured the moralization of alcoholism, painting men who today would be described clinically as having an alcohol-use disorder as corrupted, morally bankrupt individuals (Burns 2004). During my time in Chapman, while heroin was present on the streets, as was the synthetic opioid fentanyl, the throes of the opioid crisis had not yet gripped the city. For providers at Private Ambulance, like the women of the early temperance movement, it was the "demon drink" that captivated their attention: "The big one is . . . alcohol, without a doubt, the largest [type of] substance abuse that we see."

Providers' focus on alcohol consumption was not without some irony. The EMTs and medics who daily responded to calls for intoxication were not teetotalers. Indeed, many themselves drank alcohol. One evening, dispatchers rotated the crew I was with off duty briefly to attend a graduation party for the latest paramedic class at Private Ambulance. The party was one of the few times dispatchers gave crews anything like an official break. In the dark recesses of the seafood restaurant's bar, Private Ambulance's management held court. While the dispatchers did pull the crew for a call after grabbing some food from the party, we returned later to help "transport" several of the inebriated medic students back to their cars, which were a short distance away at Private's headquarters. Drinking during days off was a regular topic during shifts. These stories are not an attempt to paint Private's providers as hypocritical. To them, their drinking, even if it was in excess, was qualitatively different.

When Randy proposed bottling a fragrance called "37-Delta fresh," he invoked the most common label at Private Ambulance for discussing patients who were intoxicated.[1] Providers regularly used it as an offhand label for the patients who appeared to be drunk, without stable housing, or both. For instance, the crew of Medic 11, bored after an afternoon of girl watching, dipping tobacco, and driving around Chapman, pulled out of our post to drive into the Old Quarter. As we left, Miles took note of a person who appeared to him to be street homeless. "Yeah, we see you, you 37-Delta motherfucker," he growled as we drove past. As we sat on the bumper of the ambulance, Bruce and Miles made fun of pedestrians and commented on women who walked past. "We judge everyone, patients, people on the streets, coworkers," Bruce told me. This culture of judgment was widespread at Private Ambulance, and no group received more negative judgment than individuals who were street homeless.

Providers collectively referred to them as "37-Deltas," though no one seemed to know why. From time to time, during my interviews and observations, I would ask providers who brought up the term what it meant and from where the term originated. Providers were unanimous on its meaning but offered a variety of origin stories. During both the interviews and the observations, it became clear that few providers were completely aware of the full meaning of "37-Delta," but it nevertheless held a collective colloquial meaning among the paramedics and EMTs. During the interviews, if providers mentioned the "37-Delta" label, I asked them to define it:

> PAM: [37-Delta] . . . it is . . . I think it's the police code for an intoxicated person. So, then we use it all the time, so [37-Delta].
>
> SETH: A [37-Delta] is a homeless person in the city of [Chapman]. A "37-Delta" is a homeless alcoholic, I think, is how they define it.

Again, this displays the fuzziness providers have about the precise definitions. After all, an intoxicated person (as in Pam's definition) could be anyone from a college student celebrating the end of another week of classes to a young professional out on the town, a chronic alcoholic, or a homeless person with a substance-use disorder. More commonly, providers identified "37-Delta" as having some precise meaning for patients who were both homeless and alcoholics (as in Seth's definition).

During dinner on "Shift 99," Janelle described what ultimately was the true origin story. "Delta" is a part of the phonetic alphabet, and Section 37D refers to a specific part of the state law dealing with the treatment of individuals with alcohol-use disorders. This section of law specifically details the creation of detoxification and treatment programs. Interestingly, it does not explicitly mention the role of Emergency Medical Services. Pam's definition has a grain of truth because she connects the code to the role of law enforcement in policing alcoholism.

The term "37-Delta" was applied broadly by providers. Providers considered any individual living on the street a "37-Delta," regardless of whether the person had a diagnosed alcohol use disorder. The broadness with which providers applied this label matched its use by law enforcement in Chapman. Like EMS providers, the Chapman Police Department regularly responded to calls for service involving individuals who were street homeless. Their dispatchers labeled these calls in their Computer Aided Dispatch ("CAD") system as "37-Delta" as well. A particular part of this section dealt explicitly with police powers related to individuals who were intoxicated, requiring police to transport to a treatment facility anyone who presents to an officer or at a station who is intoxicated but has not otherwise committed a crime.

"37-Deltas" are just one more in a rich if troubling tapestry of labels applied to patients by health-care providers. Like "GOMER" ("get out of my E.R.") and "frequent flier," these labels serve to generalize about patients whom providers dislike because they are the "regular" clientele (Shem 2009; Leiderman and Grisso 1985). Providers, including EMS providers at Private Ambulance, were quick to note that these patients were what physicians sometimes call "malingerers," patients who exaggerate symptoms to receive care. They shared a range of terms for these patients, including "booze bag," "dirtbag," "creeper," and "drunk" to describe these patients.

Responding to Patients Who Were Intoxicated

Whatever the label, responding to patients who were intoxicated was a regular part of shifts. In addition to responding to the physical consequences of intoxication, such as the injuries described in the chapter's initial vignette, providers also responded to patients in states of significant inebriation. These often fell into one of several groups, including college students and patients who were living on the street because of housing instability.

Hand Drops and "37-Deltas"

On a different shift, the dispatcher sent Medic 7 for an unresponsive individual inside a transit station on a platform. Miles drove and parked the ambulance near the main entrance, and we went downstairs on the escalators into the bowels of the station. Engine 1's crew caught up with us in front of the fare barriers. Miles explained to me that the transit inspectors usually met ambulance crews there and let them through, but none were in sight. Miles waited for a passenger to come through the barrier and then jumped in, holding it open for the rest of us as we walked out onto the platform. Without any inspectors to guide us, there was some confusion about where the patient was located. However, we eventually spotted several inspectors and a transit police officer huddled over a body at the far end of the platform.

Miles had brought a device known as a "stair chair." These devices are stretchers in chair form that providers use with patients who can sit upright. Stair chairs make it easier to move these patients through tight quarters like stairwells. They moved the patient into the stair chair, where he slumped over because he was unconscious. Bruce and Miles joked around with each other as we walked back to the ambulance. They mused about letting the patient roll out of control down the platform ramp into the station's central atrium.

They continued to joke about the patient in the elevator, and Bruce described the "hand drop" technique to demonstrate that a patient is unconscious. At the hospital, Bruce described holding the patient's hand over his face and then letting it drop and hit him. He had told me about this earlier as a cure for "Hispanic panic." Women who are Latino, he told me, overreact and pretend to faint. If you hold their hand up, they will not let it drop onto their face. Our current patient, Bruce reported to me at the hospital, let his hand fall into his face and was, therefore, unconscious. He also told me the patient never regained consciousness and was registered as a "John Doe" in the emergency department, since no one could find an identification card for him. As he told me this, our dispatcher came on the air asking us to come out quickly for a call. A pedestrian had been struck by a car nearby.

Superman

Around Halloween, the dispatcher sent Medic 4 out for the "alcohol problem" in a university residence hall. After difficulty finding the building, we were met by a university police officer when we arrived on-scene. We walked up several flights of stairs with the medic bags and a stair chair, and the officer took us into a dorm room where four college-age females were standing in a semi-circle. Their friend had arrived at their room very drunk and was now in the en-suite bathroom, vomiting. We went into the small bathroom and found a college-aged student, dressed as Superman, hugging the toilet. Miles and

Sanders tried to coax him to stand up. However, he was too afraid to leave the toilet, and the medics gave him a small "emesis bag" so that he had something to vomit into if he needed it.

After they prepared the stair chair by putting a flat sheet over it to make cleanup more manageable, they tried again to coax him to stand up. The student was still unwilling, and Miles and Sanders lifted him by his shoulders and belt loops. As they did this, both medics struggled to suppress laughter. The student reached out with both arms toward the toilet. For a brief second, he was suspended in mid-air, dressed as Superman, arms outstretched in an uncanny impersonation of the superhero. They placed him in the stair chair and secured him with the seatbelts. As we left to head downstairs, the women thanked us for taking care of him. The police officer also thanked us and mentioned how annoying the students were. Miles told him, "I could do this all night. Most other people wouldn't, but . . ." and then he trailed off as he helped move the patient to the cot and into the ambulance.

Once inside the ambulance, Miles tried repeatedly to get the patient to hold onto the emesis bag, which was now partially full of vomit. Miles became visibly annoyed and grabbed a spare red biohazard trash bag. He ripped a hole in it and placed the hole over the patient's head so the young man was then wearing it like a bib. He tried to talk to the patient, whose answers were sometimes unclear or incorrect. He told Miles, for example, that he was twenty-two when, in fact, his I.D., which Miles had retrieved from his wallet, said he was nineteen. Miles gave him a hard time about lying to him as we pulled into the hospital. As we wheeled the patient inside, the staff, who were generally excited to see Miles, were far less enthusiastic. Outside, after we had cleaned the cot, Miles looked at me and said, "It is like [the staff] think they're above getting drunks."

This vignette highlights the excess providers attributed to college students but did not assign to themselves. These occurred with particular frequency on weekends: "I would say [that we see] a lot of [intoxicated] college students on weekend nights," acknowledged a paramedic, who added that these calls were for situations where "Brittany can't hold her liquor." Other paramedics admonished students during interviews for "not knowing how to drink" or complained about "blackout drunk college girls who shit their pants" because they were so drunk. These patients were occasionally acutely ill. More often, however, their condition was seen as routine by providers whose worry about containing the patient's vomit from contaminating the ambulance was the biggest priority. Providers were undoubtedly aware that acute alcohol intoxication could be severe for patients but were often dismissive, just the same.

A "Disappointing" Fall

For some calls, however, it was impossible to be dismissive, at least initially. Late one night, Medic 4 was sent by our dispatcher for a patient who had fallen off a porch. At first blush, this sounded like a minor call. However, it soon became apparent based on updates from the dispatcher that the fall was from several stories. When we arrived on-scene, the neighborhood was awash with lights from multiple police cars and fire trucks dancing off the surrounding buildings in the darkness. We parked on the main street, adjacent to the building where the call was, and were immediately met by a Chapman Fire Department medic who grabbed the cot out of our truck's rear doors. The medic asked Miles to grab backboarding equipment, which he did, dropping it on the cot.

As we walked past the building's front, there was a small group of bystanders who appeared to be in their twenties. They all seemed to be in various states of intoxication. A knot of firefighters and police officers was standing in a narrow walkway between the building the dispatcher sent us to and the building next door. The gangway between the buildings was about four feet wide. The officers were holding flashlights up, illuminating the walkway. We squeezed past them and up to where the patient lay. A firefighter told Miles she fell from the third story, possibly from the fire escape, whose darkened outline we could see directly overhead. The patient was remarkably calm as Sanders worked his way up to her and began the process of helping the firefighters backboard her.

As this unfolded, I went back to the ambulance with Miles and helped him get the truck set up for patient care. This type of preparatory work was rare for Private Ambulance medics. I saw it only during the most severe calls—typically when they had additional personnel from the fire department on-scene. Miles moved the medic equipment from its storage location into the patient compartment, "spiked" an IV bag with fluids by inserting the tubing into the bag, and asked me to set up the cardiac monitor. Once finished, we got back out of the ambulance and walked back toward the walkway. We met the firefighters, who were wheeling the cot toward us. Sanders followed with a friend of the patient's, who proved to be a bit of a distraction for Miles. Once we were in the ambulance, she continued to answer his questions to the patient, and Miles had to ask her to stop talking.

At the hospital, Miles and Sanders huddled in the triage area before a nurse sent us back to the trauma side of the emergency department. Sanders told Miles that the friend believed the patient had taken some psychedelic drugs in addition to drinking alcohol. They passed this information on to the hospital staff as we moved the patient from the cot to a hospital bed. Outside in the parking garage, as we cleaned up the ambulance, Sanders marveled at how the patient was not seriously hurt. Miles responded with a note of disappointment, noting that he "had high hopes for the call." He continued, telling us, "If she had been sober, she'd have broken her back or something." He paused, and then the disappointment returned to his voice, telling me, "Drunk people never get hurt." Miles continued, sharing a war story about a patient who took a similar fall but with more disastrous circumstances, since the patient landed on a glass bottle, which became embedded in her shoulder.

Real or Bullshit Work?

The call for the young woman illustrates why "bullshit" is an ineffective label. Given the height, it would be difficult for providers to dismiss a fall from three stories. So, the call was legitimate, but the lack of severe injury and the ties to substance use made it a simultaneously good and disappointing call to providers. In fact, all the calls described have elements of severity. The college student in the Superman costume was, perhaps, the least ill or injured. One patient had been struck in the head with a glass bottle and was bleeding, another was unconscious, and a third had fallen several stories from a building.

Miles's sentiment that he had "high hopes for the call" belies the complex nature of good versus bad calls or real emergencies versus bullshit. We cannot merely label calls involving intoxication as "bullshit" because alcohol is a part of the call. Instead, providers think in more complex ways about the types of emergencies they face. Notably, this patient fell more into the college student demographic than a typical "37-Delta" patient. If providers had responded to a fall of several stories involving one of these prototypical patients, their responses could have been different, perhaps.

Understanding the idea of "bullshit work," therefore, requires shedding providers' own beliefs about the clinical needs patients have when they call 9-1-1. "Bullshit calls" are a statement about the desirability of particular forms of calls that are partially (but not wholly) informed by the clinical complexity of patients. The patient who fell several stories was terrified about the extent of her injuries. Even if the call was disappointing, the call was undoubtedly not bullshit to her.

Other Forms of "Grunt Work"

To move away from the dichotomy between "real emergencies" and "bullshit calls," I employ the phrase "grunt work," which I borrow from a provider's description of what a "bad shift" was:

> Lots of the . . . kinda just grunt work. Picking up the homeless people off the street. We get a good amount of calls that are, kinda, make us feel like a taxi service sometimes. So, if you have a day where you just kinda have call after call and its someone with a stubbed toe or a paper cut . . . that's sorta not a good day.

This idea of "grunt work" captures a range of calls providers consider "bullshit," though with a less derisive label. I aim to capture the idea that these calls are meaningful to patients and do have clinical need indicators. At the same time, however, they do not meet providers' conceptions of what deserving patients look or act like when they are sick or hurt. In addition to calls involving patients who have abused alcohol, several other types of patients are derided by providers as not deserving of care.

Opioid Calls

Calls for opioids did occur in Chapman during my time in the field. However, they were less frequent than alcohol calls. These calls covered a range of outcomes from providers labeled "drug-seeking" to patients who were intoxicated but had not overdosed. They also included overdoses, which providers described as typically involving heroin, some combination of methadone or suboxone, or prescription opioids.

One of the distinct features of treating opioid overdoses in the pre-hospital setting is Narcan, which has the effect of "waking up" patients who have overdosed on heroin or another opioid:

> PAUL: So I mean if you're a heroin addict and you just overdosed on heroin, and I give you Narcan to wake you up, I'm not going to be mad that I had to come to this call, and say that's [not] my job. I'm going to transfer you to the hospital, the same way I would somebody that called for chest pain. You got chest pain, okay, you're going to go to the hospital. [However] I might roll my eyes, and get frustrated inside . . .

The availability of a distinct intervention that could rapidly change a patient's status made these calls more comparable, for this provider, to calls for chest pain or another medical issue. Calls for acute alcohol intoxication, in contrast, required little to no intervention. However, even the greater clinical sophistication did not stop this provider from having the same "eye-rolling" or "frustrated" response to these patients.

This "frustrated" response is part of the broader context for opioid calls. While opioid overdoses were distinct clinically and etiologically from other types of substance-use calls, they elicited the same frustrations providers reported with alcohol intoxication. As with more urgent calls for alcohol, like the patient who fell several stories, there was not a clear delineation between "good" and "bad" calls based on clinical sophistication. In other words, having a pharmacological tool for addressing a patient's symptoms did not trump other biases providers held regarding substance-use and behavioral health issues.

Moreover, though overdoses happen, they are just one part of a broader spectrum of opioid calls, many of which are not "real emergencies" to providers. For example, one of the dispatchers sent Medic 7 for an overdose in East Chapman, though when we arrived on-scene, the patient was conscious though high. Emerging from the ambulance, Luke and Barrett found the patient and his friend sitting on the stoop of a three-story building. Like many in this part of Chapman, a restaurant occupied the first floor, with apartments above. They were both handcuffed, with their pockets cut open. Next to them, police officers had cut open a dirty black backpack as well, and needles and drug paraphernalia littered the sidewalk. There were both plainclothes and uniformed officers, and the plainclothes officers were questioning the men about where they were from and what drugs they used.

One of the two men appeared far higher than the other to Luke and Barrett, and the officers on-scene gave him a choice between going with us or going to jail for drug possession. The man protested, but the officer cut him off, telling both men they could not loiter in front of businesses. The two men denied they were loitering, but the restaurant's owner was there and promised he would look out for them and call the police back if they returned. The one man who the officers had decided needed to go to the hospital opted for the emergency department over jail, and Luke helped him into the ambulance. The ride was uneventful, and Luke did nothing for the patient other than sitting in the back of the ambulance with him.

On this call and the one described in Chapter 3, the circumstances again reduced the EMS providers to the role of a medical taxi. This call also highlights a perverse set of incentives for some individuals to adopt either the social role of a prisoner or that of a patient. Though it was the police officers who gave the man the two options, the EMS providers played a critical role in this process. These are critical aspects of the idea of "grunt work."

"Psych" Calls

Much like opioid calls, mental-health calls present categorization challenges. The line between "real emergencies" and "bullshit" could be clear, particularly for the most severe calls (Prener and Lincoln 2015). When discussing what providers typically called "psych calls," one provider described a hanging they responded to as "a freak show." At the same time, her partner recounted a suicide where an individual jumped down a ten-story garbage chute into a trash compactor.

Many calls for suicidality were not as dramatic. B6 was dispatched from Eaton Plaza to a transit station in North Chapman for an attempted suicide one morning. After driving north to the station, Kyle, Liam, and I walked down to the platforms with a transit police officer holding open the gate through the fare barriers for us. Another officer joined us, asking if a couple of other providers were working today. We found the patient surrounded by several transit inspectors and more police officers. He had climbed down into "the pit" near the third rail for the trains. The patient was calm, though visibly distraught, and asked Liam during the ride to the hospital if he carried a gun. Liam reminded the patient that he was not a police officer, and the rest of the transport proceeded without incident, though Liam grew visibly nervous when the patient began playing with something in his pocket.

Outside, after transferring care to the psychiatric emergency department staff at the Mather Hospital, Kyle told me he hoped we did not have to transfer the patient. "Psych transfers," as the providers call them, were frustrating, Kyle said, because "you bring in patients like the man we just transported while working a 'twenty-four'" and you "end up being called back between two and four for a transfer." Kyle said that he did not fully understand the system, but it always seemed like hospitals decided to transfer patients to other facilities early in the morning. While providers often criticized transfer work, this frustration with the psychiatric hospitalization system had an added component of distance. Unlike with other patients, who would typically go to nearby hospitals, psychiatric facilities were fewer in the region around Chapman and so transport times could be quite long:

> It's frustrating to take a psych patient in at noon, and then you're finally closing your eyes at like two in the morning, and then they wake you up to go take that same patient down to someplace that's like an hour away.

Patients whom providers transported as part of "psych calls" were not always happy to see providers, either. Some had voluntarily consented to hospitalization, but others had been "sectioned." This is the label providers and hospital staff use to describe patients held for treatment without giving consent. B10 transported a "section" one night from the Mather Hospital to another facility. According to Alexis, the patient had attempted suicide with a mix of alcohol and prescription medications and was upset about being transported. Alexis, who sat in the back with the patient, only spoke to the patient once during the entire trip. Like the call involving opioids described earlier, this patient was caught between the labels of prisoner and patient. As before, the providers barely communicated with the patient.

Providers used a variety of labels for these types of calls, such as "whack jobs." At other points, they were derisive toward the patients. After finishing a psychiatric transfer from a university clinic to a hospital and returning to the dimly lit parking lot outside the facility, Richard looked at his partner and simply said "pussy" about the patient. He paused, laughed, and added, "Just kidding." Later, on our drive back into Chapman, Richard elaborated, telling me that "with my luck, he would have killed himself if his girlfriend had not taken him." This underscores the practice of providers to treat these far more severe, though in this case hypothetical, calls as a nuisance.

Calls for Patients Who Were Homeless

Patients who were homeless in Chapman were impossible to ignore for EMS providers.[2] During downtime in Eaton Plaza, providers frequently saw homeless individuals passing through the area or panhandling on the corner in front of the Market. Drives through Midtown Plaza, which were a regular feature of downtime during shifts, likewise brought EMS providers into visual contact with individuals who appeared or were known to be homeless.[3]

The idea that some patients would be known to providers as homeless is critical to understanding the role EMS providers play with these patients. As I have noted previously, EMS providers differ from their colleagues in an emergency department since EMS providers have a better sense of the social and spatial context surrounding a call because they are physically present at a scene. However, ED providers may have access to a patient's medical history through a hospital's electronic medical-record systems. These are not details that EMS providers have access to through their computers. Even though they pick up a patient, depending on the context, providers may be unaware of a patient's status as an individual who is homeless or someone with a history of housing instability. Therefore, providers resort to visual cues to infer homelessness, such as unkempt hair, dirty clothes, or strong body odor, which has the effect of essentializing patients and reifying negative stereotypes.

Providers felt, sometimes with cause, that patients were trying to get transported to hospitals. These attempts to get shelter in the ED were especially notable during the winter months when providers reported finding patients with hypothermia and frostbite from sleeping on the streets. The emergency department offered respite from the cold and snow, a chance to warm up, and the opportunity to get a free meal before being discharged back out into the winter weather. One provider described walking up to a bench with six homeless individuals sitting on it, noting that it could be challenging to determine which individual they had been called for, since "they all want a turkey sandwich or a place to sleep." Though Chapman offered several shelters for patients who were confronting housing instability, many individuals distrust the shelter system or are unable to get beds, particularly in the winter, when there is higher demand. The failure here is not individual unwillingness to utilize the shelter system, but rather a society who leaves individuals sleeping on the streets without viable alternatives.

Calls for hypothermia and frostbite are an excellent if tragic example of how individuals enter the EMS system. Being homeless is, in itself, not a medical problem but rather a social issue. However, it is a social issue where chronic illness often overlaps. Some but not all of the individuals living on the street or in shelters had chronic mental-health, behavioral health, and medical problems. Calls for chest pain, diabetic emergencies, overdoses, and acute intoxication were frequent among patients with some form of housing instability. So too were more acute issues that directly resulted from living on the street, like frostbite and hypothermia.

However, the first-responder system in Chapman also medicalized homelessness itself. Dispatchers often coded 9-1-1 calls for people sleeping or lying down on the street as "man down" calls. Sometimes these signaled a patient who had overdosed. Other times these were individuals who had been sleeping behind a dumpster or a business. Providers would arrive, ensure the patient had no medical concern the EMS system could address, and offer them blankets in the fall or winter. Some patients would also be offered transportation from "the wagon" down to a shelter if they wanted it. "The wagon" as a prisoner transportation vehicle was used by the Chapman Police Department to shuttle patients to homeless shelters. One of the shelters, which is discussed in greater detail in the last chapter, "Marginality," also offered some intermittent transportation for patients.

This type of interaction played out one morning after Lucy, Alexis, and I had dropped ambulances in need of service off at the mechanic around the corner from Private Ambulance's headquarters and taken a physician who had been a third rider on the overnight shift back to the Muir Hospital. Our unit, B8, was sent by dispatchers for the "man down" after the owner of a business had called 9-1-1 about a man in the lot behind his store. When we arrived on-scene, we found a man sleeping on a cardboard box under a yellow plastic sheet. He was behind a small store near a dumpster. Lucy woke him, asked him how he was doing, and told him it was not a good place to sleep. The man told her that he was cold but otherwise fine after spending the night getting high and then eating Cheez-It crackers and butter, though he was not sure why he ate the butter. A long trail of urine flowed down the parking lot from under his tarp. Lucy offered him a ride to the shelter, which he declined, and a blanket, which he accepted. She also gave him directions to the police station after he asked for them so that he could reclaim some belongings he said officers had confiscated from him yesterday.

The discussion between Lucy and the patient here is typical of these types of calls. The fundamental issue is not medical, though it is certainly possible the patient may have chronic health concerns. Instead, the sole reason for the providers interacting with him was the concerns of a store owner about the presence of a person who appeared homeless. Like other calls, providers were resentful of these interactions, framing them as outside the scope of their job. As I noted earlier, when discussing the consequences of "bullshit calls," providers focused specifically on the homeless not only because they disliked the calls themselves but because they did not want to reward them for "abusing" the system.

Other Facets of "Grunt Work"

Besides focusing on homelessness, substance use, and "psych calls," providers quickly identified other forms of daily grunt work. Most of these calls fell into the realm of "bullshit" calls, which were not seen by providers as acute. When discussing "non-acute calls" during the semi-structured interviews, providers would mention things like "minor injuries," "the flu symptoms," "nausea or vomiting," "abdominal pain," "general weakness," "diarrhea," "nosebleeds," and "a paper cut." The struggle within EMS, however, is that the flu can be deadly for some patients. Likewise, nausea and abdominal pain can signal both chronic and acute health needs requiring hospitalization. Even nosebleeds can be dangerous if a patient takes particular medications. These possibilities again challenge the notion of what providers described as "bullshit calls."

Not only does "grunt work" cover a large swath of providers' daily call volume, but it is also not necessarily dull. Around patients who were intoxicated or seemed to be suffering from psychiatric issues, providers kept their guard up. These fears were not without pretext. Instructors taught providers to defend themselves as part of their training. They emphasized it in particular when discussing patients who might be suicidal or otherwise having a mental-health emergency. Moreover, some providers had stories of being assaulted as part of their job:

> I've been assaulted, I've been punched, I've been spit on, I've been bit—everything you could possibly imagine. I've been assaulted, you know, and that's always a difficult . . . those patients are always diffi-

> cult. I believe that if somebody doesn't have their conscious mind whether or not they're diabetic, or they're intoxicated, or generally just have a bad attitude, sometimes you have to defend yourself. Whether you have to physically restrain them to protect yourself, or protect your partner, or protect hospital staff.

Not every provider had these experiences, but the risk of being assaulted was something providers were conscious of during their shifts. During the ride to the hospital with the patient who had attempted suicide in the transit station described earlier, the EMT kept a close eye on the patient when he was playing with something in his pocket. These fears add another layer of stigma to providers' views of particular groups of patients. They may be malingering and not fall into categories deemed to be "real" work by providers, but EMTs and medics also viewed these patients as potential threats to themselves or their partners. When coupled with providers' negative feelings about these calls and often stigmatized views of patients, concerns about safety add to the daily grind of these calls.

Quantifying Grunt Work

The 9-1-1 system in Chapman deserves further explanation before moving forward. Once an individual places a call to the 9-1-1 center, a call-taker records information about the call and, for most medical calls, proceeds through the Medical Priority Dispatch System (MPDS). This system, first developed in the late 1970s, consists of a guided set of questions to help the call-taker determine the appropriate type and number of medical resources. In Chapman, 9-1-1 calls all come into a single facility handling police, fire, and EMS calls. After speaking with the caller, call-takers then pass the information to dispatchers for both the Chapman fire and police departments. These personnel work next to the call-takers. They also transmit the call information to Private Ambulance's dispatchers, located several miles away at Private's headquarters for EMS calls.

Using these data, we can get a sense of the volume of calls perceived to be acute or non-acute by dispatchers (see Table 6). Of course, these designations are imperfect because dispatch information does not perfectly predict what providers find on-scene. They do provide a partial window into the volume of work that is critical, however. During the years I was at Private Ambulance, dispatchers deemed 61.18 percent of all calls as not requiring paramedics. The caller, in other words, did not indicate that these calls were "real emergencies." Dispatchers coded another 17.51 percent of calls as requiring paramedics, though the caller's information did not place these calls into the highest-priority categories. Even if every one of these calls fit providers' criteria

Table 6. Class for Service Acuity, 2011–2013

Acuity	Frequency	Percent	Cumulative Percent
Omega	236	0.76%	0.76%
Alpha	9,863	31.88%	32.74%
Bravo	8,830	28.54%	61.18%
Charlie	5,418	17.51%	78.69%
Delta	6,277	20.29%	98.98%
Echo	315	1.02%	100.00%
Total	30,939	100.00%	

Notes: Omega—calls believed to be the least acute by call-takers; Alpha and Bravo—calls believed to require Basic Life Support interventions by call-takers, with Bravo calls a higher acuity than Alpha; Charlie and Delta—calls believed to require Advanced Life Support interventions by call-takers, with Delta calls a higher acuity than Charlie; Echo—calls involving a person believed to be in cardiac arrest

of "real emergencies," it would still mean that more than 60 percent of calls did not. However, the reality is that providers do not see many of the so-called "Charlie" calls as real emergencies, either. They can originate from situations, for example, where a patient appears to have trouble breathing but is not in respiratory distress when providers arrive.

We can find a parallel glimpse of acuity in my fieldnotes (see Table 7), where I rated the severity of calls using a simple triage metric. Green calls were non-acute and did not require any interventions from a paramedic, while yellow calls required some ALS interventions. These yellow calls roughly parallel the Charlie designation in dispatch information but reflect what providers did rather than what their dispatch information indicated. Red calls were those where the patient was seriously ill or injured and approximated providers' definitions of "real emergencies." Here, just over 69 percent of calls did not require interventions on the part of providers. Conversely, only 4.76 percent of calls were for serious injuries or illnesses.

Taken together, both the calls for service data and the fieldnote data suggest, at a bare minimum, that 60 to 70 percent of Private Ambulance's calls are not acute. Based on the field observations, I believe many of the "Delta" calls, the most severe, are less severe. This difference between dispatch information and what providers find accounts for the difference between the number of "Delta" calls generally and the number of "Red" calls I observed. While we should treat neither number as definitive, they both point to the same conclusion: a large volume of urban EMS work is non-acute. Providers' feelings about "grunt work" emanate from both the number of non-acute calls and the number of calls originating as severe calls that are, in reality, less acute.

Table 7. EMS Shift Observation Interventions by Category

Acuity	Frequency	Percent	Cumulative Percent
Green	87	69.05%	69.05%
Yellow	33	26.19%	95.24%
Red	6	4.76%	100.00%
Total	126	100.00%	

Notes: Green—calls where only Basic Life Support interventions were used; Yellow—calls with some Advanced Life Support interventions, such as routine cardiac monitoring, were used; Red—calls with Advanced Life Support interventions where providers characterized the patient as seriously ill or injured.

Frequent Fliers and Structural Failures in Chapman

Another facet of this grind is the repetition in patients themselves, who were sometimes known to providers as a result of repeated contacts. One afternoon, as Alexis and Jennifer sat in their ambulance up the street from the Market near Eaton Plaza, a heavyset bearded man passed our ambulance. Alexis recognized him immediately and turned to her partner, grousing that "he's always high on something." She noted that the man "looks like shit," and he could "be mean when he's picked up." After the man passed, they talked about another man they described as homeless who recently had his foot run over by a car. He had called 9-1-1 repeatedly because he could not find his pain medications even though providers were usually able to find them in his grocery cart. Both providers laughed. They had each treated him and confirmed to each other that he was funny enough to be "worth a trip to the hospital."

One way providers build knowledge about patients is through repeated contacts like those Alexis and Jennifer described. Providers often referred to regular patients as "frequent fliers." This term is not unique to Private Ambulance. Instead, it is a common term in health care for patients who used health-care services with such regularity that, providers muse, they could accrue miles just like they would through an airline. Like other terms, like "drunk" or even "37-Delta," the term carries a particular stigma with it.

Typically, however, frequent fliers were not patients whom providers celebrated treating. One morning, the dispatcher sent the EMT's staffing B8 to Midtown for a patient with chest pain. We arrived on-scene to find multiple police cars and a Chapman Fire Department engine company already there. They were standing around two women sitting on a park bench. Next to them was a Target shopping cart with a mix of possessions and empty beer and liquor bottles. The firefighters told us the patient, "Henrietta," had been drinking. Both providers then turned to the patient and began to speak with her like an old friend. It was hard to speak with her, though, because the patient was busy fighting with the police. She was mad because Chapman Police Department officers took her "nips" last night (small, single-shot liquor bottles). The officer told her that she could not have them in Midtown Plaza, and the patient responded angrily, "Where are we supposed to go?" The officers responded that she could have them anywhere but Midtown Plaza. Lucy and a firefighter got Henrietta's attention again long enough for her to refuse any care. The police departed, warning her if they received another call for her, they would "P.C. her" (place her in protective custody).

Back in the ambulance, Lucy and Alexis told me they had met the patient before, though they had not met her partner. Lucy told me, "I don't mind them [the patient and her partner], I'd rather deal with them than 'Amanda,' Amanda gets belligerent, or the drunk Mexicans." All these patients, including the two women we had just seen, had achieved a certain degree of infamy among Private Ambulance's medics, who treated them or saw them during downtime regularly. "The Mexicans," alternatively referred to as "the three amigos," were a group of men notorious among providers for their alcohol consumption.

We saw the women two more times on our way to other calls in Midtown during our shift. The first time, the Target cart was lying upside down in a park with its contents strewn everywhere; the two women were asleep near it. Later, on our way to another "man down" call, we passed our patient again, sitting next to her Target cart. A short time later, after the police took our patient from this call to a shelter, our dispatcher sent us to the assault in Midtown. It was Henrietta, who was leaning up against the exterior of a drugstore and crying. She told Lucy that her partner, whom we had seen her with earlier, had beat her up. The police told her there was nothing they could do since her partner had left the area, and they needed to stay away from each other. The patient alternated between crying and yelling at the police. Lucy and Alexis reiterated the officers' advice to stay away from her partner, and Henrietta refused help. As we put our bags back into the ambulance, the police wagon arrived to transport this patient to the shelter, too.

This woman and the other patients providers identify as "Amanda" and "the Mexicans" are examples of what providers call frequent fliers. In many cases, though not all, the patients seen regularly that Private Ambulance providers were most critical of were individuals who had some form of housing instability along with known substance use. Often, this was alcohol, and so the patients were labeled not just as frequent fliers but as "37-Deltas," as well. The identification of these patients is critical for understanding the broader context in which EMS providers work daily.

The experience of "frequent fliers" is perceived as if everyone is on a treadmill or stuck in a revolving door. The patients keep coming back time and time again, with the same three possible dispositions. Providers either leave them on the street, request transport to a shelter for those who are street homeless, or transport them to the hospital. In Chapman, few of these patients found themselves arrested as an alternative. If providers transported them to the hospital, there was a perception that they would often remain in the emergency department for a few hours only for the hospital staff to discharge them back into Chapman. Being discharged sets these patients up to begin another cycle, sometimes multiple times within a single day or even a single shift.

The cyclic nature of frequent fliers raises a critical question: Why is it that EMS providers treat these individuals to begin with? If we take providers at their word, these calls are not the type of work they should spend their time doing. The answer lies in a massive shift that was gripping American health care when EMS was transitioning from its proto phase into the modern system we have today, a transition known as deinstitutionalization.

As with EMS itself, the roots of the movement to end the confinement of individuals with mental illnesses were laid in the nineteenth century. Activists opposed to state mental hospitals began to argue that the hospitals were cruel, inhumane, and in need of reform. By the 1960s, hopes had risen among mental-health-care providers that other forms of treatment, like prescription medications, could be more successful at addressing patients' needs. These massive facilities, built in an earlier era, were also falling into disrepair and were expensive to operate. The moment was ripe to shift mental-health care into the community.[4]

However, the shift toward community mental-health care did not progress smoothly. Austerity and privatization have characterized contemporary outpatient mental-health care, and the demise of state hospital systems has left some individuals with no other options to seek care. The fundamental failure here was not deinstitutionalization itself. Indeed, many of the criticisms levied against these hospitals were manifestly correct. Instead, it was the failure to equip communities to care for their neighbors (Lamb and Bachrach 2001; Mechanic and Rochefort 1990). At the very moment when this particular patient population found itself falling through the cracks, emergency departments and EMS systems were becoming more formalized. Without reliable community services and a robust social safety net, the ambulance and the emergency department became the only alternatives to jail and prison for some. This choice quite literally occurs on EMS calls, when police officers present individual patients with the choice of "jail or hospital." Reporting that local jails, like Cook County Jail in Chicago, are now the largest de facto psychiatric hospitals in America underscores this trend (Ford 2015).

Not only has our collective failure to offer treatment in the community for everyone affected options for patients, it shapes what happens next for EMS providers and patients alike. Psychiatric emergency services have also suffered cuts both in terms of the availability of emergency departments and in-patient units. In and around Chapman, there are fewer options for patients in both settings. This shift translates to longer transport times that EMS providers have to endure and more frequent boarding of patients in psychiatric emergency departments. At the same time, providers wait for in-patient beds to become available. The Mather Hospital is symbolic of this. Once home to a large in-patient psychiatric facility, cuts meant that the vast majority of those beds were no longer available to patients by the time I arrived at Private Ambulance.

More generally, though, so many of the calls providers respond to in Chapman have their roots in failed systems to provide community care for a range of illnesses and social issues. Patients with substance-use disorders, for example, cycle in and out of emergency departments like the Mather Hospital's ED without any apparent alternatives to breaking this revolving door of care. Since EMS providers are unable to refuse care, they have few options for breaking this cycle themselves. Emergency departments similarly lack the mission, the resources, and the influence to interrupt the cycle fundamentally. There may be mental-health services available, for instance, but in many cases, the providers' attitude at the Mather Hospital was to place patients who were "37-Deltas" in "the tank" and discharge them as soon as possible.

The presence of many calls for minor health issues raises a similar concern if we expand this outward from just focusing on patients with mental- or behavioral health needs. The opportunities to obtain care are limited in many American cities, particularly given the nature of insurance access. Even patients who can gain some level of care through emergency departments can have poor outcomes. On two different occasions, I was present as Private Ambulance providers treated the same man, living in public housing, who could not speak English. On the first call, for tooth pain, Thomas was visibly irritated about everything from the language barrier to the rooms tightly packed with furniture and the reason for the call itself. Later, when I returned to the apartment with Bruce and Miles, it was for chest pain. While the patient was not having a cardiac event, the tooth from the first call was now abscessed, and the patient's body was struggling to fight the infection. After the call was over, Miles described checking the patient for sepsis as he transported him to the hospital.

This patient was not a frequent flier as far as any of the providers knew. Yet he still cycled through two emergency department visits, the first visit not leading to a resolution and resulting in a second and far more severe visit to a different hospital. After we were back outside the ambulance entrance to the emergency department, Bruce ruefully complained that "we've had all the poor people" on this shift. Though he was bemoaning this fact, it is a prescient observation. Private Ambulance's EMTs and medics spent much of their shift responding to systematic failures with primary care, mental-health care, addiction treatment, and housing policy. Instead of fast-paced, heart-racing action to treat critically ill patients, the daily grind of shifts meant providers spent far more time mopping up for broken social systems.

Treating Marginality

While the call volume at Private Ambulance reflects these structural failures, providers' base frustrations rested on the dichotomy between "real emergencies" and grunt work. As one medic told me:

> They tell you in school that "you're there to take care of sick people" and "you're there to keep people alive until they can get to the hospital" and that kind of falls out of the model to say "you're here to take care of people who are having severe mental illness symptoms" because in our mind you're not dying from that.

This provider frames the distinction in terms of clinical deservingness. However, the antithesis of "real emergencies" is not just "bullshit calls" but instead calls for patients whom providers do not see as *socially* deserving of care. The fact that the provider, like others at Private Ambulance, focused on patients with mental-health issues is not accidental. The infrastructure around Private Ambulance, such as the psychiatric emergency department at the Mather, suggests that there is a place for emergent psychiatric care. Overdoses and acute alcohol intoxication likewise can be severe, even if they do not rise to the status of "real emergencies."

The role of social deservingness in EMS care is particularly crucial because providers cannot control their workflow. This lack of control is an essential aspect of EMS work's marginality. For example, primary-care providers can opt not to accept Medicaid if they are uninterested in serving patients who use it for insurance. Emergency departments can place patients in waiting rooms, sometimes for hours, if the issue a patient presents is not critical. EMS providers have no such luxury.

The social deservingness of patients and the stigma associated with grunt work are both cultural facets of EMS work that inform how providers think about the entirety of their jobs and undertake them on a daily basis (see

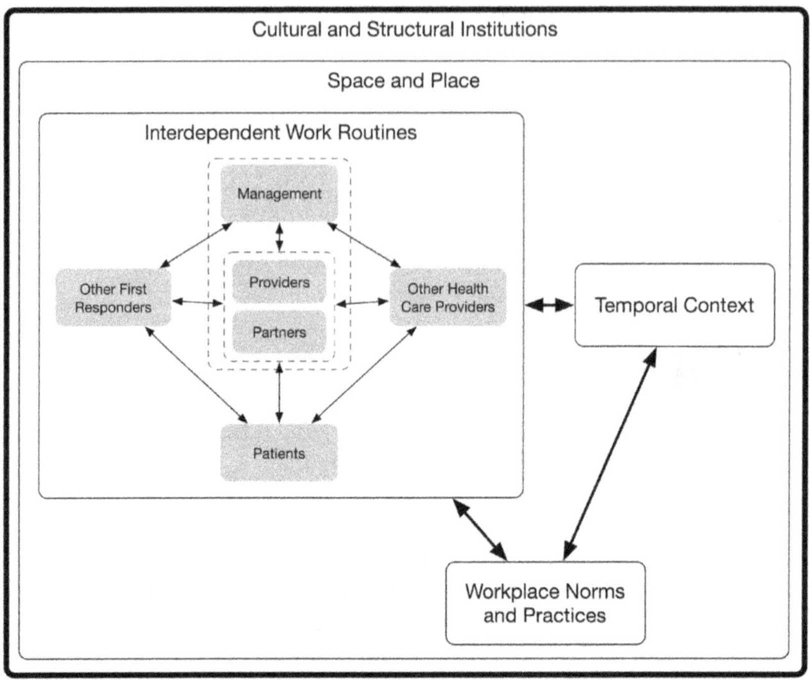

Figure 13. Evolving Theoretical Model—Integrating Cultural and Structural Institutions (graph by author)

Figure 13). They are also part of the broader orientation health-care providers have toward patients. EMS providers are not unique in their disposition toward patients who have psychiatric illnesses, suffer from housing instability, or have substance-use disorders. Researchers have found similar stigmatized views among other health-care providers. It is perhaps unsurprising that health-care providers would have a more complex view of deservingness than the Hippocratic Oath would lead some to believe. Providers reflect the undercurrents within American society about what "legitimate" mental and physical health concerns are.

Providers' views of patients form a critical aspect of the norms and practices of EMS work itself. However, stigmatized views of patients run deeper within EMS work. They permeate providers' interdependent work routines by affecting how they interact with patients, other health-care providers, and other first responders. The idea of "frequent fliers" is also a facet of the temporal context of EMS work. It is a nod to the repetition providers experience at multiple levels within and between their shifts. The iterative model of EMS work that we have developed over the previous chapters, therefore, locates the cultural forces shaping EMS work as an institution within which the entire milieu of pre-hospital care sits.

When providers question why these calls are their job at all, they are pointing to the structural failures pushing patients into the EMS system. Modern EMS work cannot be divorced from the other institutions that form the social safety net in the United States and in Chapman. When providers interact with patients who have housing instability, they come into contact with a process that numerous other institutions, including shelters, harm-reduction groups, street outreach teams, and law enforcement also engage with regularly. When providers treat patients living in poverty, they are similarly engaging with a community also served by safety-net hospitals, public housing, Medicaid, and other means-tested programs.

This web of institutions is crucial to understand because a failure at one point can cascade through other institutions, ultimately stressing the EMS system and the providers who staff it. The connectivity between these social institutions is not always well understood, nor is the EMS system's role in it often acknowledged. When we think about the connections between a patient's home in a shelter, public housing, or on the street and how the individual accesses care, it is often the EMS system providing that link. For patients who do not have family or transport to take them to dialysis appointments, the EMS system steps in to provide transportation. When shelters become full, dialysis companies change policies or locations, or legislatures cut back safety-net services under the guide of austerity, it is the EMS system that becomes the service of last resort.

Crucially, though cultural and structural institutions sit behind all of the processes shaping EMS work, they often find themselves in diametric opposition. As I have argued, EMS culture rejects the role of a safety-net service it so often finds itself pressed into because of these structural failures. When Bruce lamented that "we've had all the poor people" during a particular shift, he was capturing both points. Like other providers, Bruce rejected this work despite understanding that he could do nothing to stem the flow of these patients. The "grunt work" providers engage in is also not evenly distributed within Chapman. This maldistribution of EMS work is where we turn our attention to in Chapter 6.

6
Stigma and Space in Midtown

"[The dispatcher] fucked it up—the call in Midtown is going to be bullshit obviously . . . probably some drunk." (Bruce)

An Assault at the "Wet Shelter"

One afternoon, our dispatcher sent the crew of B6 to the "wet shelter" at the southern end of Midtown for the "traumatic injury." The "wet shelter" was notorious among providers. The shelter operated on a harm-reduction principle, with individuals who were using alcohol or other drugs able to stay there. Other shelters in Chapman were "dry," meaning that individuals had to be sober while they stayed there. When we arrived on-location at the "wet shelter," we found a Chapman Police Department officer already there, though it turned out not for the call our dispatcher sent us to the shelter to address. A staff member buzzed us through the door past a woman standing outside who tried to chat with Kyle and Liam. Once inside, another staff member escorted us into the shelter's clinic, where a clinician and a man who turned out to be the patient were standing. We had to wait while the clinic staff worked to move another individual, who the clinician told us assaulted our patient, out of the front door's common area.

While we waited, another clinician brought over the Chapman police officer. The patient, who had been talking with us and the staff member, immediately stopped talking, and Kyle and Liam had to discontinue their assessment while the officer was there. They were eager to get back out to the ambulance, but the shelter director came over and stopped them. The director told the patient he needed to call the shelter from the hospital and not come directly back. The patient got upset, believing he would not be allowed back into the shelter because he did not want to report the assault to the police. The shelter director assured him he would be allowed back, and the patient told him he did not know the number and asked if the hospital did. The director smiled and said, "Oh yes, they have" to the patient, drawing out "oh" in a knowing, slightly sarcastic way.

We finally got the patient out to the ambulance, and Kyle was able to obtain a more precise story, since the shelter staff and the police officer were no longer there. Kyle worked to bandage the patient's minor injuries while Liam drove us over to the Mather Hospital. Though we had picked the patient up from the "wet shelter," Kyle told me later that the patient denied any current substance use. When we arrived at the hospital, two patients were screaming from "the tank," the four-bed holding room across from the nurses' station where patients who were intoxicated, or who staff believe were street homeless, often were directed by the hospital staff. One was upset because the other would not talk to him.

Locating Grunt Work

In Chapman, grunt work is not just a cultural and institutional phenomenon. Grunt work is also a *spatial* phenomenon. EMS work's spatial nature is perhaps the most significant difference between it and other forms of health care. With ambulances, the health-care system comes to patients rather than the reverse. Providers get to experience the sometimes chaotic realities in which their patients live or find themselves. Such was the case with the call at the "wet shelter," where providers entered what for most Chapman residents is typically a "backstage" location most people do not get to see. The way providers experience this chaos becomes part of how providers contextualize their patients' clinical condition. During their Private Ambulance careers, providers develop a depth of spatial knowledge about places where they can spend downtime and where specific calls occur. They learn the streets, neighborhoods, and locations of businesses. These form the basis of particular frames informing how providers view the city and the dispatch information dispatchers pass to them before each call: the patient and the place where providers find them become inextricably linked.

Provider Perceptions of Where Grunt Work Occurs

For providers at Private Ambulance, no city area was more salient in terms of "grunt work" than Midtown. All the providers discussed it during their

Table 8. Sketch Map Descriptive Statistics

Type	Frequency	% of Respondents	Mean *n* of Clusters per Respondents	Moran's *I*
Frequent Calls	105	100.00%	3.50	0.471
Substance Use	93	100.00%	3.10	0.503
Homeless Patients	80	100.00%	2.67	0.404
Chronic Illness Calls	36	50.00%	2.00	0.358
Non-Acute Calls	36	43.33%	2.77	0.510
Psychiatric Calls	36	56.67%	2.06	0.605

Note: All Moran's *I* values shown have values that are less than 0.001.

interviews and raised it on many shifts. The city of Chapman has official neighborhoods, though Midtown is not one of them. Instead, it is one of several "plazas" sitting at the intersection of major thoroughfares. Midtown rests between the "Fulmore" to the west and "Mid-Chapman" to the east. For most providers, these plazas were the most salient way of describing Chapman's geography. I asked each provider to identify areas on a map where particular work types took place during interviews. This exercise, called "sketch mapping," included questions about where various calls occurred regularly.

I asked providers about several different calls: those involving substance use, calls where patients were homeless, "psych calls," calls providers did not believe were acute, and calls for chronic illnesses. I also asked providers where they responded to frequently. Every provider identified areas within Chapman where they frequently responded and spaces where calls for patients who were homeless and calls involving substance use were frequent (see Table 8). A smaller proportion of providers, approximately half, identified areas where "psych calls," calls for non-acute issues, and calls for chronic illnesses occurred.

When we look at these responses together in Figure 14, we can see readily observable patterns in providers' perceptions of where work occurs. In the maps for frequent calls, patients who are homeless, and substance-use calls, we see the highest number of clusters focused on the Midtown area. There are secondary clusters in each map to the north, in the "Old Quarter" area of the city, near where Eaton Plaza sits. Providers distinguished homelessness there, focusing on a younger group of individuals they called "gutter punks." In particular, on the substance-use map, there are also higher frequencies in East Chapman. One provider scribbled out a syringe on his sketch map when describing responding to overdoses there. The maps for both "psych calls" and

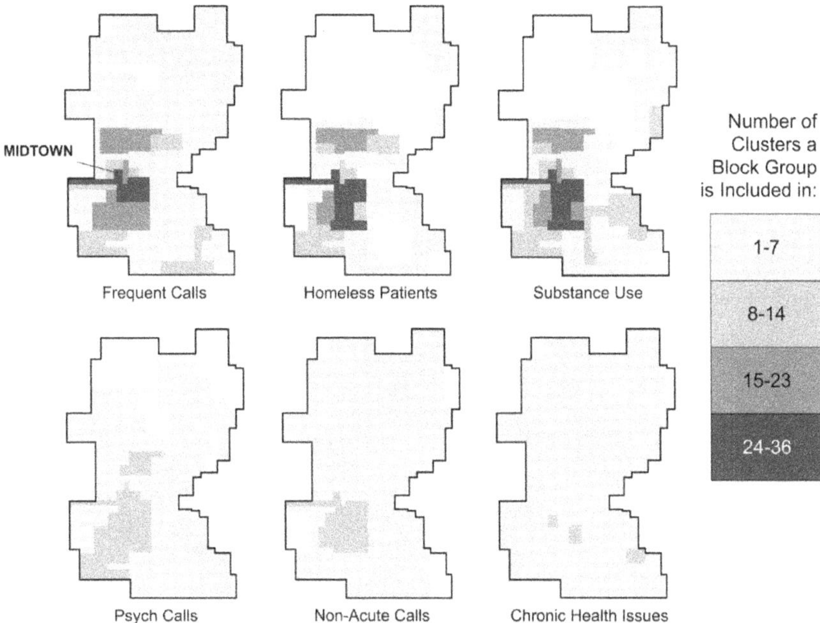

Figure 14. Provider Perceptions of Grunt Work in Chapman, Frequency (graph by author)

non-acute calls, despite having an overall smaller number of frequencies, also show clustering in the Midtown area.

We can quantify these clusters in several ways. Table 8 includes Moran's I measures for these data. This statistic measures spatial autocorrelation, the degree to which mapped data cluster near each other. Each of the sketch-map data sets has a positive value, with most between .4 and .6, indicating some moderate clustering. We can further illustrate Midtown's focus by using a spatial statistic called the Getis-Ord GI* (see Figure 15). This technique identifies areas with a high frequency of a particular phenomenon that are surrounded by other areas with similar high frequencies. With provider perceptions, we can use this technique to identify "hot spots" where patterns are shared across providers' responses to the sketch-map prompts. All six of these prompts show "hot spots" in the Midtown area and "cold spots" across a swatch of North Chapman above where the Old Quarter is located. These "hot" and "cold" spots are areas of high and low numbers of marks made by participants, respectively, that are also surrounded by other areas of high or low endorsement. These clusters help us identify crucial patterns in the sketch-map data highlighting where providers' attention is collectively focused.

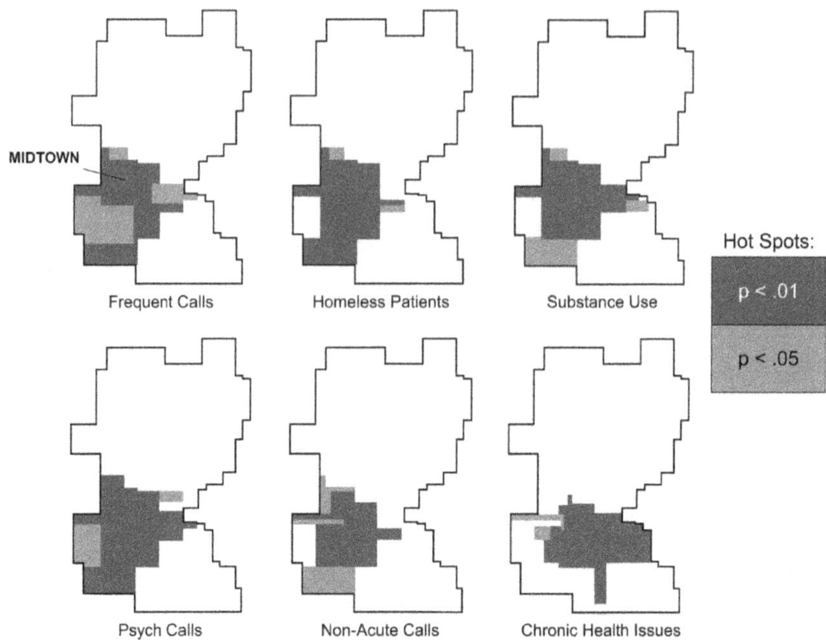

Figure 15. Provider Perceptions of Grunt Work in Chapman, Getis-Ord GI* Results (graph by author)

Shared Perceptions and Misconceptions

It is crucial to remember that the sketch maps represent providers' *perceptions* of where their work occurs. Perceptions are essential for understanding how providers view the work they collectively engage in daily. However, they also differ in systematic ways from more objective measures of where EMS work takes place. These differences do not mean those perceptions are wrong. Indeed, differences between providers' sketch maps and other measures of where EMS work occurs can be revealing.

The bi-variate map shown in Figure 16 provides one such comparison. It compares a total number of EMS incidents per Census block group to the number of times a given block group was included in providers' sketch maps for the prompt asking them where they respond to frequently. The map therefore compares a subjective measure of frequent responses to a more objective measure of where this work occurs. Areas of agreement are colored white, while areas where providers' perceptions and the count of EMS incidents differed are highlighted in gray on both panels of Figure 16. In responding to the sketch-map prompt, providers underemphasized their work in East Chapman and North Chapman (see the

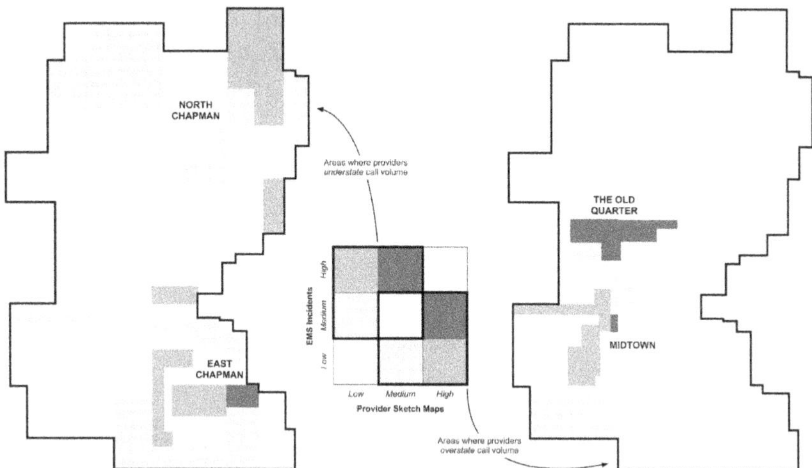

Figure 16. Bi-Variate Map of Provider Perceptions and Dispatch Locations for Grunt Work (graph by author)

left panel). On the other hand, they overemphasized responses in the Midtown and the Old Quarter areas of the city (see the right panel).

These differences between the perceptual data collected during the sketch-map exercise and the calls for service data are not especially surprising. Indeed, we can interpret them as a spatial variant of what is known as "the clinician's illusion" (Cohen and Cohen 1984). This concept captures site-specific effects driving providers' perceptions of the patients they treat. Since there is no process of random assignment for patients to health-care facilities, providers often end up with a biased sample for particular illnesses. For instance, they may find that their patients with diabetes have significantly worse outcomes than patients with diabetes as a whole. If they were erroneously to conclude that diabetes has a particular trajectory, these providers would be invoking the clinician's illusion based only on their biased sample of patients.

A similar parallel has been found, for example, in residents' perceptions of disorder in neighborhoods. The actual incidence of disorder does not predict these perceptions well. Instead, other factors such as the percent of African American or immigrant residents of a neighborhood are far more predictive of how residents perceive disorder in neighborhoods. As with the clinician's illusion, it is the perception of these communities' distribution and not the reality that matters. Sociologists have long called this broader notion that perception matters more than reality the "Thomas theorem" (Merton 1995) after Dorothy Swaine Thomas and W. I. Thomas, two sociologists connected with the Chicago School during the 1920s.[1]

For EMS providers, their perceptions are not just of what type of clinical issues they confront but where these issues manifest. Just as the clinician's illusion has the effect of misrepresenting a clinical population's key characteristics, providers' illusions reflect not the population distribution but rather the biased sample they experience during their shifts. Recognizing EMS providers' perceptual patterns in their work and identifying where those patterns occur is not about painting providers as incorrect. Instead, it provides an opening to understand the salient factors influencing providers' focus on specific populations or neighborhoods at others' expense.

Midtown

At the heart of EMS providers' own "clinician's illusion" is Chapman's Midtown area, which stands out across all three of the figures presented earlier in this chapter. Midtown is not one of the city's officially designated neighborhoods, four of which come together in the area providers' label as Midtown. This intersection of neighborhoods occurs at a literal intersection, where two major thoroughfares, Main Street and Riverside Avenue, come together. Known as "Midtown Plaza," commercial businesses of all varieties surround this routinely busy junction. There are banks, restaurants, coffee shops, concert venues, a Starbucks, a 7-Eleven, and several small local markets. The Midtown transit station includes three extensive collections of bus shelters serving several bus lines connecting Midtown to Chapman's other neighborhoods and the surrounding metropolitan area.

At the heart of Midtown Plaza is the Plaza itself, an ample concrete space on the southwest corner of Main Street and Riverside Avenue. "Park" would perhaps be too generous a word. There is no green space here, though a small park a block to the west on Riverside Avenue does offer some. The Plaza stretches a block in width along Riverside Avenue. Near Main Street, the Plaza is about fifty feet in width. Benches around several large concrete planters that have trees planted in them adorn this portion of the Plaza, which sits in front of a bank branch. The other end of the Plaza is narrower, about ten feet in depth, without benches or other amenities. This portion of the Plaza serves as one of the bus shelter hubs, which sits in front of a corner store and a sandwich shop. At this end, there are no benches or other amenities.

On the same side of Main Street, just to the south of the Plaza, is a large chain drugstore. As one walks south along Main Street past the drugstore, several retail stores include a chain coffee shop and a liquor store. A second liquor store sits across Main Street and slightly further south. Trash, including discarded "nips," small, single-serving liquor bottles, lies discarded in front of the businesses. Urine trails sometimes run over the sidewalk here and mix with the smell of fast food, body odor, and diesel engines from passing trucks. Like many dense urban crossroads, Midtown Plaza is also a cacophony of the city's sounds: honking, car and truck engines, pedestrians' chatter, helicopters flying overhead, and the sound of sirens from ambulances and other emergency vehicles.

The Plaza itself was the primary focus of providers' attention during downtime when we would cruise through the major intersection and providers would look for individuals whom they knew from past calls. However, it was only one of several locations that are particularly important for discussions of homelessness and substance use in Midtown. Across Riverside Avenue sit additional wooden park benches. Down Riverside Avenue to the left are two park-like areas, one on each side of the street, adorned with benches and a small area of green space. Near these parks are two social-service facilities that provide services, including needle exchange and other harm-reduction services to both the homeless in Chapman and individuals with substance-use issues. All these locations are within a block's radius to the north and west of Midtown Plaza.

Outside of the Plaza, the neighborhood unfolds from either side of Main Street, which bisects the Midtown neighborhood from north to south. For much of its length, five- and six-story structures line Main Street. Most of these buildings have retail establishments, restaurants, or bars on the first floor and then a mix of commercial and residential units on the upper floors. Along this strip are additional services and businesses that cater to a wide range of low-income residents and the homeless, including several "dry" shelters, a check-cashing business, and a used clothing store. Main Street's strip has had a long reputation for being a bohemian neighborhood within Chapman, replete with bars offering live music and several larger music venues, as well as vegetarian restaurants. The neighborhood's reputation includes a degree of tolerance toward homelessness and substance use. These characteristics have been noted in the local media and lamented by city politicians and neighborhood groups seeking to "clean up" Midtown. One local media article about the Midtown neighborhood, published during this book's fieldwork, interviewed a longtime local business owner who described the neighborhood's past reputation for drug sales and sex work.

Recent reports made public by the Chapman Police Department describe Midtown as one of several critical areas for Chapman's homeless population. One report, which corresponded with the timing of the EMS shift observation phase of data collection, described Midtown as "gritty" and the homeless individuals who frequented the area as "more hardened." The report described the population as consisting primarily of older individuals who have been homeless for an extended period and have a history of incarceration and alcohol-use issues. This report suggests that some of Midtown's former grit remains despite significant changes in recent years. These have occurred primarily across the southern swath of Midtown, which has seen considerable development, as one paramedic noted:

> TIM: Midtown Plaza has changed a lot, actually. It's much cleaner and safer now. Midtown Plaza was way more dangerous ten or twenty years ago. It's kind of . . . and it's changed a lot. [Technology] companies have come into Downtown Plaza. It's a huge amount of money so that's changed a lot. There used to be a lot of vacant dirt lots in Midtown Plaza and Downtown Plaza and that doesn't exist anymore.

These vacant lots, the site of old factories and business lost to deindustrialization during the 1960s and the 1970s, have been rebuilt as Chapman's knowledge economy has expanded. Midtown's southern part is now home to science firms and technology startups where ironworks and factories once stood.

Outside of these two commercially focused areas, to both the east and west, are residential zones. They are especially dense, particularly in the blocks just west of Main Street. These blocks include numerous apartment buildings and a high-rise building operated by the city of Chapman that is open to individuals receiving Social Security retirement or disability payments. Further west and east from Main Street, the apartment blocks give way to densely situated multifamily homes, many of which are two-and-a-half- or three-story homes subdivided into apartments. There is little commercial activity in these parts of the neighborhood save for the occasional corner store.

Further to the south, at the edge of the neighborhood, are both a "wet" and a "dry" shelter. The "wet" shelter, as I noted, allows individuals who are currently using substances to stay there. These types of shelters embody a harm-reduction strategy focused on housing first rather than sobriety. The other shelter along Main Street, and a shelter for women to the north of Midtown Plaza, are both "dry" shelters, meaning sobriety is a condition of housing. While providers did respond to Chapman's shelters, it was the "wet shelter" they described as responding to most frequently.

The Multiple Stigmas of Patients, Illnesses, and Place

The focus providers bring to Midtown, which is evident in the sketch maps they do and the frequent discussion providers had about the neighborhood during both the fieldwork and the interviews, is what I term here the "Midtown effect." It has an overwhelming focus on one neighborhood to the exclusion of everyday work elsewhere in Chapman, and it is rooted in a stigmatized view of how grunt work intersects with particular places. The neighborhood comes to be defined in providers' minds by the "frequent fliers" who spend time there and their stigmatized social and health statuses.[2] The perception that these patients are found overwhelmingly in Midtown forms the basis for providers' overall evaluations of the neighborhood. These assessments are at the root of a neighborhood stigma above and beyond the stigmas of mental health, substance use, and homelessness.

Responding into Midtown: Grunt Work and Frequent Fliers

Riverside Avenue runs from the Plaza west to the river, which forms a portion of Chapman's city limits. One afternoon, dispatchers sent Medic 6 to an area just west of the Plaza to report a patient having seizures. Thomas and Amanda were inside the hospital, and they quickly went out to the ambulance, with Amanda jumping into the driver's seat and asking if the call was on the Midtown Plaza or river end of Riverside Avenue. The dispatcher directed them to the small park just to the west of the Plaza itself, and the police officers who were already on-scene motioned excitedly for us as we approached the scene.

The patient was having grand mal seizures that resulted in convulsions rippling up and down her body. As she seized, her boyfriend stood to the side. Thomas questioned him about what drugs she had taken, finding out only that she had been consuming alcohol. The boyfriend continued to try to hand Thomas the patient's suitcase with her belongings, telling him to bring it to the hospital himself. The boyfriend said he was not sure if he would go with them. Thomas told Amanda he wanted the patient in the ambulance as soon as possible. As we moved the patient into the ambulance, she stopped seizing. Thomas tried to hook her up to both the cardiac monitor and oxygen, but the patient at first refused these measures. After some back and forth, the patient relented, but then began seizing again. Thomas tried to ask her to calm down and laid her down from the sitting position she was seizing in. As he did this, he shouted for Amanda to head for the hospital.

Unlike the assault described at the "wet shelter" at the beginning of the chapter, this call illustrates the more severe end of the spectrum of calls providers responded to in Midtown. The call at the "wet shelter" represents the other end of this spectrum, a call for which EMS providers did little for the patient. These bookends highlight the reality of work in Midtown for EMS providers as they experience it. Calls are sometimes particularly acute, as with the patient whose active seizures presented an acute health issue for her. Nevertheless, even there, the specter of "grunt work" remains close at hand. Unlike critical calls in other areas, providers felt that even here, it was just sicker versions of their "regular customers."

This notion of regular customers, which Chapter 5 termed "frequent fliers," was expressed more strongly in Midtown than in any other neighborhood in Chapman. Providers reported responding to the same patients multiple times in a single shift here, such as in the experience of Lucy and Alexis described in Chapter 5. During that shift, they had responded to two calls for the same patient and, in the intervening period, passed the patient and her partner on the way to a different call. Many providers shared similar stories, describing responding to the same patient and sometimes transporting him or her to the hospital, only to have to treat the individual again in a few hours. In providers' minds, these stories were not just stories about the patients themselves but about Midtown.

Stigmatized Views of Patients and Illnesses

The result of these interactions with patients in Midtown can be real, visible frustration on the part of providers. Paramedics would sometimes look defeated or angry when they heard the dispatch information go out for a call in Midtown. When asked what it was like responding to these sorts of incidents where the paramedic knew or thought he knew who the patient would be, one provider responded:

> CHARLIE: It's day to day . . . it depends. Some of them, some days they're nice and if they're nice I'll be nice to them. It's a . . . are they yelling when you roll up? Are they yelling at the cop? Are they yelling at you? Are they yelling at bystanders? Are they so gorked out of their mind that they're taking a leak in the middle of [Riverside] Avenue? In the middle of the day? It can be frustrating. If they're being nice, I'll give them the benefit of the doubt. I believe every day is a new day. . . . [But] it can be draining. It can be wearing, though. If you seen them multiple times in a shift it can be draining.

There is frustration, then, with specific instances of patients who are yelling, potentially violent, or otherwise participating in something deviant like urinating in a street that runs directly through Midtown Plaza.

However, providers also hold more deeply rooted frustration with system-use patterns and "abuse" they perceive (Prener and Lincoln 2015). The net effect of repeated encounters with "frequent fliers" is the development of intersecting stigmatized attitudes about homelessness, substance use, and mental illness that result in a more fundamental aversion to this patient population. This attitude appears in Charlie's quote when he says, "So and so has been drinking, he doesn't have any medical problems, doesn't need to go to the hospital." This distinction of alcoholism from being a "medical problem" frequently occurs when discussing "37-Deltas" with EMS providers at Private Ambulance.

Many of the providers, then, have negative feelings about working with patients who are substance users. When asked about this population, one provider noted, "Well, I don't have many positive things to say." Providers construct these patients as lacking a medical need and as active "abusers" of the EMS and social safety-net systems. Identifying patients as "abusers" is a separate distinction from labeling patients as "substance abusers." Instead, "abusers" in this context are patients who misuse the availability of EMS resources:

> CP: What's it mean to be an "abuser"?
>
> JOE: Um I would say, drinking multiple pints of ["Rossiya"] every day and calling EMS for a transport because you're not feeling well. That's an abuser of uh the money that you're given by the government and the public services that we give.

"Rossiya" is a locally produced, cheaply priced, foul-smelling vodka available in pint bottles for just a few dollars. When asked during interviews what the types of alcohol they saw abused, over half the providers answered that it was "cheap vodka," with approximately a third of all providers naming "Rossiya" explicitly. During visits to the Midtown area at several different points in the study, I noticed the clear plastic bottles it comes in discarded on sidewalks and in gutters. "Rossiya," like "37-Delta," was therefore used as a label to indicate a particular population. As one provider put it, "It's mostly your high-octane low-cost stuff, so we're not talking about our craft beers here. We're talking about like cheap vodka. The stuff that would pass as motor fuels in most other countries."

Like "37-Delta" and other terms discussed earlier, "abuser" and "substance abuser" are two examples of ascriptive labels applied to patients. "Rossiya" is a powerful adjunct to these labels. Its reputation becomes symbolic of the frustrations providers have with responding to substance use. Moreover, the comparison of Rossiya to craft beers belies a class analysis on the part of the providers. EMS providers present themselves as working- and middle-class individuals, and casting dispersions toward alcohol "that would pass as motor fuel" can distinguish themselves from their patients. What is critical here is framing patients as socially inferior "abusers" of the EMS system and, by extension, society at large.

Providers gave similar accounts of homelessness, describing those patients as attempting to game the system to get a warm bed to sleep in or a meal at the hospital: "three hots and a cot," as one provider put it during an EMS shift observation. Providers believed patients who were homeless would lie about or exaggerate their symptoms to get these things:

> Nora: And they really, probably not, I shouldn't say they're lying, but sometimes there's many that you work up for chest pain, if they said they have chest pain, they have chest pain. But they're trying to get. . . . They'll admit it. They'll say well I want a sandwich, you know, whatever. Sure, I bet you do. You know what I mean?

Another provider noted a similar phenomenon with homeless patients in Midtown:

> Charlotte: Most of them are intoxicated. . . . If they're not intoxicated, they were intoxicated. And now they want to go to the hospital, for generally a reason, an ailment that they describe that isn't real. You know, whether it's shortness of breath, or chest pain, or diabetes, that's what we get. They're not really having those symptoms, we can't tell them that, but when you bring them into the hospital and they check them all out and they realize that you're not, this isn't real, that's when we find out that person really didn't have a blood sugar of thirty or something.

The homeless, then, are constructed as individuals who will do anything, up to and including lying, to gain access to shelter and food.

These views inform providers' overall responses to individuals who have either substance-use disorders or who are homeless, but providers' responses are magnified when it comes to patients labeled as "37-Deltas." One provider described working with patients who are substance users; the conversation drifted to patients who are frequent fliers, and the paramedic told me:

> Ed: When I'm taking the same patient four times for the same exact thing and it's . . . a layperson can understand that it's bullshit every single time, it's the most frustrating, infuriating feeling in the world. Because you, they're wasting resources. And it's not like we have something better to be doing like a cardiac arrest that's not getting help because we're helping you. No, it's just wasting my time because I do it every single day, and you never change, and you never follow the programs that are set up, the social programs for you. And that makes the other wave of compassion just disappear. And it's just due to the sheer volume of how many times you see these patients. I see patients more times in a week than I see my family in a year.

For this paramedic and others, patients' inability to get sober or get off the street are further evidence of their own personal failings. This is a viewpoint that again repositions providers' attention from alcoholism as an illness toward alcoholism or homelessness as the product of personal, internal failures not requiring medical attention. Patients labeled as "37-Deltas" are not just individuals whose behavior (being intoxicated in public, urinating in the street) stands out to providers and individuals who have personally failed.

Providers also had a strong physical response to these patients. The smell of patients, described at the beginning of the introductory chapter, is an essential stigmatizing facet of "37-Deltas." Work with the "37-Deltas" who are "frequent fliers" fits both this broad sense of "grunt work" and the conceptualization of "grunt work" as dirty work. The "37-Delta" patients had a reputation for the smells that often accompanied them, including "urine, or feces, or alcohol . . . [or] body odor." Another provider told me, "They smell, they usually smell," before going on to describe the smell like a "football locker room with socks in there for years" and warning that removing these patients' shoes was a bad idea. During the EMS shift observations, some patients smelled so strongly of feces that providers gagged as they neared the patients. Other providers described "37-Delta" patients who defecated on the floor of the ambulance. The olfactory experience of working with "37-Delta" patients and the need to air out and disinfect significantly soiled ambulances gave these calls a reputation of literal "shit work."

The stigmas providers held about homelessness and substance use were the product of several different frames. Providers see these patients as generally undeserving of care because, as I have noted before, these are calls for issues that do not fit with EMS's definition as an acute-care system. Beyond this dissonance, providers view both chronic substance use and homelessness as the products of individual failures of patients who are willing to "abuse" EMS and emergency department services. When combined with these calls' dirty nature and the association with disorder (such as public urination), these frames emphasize this work's particularly problematic nature for providers.

The Social Production of Neighborhood Stigma

The overwhelming focus providers have on the Midtown neighborhood is the product of several intersecting stigmas about substance use, homelessness, and the negative characteristics associated with "37-Deltas" and patients who drink "Russiya." These overlapping and intersecting stigmas (Logie et al. 2011) collide on a single neighborhood, with providers associating this particular population of patients with Midtown in ways that generate a spatial stigma as well—in other words, a notion that Midtown is somehow spoiled as a neighborhood.[3] During the semi-structured interviews, a paramedic who lived in

Chapman described the neighborhood she lived in as ideal because it was far away from "the homeless," describing the "bad parts" of Chapman as the "drunk shelter" (i.e., the wet shelter) and Midtown. Several providers described avoiding the neighborhood if they could to not run into some of their "regular customers during off duty hours," a reference to frequent fliers.

Providers contrasted the patients they found in Midtown with other city areas, particularly the Old Quarter. Like Midtown, providers regularly interacted with patients who they believed to be homeless in the Old Quarter. However, providers stratified their understanding of homelessness between these two neighborhoods:

> RYAN: The homeless typically that we deal with are the ones that kind of reside in [Midtown Plaza]. Those are more of the substance abusers. If I had . . . geographically to tell the difference between homeless in [Midtown Plaza] and the homeless in [University Plaza], the homeless in [University Plaza] homeless patients are typically not—you're not finding those as substance abusers. They're just kind of more of the strange folk that live around that area. They don't really tend to bother anybody.

This contrast between the communities of individuals who were street homeless in Midtown and the Old Quarter, the neighborhood encompassing University Plaza, is an important one. It speaks to differences between the perceived distribution of homelessness noted earlier and the Chapman Police Department's data calls for service data. For providers, the most salient difference was substance use: "A lot of time in [Midtown Plaza], it's all drug- or alcohol-related; and most of the time, homeless."

During shifts, providers used dispatch information that located calls in the Midtown area as a critical piece of information for anticipating the type of call they would see. The dispatch information transmitted to Private Ambulance was often sparse, directing ambulances to respond to an address for what was often a two- or three-word description of what may have been wrong with the patient. In particular, providers assumed, given a particular set of dispatch information such as for the "man down" in Midtown, they would be seeing one of their frequent flier "37-Delta" patients:

> CP: What clues you into . . . [thinking you know who the patient will be]?
>
> RACHEL: The region. If I hear that it's going to be a 47-year-old female in [Midtown Plaza], you know, who's down on the ground, I can with pretty much 90 percent accuracy guess who exactly the patient is. If it's in that area, I'm almost positive that [the caller] is, it's a bystander who doesn't know the area very well, sees someone there, and doesn't

> understand that we have this homeless population that are a bunch of alcoholics, and who are very, almost all the time drunk. So they don't know that this is regular for us, and that we see that. So when I hear that, then that to me, it's the region that I know that it's not going to be the person who is unconscious for some strange, weird reason. They're probably just drunk and don't want to wake up.

Beyond the repetition of the "just drunk" argument, this quote underscores Midtown's association with homelessness and substance use. Midtown suffers, then, from the convergence of two stigmas, homelessness and substance use, on a particular geographic area providers identify based on this convergence. Midtown, for EMS providers, is analogous with homelessness and substance use. This identity leads to forming a third form of stigma, this time aimed at Midtown itself. Like a person who is homeless or has a substance-use disorder, Midtown suffers from a "spoiled identity" (Goffman 2009) with consequences for both EMS providers and patients.

Structural Forces and Disordered Space

The convergence of homelessness and substance use in Midtown is not accidental or random. Indeed, Midtown's earlier description noted the variety of services available to individuals with housing instability or substance-use issues in Midtown Plaza's immediate area. These included a social-services building with services aimed at these populations, a harm-reduction program, liquor stores, and other businesses (a chain fast-food burger restaurant and convenience stores) offering low-cost food. The main area of Midtown, situated along Main Street, also housed several shelters for both men and women. These shelters nearest to Midtown were "dry" shelters.

However, Midtown itself was known by providers for a different facet of the homeless population, the "37-Delta" individuals who used a different shelter. The impact this shelter had on the neighborhood is essential, mostly since it sits at the very fringe of Midtown. Providers described Midtown Plaza as being along the walking route between the "wet shelter," the Midtown Plaza area, and the "Mather Hospital," where many of the "37-Deltas" would find themselves after an ambulance trip. Patients, according to providers, would stay in the shelter and then spend the day drinking in Midtown Plaza. When they had become so intoxicated that they could not walk, Private Ambulance would transport them to the Mather Hospital's "drunk tank," where they would sober up, and the hospital staff would discharge them. Shortly after, providers would report finding these individuals in Midtown again.

One provider described this congregation of patients at Midtown Plaza as a "pack," another as a "pack of wild dogs." The result is what providers see as a near-constant state of disorder. One provider described Midtown:

> Paul: I mean you've got people that have nothing, or they're on drugs, or they want to be on drugs, so they want a fix. Now . . . they're mixing in with professional people, or people that are going to work, or have money, or have things that they want. And I guess sometimes, that's where you see bums, you see robberies, we do get those. There [are] assaults down there. Them fighting with each other, or fighting with other people.

Other providers described individuals sleeping and relieving themselves in plain view in the public spaces in and around Midtown Plaza. When these behaviors result in contact with law enforcement or a bystander who calls 9-1-1, Private Ambulance providers would respond to assess the patient and potentially transport the individual to the ED.

This pattern represents two cycles for "37-Delta" patients. One of the cycles is through the social- and emergency-services systems, with individuals moving between these various institutions multiple times per day. This "institutional cycle" is vital because the EMS system is the physical, connective link between these institutions. They are often the gatekeepers who decide whether a patient can walk ("ambulate") well enough to be funneled back into the shelter via transport provided by the homeless outreach workers or the Chapman Police Department. Similarly, Private Ambulance provides a means for accessing the emergency department at the Mather Hospital.

The second cycle is a spatial one. As individuals who are labeled as "37-Deltas" move through the institutional cycle, they navigate several different neighborhoods (sometimes on foot, sometimes as passengers in an ambulance or one of the vehicles used by homeless outreach workers) that intersect at Midtown Plaza. The Plaza is, therefore, an inflection point between the two major institutions that serve individuals who are "37-Deltas": the "wet shelter" and the Mather Hospital. This spatial cycle is essential not only because of the real consequences it has for EMS work in Chapman but also because it illustrates the importance of thinking about how inter-neighborhood institutions link neighborhoods together in cities (Sampson 2012). These linkages have not been traditional foci in the neighborhood-effects literature, but the spatial cycle described here illustrates the importance of these on the daily reality of EMS work in Chapman.

These cycles represent not just the daily patterns of usage occurring in particular spaces; they also represent connections between different facets of the social safety net: shelters, harm-reduction programs, and medical centers. At the same time, they intersect with connections between deleterious institutions, like liquor stores and pharmacies, where individuals can purchase liquor and substitutes for alcohol, and public plazas, where they can spend time. This diverse, tangled web of institutions is itself a by-product of deinstitutionalization. They provide the treatment and housing services that, in an earlier era, would have been made through a state hospital. Even the Plaza and the liquor stores have a role, providing a substitute for missing day programs and a coping mechanism for managing the reality of living on the street. They also do so in an incomplete way, a victim of the unfulfilled promises of providing care in the community. The incomplete linkages between these institutions create gaps for patients to fall through, and they have consequences for EMS providers.

The Consequences of Midtown's Stigma

Analyses of the qualitative data collected during the EMS shift observations and semi-structured interview phases of data collection identified two broad consequences of the overwhelming focus on Midtown that providers describe. The first, the practice of "informal exclusion" is an expansion of the role of other first responders (i.e., the police) in "moving" and "pushing" the homeless into certain areas of cities (Stuart 2014, 2016). In Chapman, the EMS system participates actively in this process of managing homelessness in Midtown. The second consequence is what providers call "getting burned," misattributing or writing off signs and symptoms of a real illness as the consequences of homelessness or substance use. This section describes both consequences, beginning with the EMS system's role in enforcing exclusionary policies to limit homeless individuals' activities in Midtown Plaza.

Informal Exclusion

The first consequence of note is a shift in EMS providers' role from treating medical issues toward managing the use of space.[4] Midtown Plaza is an example of a prime space that is primarily occupied and utilized by "mainstream society" (Stuart 2014, 2016). The bulk of the literature on prime spaces and the geography of homelessness has focused on the role police play in "rabble management" (Stuart 2014), yet in Chapman, the EMS providers play an essential role in this process as well.

> Noah: [Main Street], [Midtown Plaza], mostly where the homeless are, people are homeless if they're sleeping on a bench, they're sleeping in

> day camps. They usually call us to come move them or take them if they can't walk. If they're too intoxicated, we take them to the hospital. If they can walk, they walk away and we move them to another area. Or if they want to go to a shelter, we'll get them transportation to a shelter.

This quote summarizes the patient disposition options available to providers earlier, but vitally highlights the role EMS providers play moving certain people along—interactions with the homeless often including admonishing individuals for spending time in Midtown or other prime spaces. For example, the interactions over multiple calls described with "Henrietta" in Chapter 5, included a police officer's comment that the patient could have alcohol anywhere but in Midtown. One potential side effect is that this advice incentivizes patients to seek other "marginal spaces" to drink, sleep, or pass the time (Stuart 2014, 2016).

Providers' approaches could be more confrontational. One night, Medic 11 was dispatched for the report of a "man down" in Midtown. As we arrived on-scene, a Chapman Fire Department engine company and a Chapman police officer were both on-scene with the patient. The patient was in a fifty-foot stretch of sidewalk near a transit station and some bus shelters. Numerous people walked past on the sidewalk, staring at the patient and us. It was dark out, but the lights from the street and nearby businesses lit up the scene. Empty liquor bottles and bottles of hand sanitizer lay discarded nearby.

The engine company's members told us that the patient had not been cooperative. Dave talked to the patient, "Rhonda," and explained he was concerned about her because the caller stated that she had been losing consciousness. Rhonda became frustrated with the providers and eventually tried to walk away as she insisted that she was fine and just hungry. They asked why, and she explained she had not eaten that day. Her real frustration was that the wet shelter staff had banned her from the facility. Moreover, she told the providers that the police kept some of her property after being arrested on outstanding warrants earlier in the week. The CPD officers confirmed the arrest and indicated that they recognized her.

Another CPD officer arrived. She told us that the patient has a history of substance use, called her a "junkie," and said that Rhonda must wait until Monday to get her property back. However, the officer did call down to the shelter and confirm that the patient could stay there in theory. It was a theoretical issue because the shelter was already full for the night. Dave told the patient she could stay in Midtown because "it's not safe for you here." Dave stated that he "would feel better if you went to [the shelter] or to the hospital," though the shelter was not an option, and the patient refused to go to the hospital.

Dave was becoming more frustrated and warned the patient, "If we come back for you again you won't have a choice" about going to the hospital. Rhonda was agitated now, too, insisting that her problem was that she had not had enough to eat and did not need to go to the hospital. Jeffrey told her, "We can't tie up trucks for this." He meant that ambulances had other, more essential calls to attend to and they could not be distracted with this sort of discussion with patients. As Jeffrey explained this to the patient, Dave obtained an "against medical advice" ("AMA") signature from her, noting that she was refusing transport to the hospital. With the signature in hand, we packed up and left the scene.

A short while later, after driving north into the Old Quarter to take care of an errand involving a patient recently receiving routine care from Private Ambulance, we were again called back to Midtown by dispatchers. Again, the call was for the same "man down" description and in the same area as the prior call. Both providers reacted immediately with frustration, assuming that this was the same patient as before. They reiterated their insistence that she would be transported to the hospital this time. We arrived on-scene at the same place where we left Rhonda beforehand. This time, the officers stood across the street and did not respond with us to talk to the patient. Dave and Jeffrey both got out of the ambulance and immediately insisted that Rhonda come with them. They told her that someone saw her passed out again; Rhonda insisted that she was sleeping. She asked where she was supposed to sleep, and Dave responded, "Somewhere where people won't call 9-1-1." She asked where such a place was, and Dave said, "I don't know, I don't have that answer for you, you gotta be responsible for that."

The back and forth continued, with Dave telling Rhonda she had to go to the hospital. They got the cot out and picked the patient up and placed her on it. The patient protested loudly, but they placed her in the ambulance over her cries. Rhonda insisted that she did not know where to sleep as we drove to the hospital. Dave responded just as insistently that the patient couldn't sleep in Midtown because people would see her and call 9-1-1. Once we arrived in the emergency department, Dave communicated to the hospital staff that they had seen the patient twice that evening and that people had kept calling, telling 9-1-1 the patient was passed out on the sidewalk. The patient continued her strident protests that she was just sleeping, and the hospital staff admonished her, telling her that "college is back in session now and we can't have people sleeping out [in Midtown]."

This story is but one example of providers mentioning to patients that their behavior was "not allowed" in Midtown. Enforcement of this informal prohibition on certain behaviors is first attempted by threatening patients, sometimes with protective custody by the police or sometimes with transport to the hospital, as in the previous example. Providers will often remind patients that they cannot be in a particular area. In both previous examples, patients asked where they could go, and providers did not provide a clear answer. The response in these cases and others was along the lines of, "I don't know where you should go, but I know it's not there." In the example involving Rhonda, the paramedic invoked the notion of personal responsibility, adding that it was up to the patient to find a suitable location to spend time out on the street. However, these interactions occurred elsewhere, though with far less frequency than what providers engaged in near Midtown.

Getting Burned

For providers, "moving [patients] along" presents a risk. If a patient is not malingering but instead has a medical need, but that need goes ignored, there is a risk of an adverse health outcome. First and foremost, this is a risk for patients. It also opens providers to both immediate risk at work and longer-term legal risk. Each interaction for providers, then, results in a decision-making process for the providers about the appropriateness of the chosen disposition. In the example from the previous section, the paramedics had the patient sign an AMA form after their first contact with the patient. The form advises the patient about the risks of not being seen at an emergency department and is meant to provide legal coverage to the providers.

Making the wrong decision can result, as providers call it, in "getting burned." One provider, James, recounted an experience of getting burned from several years before the interview:

> JAMES: [We] got called to [Midtown Plaza] one of the ATMs, for the seizure. And, um, walked in and there was a male who looked like your typical homeless man, ya know person, kind of raggedy clothes, he smelt bad, um, unshaven, just didn't look like a guy who took care of himself. He was laying in the ATM. And I was like kind of like yeah "get up," I assumed he was drunk, just passed out in the ATM. And I'm trying to drag him out, he could barely walk. And I'm like "come on, come on." Get him in the ambulance, drive him to the hospital. Get his name, the whole time in the back he kept holding his head "I don't feel good, I don't feel good." I just wrote him off as a drunk. Got to the hospital, gave a shitty report: drunk guy in [Midtown Plaza]. Came to find out he was in renal failure and hypotensive and he went to the ICU. So ever since then, well I left [Private Ambulance], I took a break. Um so every time now, when I go to [Midtown Plaza] and I go "this is bullshit," I'll take the time to do my job, so just to make sure they're not really sick.

This experience, in which James assumed that a patient with low blood pressure and kidney failure was "your typical homeless man," represents a cautionary tale for many providers. James connected the experience of getting burned to the larger associations providers make between patients with substance-use disorders and homeless patients. He also noted the ease with which providers label the symptoms of patients originating from Midtown Plaza as "bullshit." In particular, he noted how easy it was to pass symptoms off as patients "just being drunk" when they had more complex medical issues:

CP: And what's it like when you show up and you do know the patient?

JAMES: Um, you . . . when you get there and I see him I just go oh it's so-and-so I'm not too worried about it. Ya know unless they do have a specific complaint, like short of breath. Ya know I'll take the time and really, ya know, really assess them fully to make sure I don't get burned and miss something.

CP: What does getting burned entail?

JAMES: Say you're picking up the same person three times a day, almost every day, and they could say "you know I'm short of breath" but they're talking, ya know speaking to you in full sentences and showing every sign that they're not short of breath, but the day they are short of breath you're fed up, mostly because they start to wear on you. Or you're kind of like "yeah yeah come on to the hospital," and you just kind of sit in the back and ignore them, cause they're being themselves, but they can actually be having a medical problem and you miss it when you bring them to the hospital. You pass it off "yeah it's the same thing he's been drinking" and then the hospital will do a full assessment and find something wrong, like he was having a heart attack or something.

James singles out the experience of treating "frequent flier" patients, particularly those who have a reputation among EMS providers for exaggerating symptoms, as a particularly risky group for "getting burned." This provider also notes the frustration that providers struggle with when dealing with "frequent flier" patients by describing these interactions as ones that "start to wear on you."

Other providers recognized the risk "frequent flier" patients posed to providers' decision-making. In particular, for these patients, there is a sense that they are like "the boy that cried wolf," as one provider put it:

HARRISON: The boy that cried wolf thing fits into this hugely because we get sent to the chest pain at [University Plaza] so many times, and you get there and it's the same guy who knows that if he says he's having chest pains, he's going to the hospital, no questions asked. So you get

> this kind of mentality in your head that it's a poison that you can't let it get in your head, but you're like oh here we go again, just another drunk.

Misdiagnosis is, of course, a risk in any medical interaction. However, for providers who treat the same patients over and over again for issues providers characterize as "bullshit," "crying wolf," "abuse," or manipulation, it can be challenging to maintain focus on the reality that each interaction could be the result of a severe medical issue. One provider described this difficulty:

> DREW: It's very hard sometimes to, like, maintain a level of attitude with them. You don't want to get complacent in dealing with them because 9 [times] out of 10, they are just drunk. But that 1 out of 10 [times, they] could have a real medical emergency. But because [of] those other 9, like the boy who cried wolf . . . they were just drunk those nine times you can, it's hard to fight the urge to just say, ah here you go again it's another drunk, let's just transport him. He could actually have a real medical problem.

Therefore, getting burned is a particular risk with these patients because providers become inured to them over time. When combined with the stigmas providers associate with substance use and homelessness and the overarching assumptions providers make about patients in Midtown, the tendency to make assumptions about patients can be especially dangerous.

Such assumptions can result in delays in care, as in the example from James at the beginning of this section, or unnecessary interventions. During the field observations, the crew I was with one night was asked by the Mather Hospital emergency department staff to stabilize a patient brought in by another Private Ambulance crew. The patient was a "frequent flier" who regularly spent time in Midtown according to the providers I was with and had diabetes complications. The ambulance crew who initially treated the patient had assumed the patient had just been drunk and had not investigated the individual's altered level of consciousness further. The result was several interventions by ED staff that would have otherwise been unnecessary had the low blood sugar been identified sooner. Adverse health outcomes such as this are the ultimate consequence of "getting burned."

Stigmatized Place in EMS Work

Midtown represents the collision of two significant forces in EMS work, the spatial regimes that locate interdependent work routines in cities and the cul-

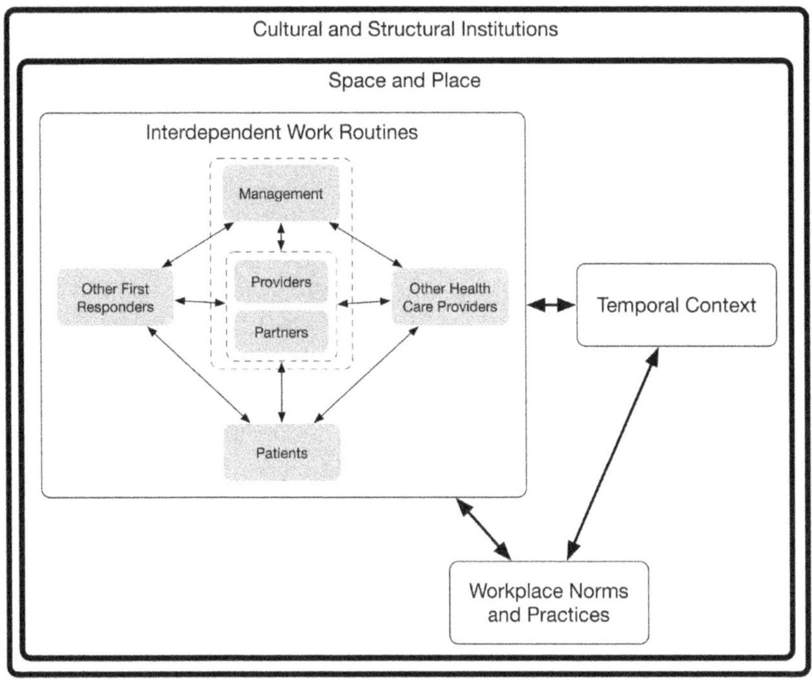

Figure 17. Evolving Theoretical Model—Highlighting Space and Place as well as Cultural and Structural Institutions (graph by author)

tural and structural institutions that shape the way EMS providers think about their jobs (see Figure 17). These represent the outer layers of the EMS work model we have developed over the preceding chapters. When providers respond to calls in Midtown and engage in the fundamental tasks associated with their work routines, they do so with a wealth of prior experience but little concrete knowledge about what they will find when they arrive on-scene. Small bits of information, like the patient's reported age, gender, location, and dispatch information, all become salient details despite their vagaries. Providers' responses to these patients build on how they think about "grunt work," their sense of Midtown's geography, and the cast of patients who make up their mental rosters of "frequent fliers."

These preconceived frames for viewing Midtown are more durable than elsewhere in the city. Midtown occupies an outsized place in providers' consciousness about their work. Midtown also provides a concrete example of how individuals develop stigmatized frames about particular places in their orbit. As in Midtown, it is the marriage of stigmatized social conditions with the belief, correctly or otherwise, that these social conditions are present in exceptionally high numbers in a given place. As the quote at the beginning of this chapter captures, providers start from an assumption of bullshit until proven otherwise: "The call in [Midtown] is going to be bullshit obviously."

Midtown also captures the consequences of these frames for patients who come into the EMS system. Like police, EMS providers in Midtown take an active role in managing space and enforcing informal exclusion by moving patients along. The assumption of preexisting bullshit puts providers at risk of "getting burned" if they misdiagnose or fail to take a patient's concerns seriously. However, these can be sick patients with "legitimate" medical needs, several providers conceded. "Getting burned" entails a mistake whereby providers misattribute a patient's symptoms as the consequences of substance use when they reflect a different medical issue, such as low blood sugar. Therefore, these dominant assumptions put providers' careers and patients' safety at risk if providers become inured to the constant exposure they have to specific "frequent flier" patients.

Conclusion

Beyond both institutional and occupational marginality, EMS work in Chapman revolves around working with marginalized patients. This overlap with marginalized communities represents the third form of marginality that defines urban pre-hospital medicine. "Grunt work" comes in many varieties, including treating patients with long-term consequences from chronic illnesses. These can include chronic physical diseases like diabetes and chronic mental and behavioral illnesses, including substance use. It also encompasses responses that are primarily driven by social conditions, like extreme poverty. I want to be careful not to medicalize homelessness. However, providers at Private Ambulance will be quick to point to the various comorbidities they treat and the potential mental-health consequences of living on the street and injuries like frostbite. Those issues aside, providers regularly interact with patients whose social circumstances, and not their health status, are the pretext for them interacting with the EMS system. These calls form the crux of "grunt work."

Nowhere is this work more present in Chapman than in Midtown, where providers regularly respond during shifts to treat patients with some form of housing instability. Very often, they also have been using alcohol or other substances. In Midtown, Private Ambulance providers are stuck in a cycle of patients who are between shelters, public spaces like Midtown Plaza, and the hospital. Often, the ambulance crews themselves provide the connective tissue between the shelter or plaza and the hospital itself. They may see the same patient multiple times during a shift or see them in the hospital and then again later on the street near Midtown. These "frequent fliers," as providers know them, become a defining feature of how providers view their work. Their very presence is a symptom of another marginality, the failure to address the consequences of deinstitutionalization and create adequate options for offering housing, health care, and social services to individuals who experience housing instability as well as mental and behavioral illnesses.

The focus I place on Midtown represents a unique look at the spatial aspects of EMS work, including both *where* it is located and *how* providers view these spaces. There has been some acknowledgment of EMS work in underprivileged neighborhoods and an acknowledgment that EMS work often entails work with vulnerable patients. However, the ways in which providers simultaneously construct their work and locate that work in particular neighborhoods have not been explored in the social-science research on EMS. Moreover, studying the social construction of neighborhood stigma itself is still a field in its infancy. These chapters therefore speak to pressing issues both inside and outside the ambulance.

Providers' emphasis on Midtown is part mirage, a spatial version of the classic "clinician's illusion." It is so jarring for providers because it represents a distinct departure from how they view their work. As I argue in Part I, it is "real emergencies" that captivate them. They train extensively for these calls. Patients who have consumed too much alcohol but remain conscious or are experiencing symptoms of mental illness do not fit into providers' views of these "real emergencies." Even though working with patients who do not have "real emergencies" is most of what providers do, their concept of EMS work is sharply discordant from this reality. Addressing this gap is the subject of the concluding chapter.

Marginality, Stigma, and the Future of Pre-Hospital Medicine

"Let's try this again." (Thomas)

The Last Call

Late one night, the dispatcher at Private Ambulance sent Medic 6 to a report of "trouble breathing" in North Chapman. The crew had been trying to return to Private Ambulance's headquarters, but calls had prevented them from doing so. Thomas needed the GPS unit in the ambulance to find the address, following its instructions as he drove toward the call location. While Thomas drove, Amanda worked on her paperwork from the previous call, a vent transfer. When we arrived on-location, an engine company from the Chapman Fire Department was already there. Thomas parked behind them and checked out the gravel path that led back to the home, which sat back from the street behind another structure. Thomas told Amanda he did not think we could get the cot back there, so they stacked the cardiac monitor and equipment on the stair chair and walked back along the dark driveway to a door, where firefighters met us.

One of the fire department's EMTs was in the back of the house with the patient, an older man named "Rodger." The rear room was dark, cramped, and impossibly messy. The firefighters got to work moving furniture around so Thomas and Amanda could maneuver the stair chair through the house. This was a challenging task, as the rooms were cramped, and Amanda and Thomas would have to move the patient through the small living room that separated the front door from the room where the patient was. The living room was next to a small kitchen, where the sink and counters were piled high with dirty dishes.

Rodger had cancer, Thomas told me, and was having trouble breathing. His primary-care provider had instructed him to go to the hospital, and Amanda started to help move him to the stair chair as she asked him questions about his condition. Once they loaded Rodger onto the stair chair, Thomas and Amanda worked together to move the patient back out toward the ambulance. Outside, the headlights on cars illuminated the street as they lined up behind the ambulance, unable to pass it on the narrow North Chapman street. They waited as Thomas and Amanda loaded Rodger into the ambulance. Inside the patient compartment, Thomas connected the patient to the cardiac monitor and learned more about the patient's medical history as we made an uneventful drive into Chapman to the hospital the patient had requested. After we were given a room by a nurse and had dropped Rodger off, we remade the cot and transferred the cardiac monitor data to the laptop. When the data transfer finished, Thomas looked at Amanda and me and said, "Let's try this again." It was time to make another attempt to return to headquarters for the night.

Context and Contradiction in EMS Work

Taking "Rodger" to the hospital was an uneventful call at the end of a long day for Thomas and Amanda. Together on Medic 6, they had attended multiple ALS interfacility transfers, including a vent transfer, and multiple calls in public housing complexes. Their calls included falls in a sober living home and an assisted living center, a cyclist injured after falling off his bike, a call for a patient who was homeless and having seizures in Midtown Plaza, and a person choking in an Old Quarter restaurant. Thomas, speaking in his typically understated manner, looked at me after the call at the sober living home and remarked dryly that this "hasn't been a [typical weekend shift]." These calls ranged across the spectrum of work that EMTs and paramedics at Private Ambulance engage in regularly. Several calls were on the more severe end of the spectrum of patients. These included the patient who was seizing and the call for the man choking, though fortunately, the man's airway was partially clear by the time we arrived. At the other end of the spectrum, the calls for falls were not serious whatsoever.

What was notable about this shift, aside from how busy it was for a Sunday, was the calls that originated in systemic failures in how we care for our neighbors in the United States. Both falls occurred at facilities with professional staff, but in neither facility could they provide first aid. The fall at the assisted living facility was not even a fall. The patient slipped out of a chair and just needed Amanda and Thomas to lift him back into it. Since the staff could not lift the patient back into the chair under the facility's rules, they called 9-1-1. The calls

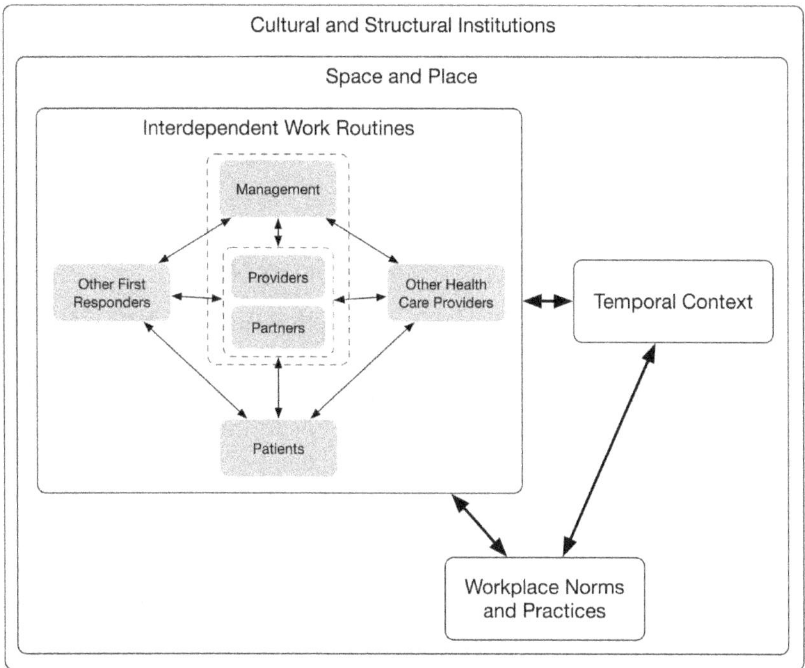

Figure 18. Full Theoretical Model (graph by author)

in public housing, the call for seizures in Midtown, and our nighttime trip with Rodger all took place for people living on the lower end of the socioeconomic spectrum. Not all were living in extreme poverty, but all were living with some form of precarity. While providers frame these calls as "bullshit" and focus on a patient's behavior, the calls also reflect structural failures well beyond any patient's control.

Providers wrestle with this precarity daily. Each shift is an exercise in navigating the theoretical model this book develops (see Figure 18). The providers work with each other, with firefighters on-scene, and with patients, all of which involve emotional labor that speaks to EMS work's interactive nature. The desire for downtime and the unrelenting pace of their shift speak not just to the norms of a weekend shift but also the temporal context of their work. Then there are the daily struggles EMS providers wage against larger structural forces. These reveal the connectedness (or lack thereof) of EMS to the health-care system and the broader ways in which space, place, and social institutions affect the experience of treating Rodger's trouble breathing that night. The experience of Thomas and Amanda throughout their weekend shift highlights two other critical facets of EMS work. First and foremost, the EMS system's role is split between a formal mandate to provide critical care and a practical mandate to fill gaps within the social safety net. This role means that providers spend a significant portion of their shifts connecting individuals and health-care institutions, emphasizing not just *where* EMS work takes place but how EMS providers serve as an *inter-neighborhood institution*.

Institutional Context: EMS and the Social Safety Net

There are two dominant approaches to conceptualizing the social safety net. Both emphasize the role particular institutions play in sustaining the lives of the most marginalized individuals. One is to focus on programs and institutions providing social benefits. These are the core institutions of the modern welfare state, though countries have privatized many of these programs under neoliberalism. In America, these institutions include programs like Temporary Assistance for Needy Families (TANF; "welfare") that provide cash benefits to families. They also include programs like Supplemental Nutrition Assistance Program (SNAP; "food stamps") and Special Supplemental Nutrition Program for Women, Infants, and Children (WIC), which subsidize families' grocery budgets.

Focusing on health-care institutions serving individuals living in or near poverty has been an alternative way of conceptualizing social safety nets. These can be insurance programs, including Medicaid in the United States, whose primary eligibility requirements revolve around a relationship to the federal poverty line. There are also "safety-net hospitals" that provide a disproportionate amount of care to patients who are in some way marginalized. While there is substantial agreement on the broad terrain of this definition, which originates from an Institute of Medicine report in 2000, there is little consensus on the specific way to operationalize what it means to be a safety-net hospital. Historically, these may have been public hospitals. However, they also encompass private institutions that treat many individuals living in poverty by either mission or location.

Despite its importance, we have continually whittled away at the social safety net. As I have argued elsewhere, much of that has come under the guise of neoliberal economic policies of austerity and privatization. Deinstitutionalizing, another force I describe, occurs alongside these broader shifts. The EMS system originated in a period of significant transition for American health care. General practitioners were moving away from house calls, extensive in-patient facilities for treating mental and behavioral health were being closed in favor of treatment in the community, and public services became privatized. Shifts away from house calls and deinstitutionalizing were necessary in many respects, which is crucial in this discussion. However, the promises of community treatment and the private market offering sufficient opportunities for care went unfulfilled in many cases. This failure to replace aging and inadequate institutions with new ones up to the task is the crucial point of failure.

The consequences of the dual forces of deinstitutionalization and privatization have meant that patients' opportunity structures for seeking care are now constrained. What is left of the social safety net can be difficult to navigate. Calling 9-1-1 becomes a catch-all way to access care without wrestling initially with the modern American health-care system's complexities. The EMS system's openness and accessibility are also its undoing. While EMS providers can respond in minutes to a patient in need, they often lack the tools to address the non- and sub-acute illnesses prompting the call in the first place. EMTs and paramedics are not a facsimile of the general practitioner, nor are they trained as social workers. Therefore, patients cycle through the EMS system and emergency departments without having their underlying conditions addressed and resolved. Providers' frustration with "bullshit calls" and "grunt work," discussed throughout Parts I and III of this book, captures their orientation toward the reality of working in a safety-net institution. It speaks to the EMS system's continued role as "street-level social workers" and the EMS community's fractured divide over this work.

Spatial Context: EMS as an Inter-Neighborhood Institution

These struggles with patients speak to a second fundamental misunderstanding of first-responder work. For a time, in the middle of the twentieth century, an urban myth of sorts developed about emergency services' availability in American cities. It was not a full myth. Like New York, many American cities struggled under the weight of decreased revenues after recessions during the 1970s. Cutting first-responder services was one easy way to decrease costs, and the language of austerity drove significant structural changes to police, fire, and nascent EMS services. These cuts are a piece of what some refer to as the "retreat of the state" during this period (Wacquant 2009). Austerity also drove deterioration in public housing, where maintenance budgets meant lights, elevators, and even doors broke and went unfixed (Venkatesh 2009).

Residents in public housing and elsewhere complained that 9-1-1 calls went unanswered, and undoubtedly intentionally dropped calls occurred to some extent. Computer-aided dispatch systems and other elements of the "digital panopticon" discussed in this book ensure that calls cannot be ignored or dropped by services. Of course, these innovations do not mean that EMS response times are always appropriate or systems do not struggle to provide adequate services. It does, however, illustrate that the first responder never entirely retreated from urban neighborhoods. Indeed, the EMS system was and is the thread that ties together different neighborhoods, particularly for individuals living on American society's margins. EMS work occurs in every neighborhood of the city of Chapman, but calls occur in some places with far more frequency than others.

Thus, while the EMS system theoretically connects every neighborhood to a set of health-care institutions (namely, emergency departments), certain areas of the city have particularly strong connections between place and the EMS system. Moreover, Midtown's case illustrates how other inter-neighborhood institutions, particularly the social and health-care agencies that serve homeless individuals and those with substance-use issues, shape the EMS system. It is not just that Midtown, and Midtown Plaza in particular, represent concentrations of "37-Deltas" who are "frequent fliers" in the eyes of EMS providers. Midtown is the inflection point between these various services. Place effects in EMS work, therefore, illustrate the importance of thinking beyond neighborhood borders.

For social scientists and public-health researchers, questions about neighborhood effects on health have been at the forefront since the 1920s (Sampson 2012). A fundamental debate is whether neighborhoods with social problems or poor health have these because they comprise people living in poverty, for example, or because of something independent of the individuals living there (Oakes 2004). EMS and other inter-neighborhood institutions are not endogenous aspects of neighborhoods, however they may be operationalized. EMS's spatial organization is a product of both the spatial heterogeneity of communities and the connections across and between neighborhoods. Chapman's EMS responses reflect these connections and aspects of individual neighborhoods, making the EMS system (and other inter-neighborhood institutions) a useful barometer for the spatial organization of urban social problems. In the case of EMS work in Chapman, the system, therefore, reflects the spatial organization of extreme poverty (in the form of homelessness) and the spatial contours of other social problems such as heroin and alcohol abuse.

However, the EMS system also has a hand in responding to and treating these social problems. Providers' responses to these problems and the patients that have them may, therefore, reify not only the problems themselves, but particular neighborhoods as "marked" spaces. Thus their ability to "move patients along" by enforcing informal spatial exclusion may help shift a neighborhood's reputation. Likewise, the failure to respond adequately to patients (what providers term "getting burned") may only seek to entrench further the perception of a neighborhood as a "sick" community if those patients return there after their release from the hospital. Thus, by focusing on inter-neighborhood institutions, it becomes possible to understand both the spatial occurrence of social problems and the varying degrees to which institutions respond to these phenomena.

What is interesting about this duality—where the EMS system both reflects and shapes the social problems endemic in Chapman—is that it further complicates the notion that the state has "retreated" from the most marginalized communities in cities (Wacquant 2016). On the one hand, the regularly repeated involvement of these communities with the EMS system challenges the idea of the retreat of the state (Squires and Lea 2012). On the other, the privatization of EMS services speaks to the very neoliberal conditions that are part and parcel of the broader retreat of state institutions that scholars like Loïc Wacquant refer to when discussing retreat.

Such a retreat refers not just to a literal decline in services but also to the state's lack of involvement in providing these services. It also speaks to the profound need to take space seriously. Spatial context is not just a question for urban sociology; instead, it is something whose influence cuts across the plethora of research interests that make up sociology (Fuller and Löw 2017; Logan 2012). Despite sensitivity to space in some quarters, specific subfields of sociology, including the sociology of work, often fail to situate their research sites within their broader sociospatial context. In particular, there are trends within firms to work remotely or in reconceptualized office spaces meant to foster creativity. Collectively, firms also seek to locate themselves in "innovation centers" (Storper 2013). They may do so for many reasons, but the desire to locate in Silicon Valley, Boston's Route 128 corridor, or downtown Manhattan has implications for their employees' relationships with firms and work itself. Greater attention to how spatial context shapes work, not just social and health services' work in cities, is necessary.

The Social Production of Stigma

Space is not the only contextual factor that the emergent theory I present here contains. The social context within which care unfolds is also essential to understanding the EMS system. We frame ambulance work in the United States as a part of the acute-care system. However, providers in Chapman and elsewhere routinely respond to what is perhaps better described as "everyday health crises" (Prener and Lincoln 2015). Providers' frustrations with these calls result from what I characterized as "intersectional stigmas" involving negative opinions about a range of social and medical problems, including mental illness, substance use and abuse, and homelessness. These frustrations are essential in their own right, since provider frustrations can impact the quality of care delivered (Glisson and Hemmelgarn 1998; Glisson and Durick 1988). However, they are also vital because they provide a mediating link between place and individual-level health outcomes that explain how the EMS system affects patients.

Shared Perceptions and Occupational Community

I have described three sets of perceptions that are held by providers: (1) perceptions about the work that they do; (2) perceptions about the people they work with; and (3) perceptions about where that work takes place. The data presented throughout this book suggest that Private Ambulance's emergency medical technicians and paramedics share these perceptions widely. We cannot explain these perceptions away as products of prior experience. Many of the Private Ambulance providers who participated in this study had not worked elsewhere and had not been exposed to Chapman for any significant period before beginning their employment. These perceptions, then, are generated by providers' on-the-job experiences and their interactions with colleagues.

In Chapter 5, the discussion of socializing and community centered on the spatial constraints on these activities. Despite the spatially diffuse nature of downtime and the physical constraints that come from limited access to parking in "frontstage" areas of the city, providers build a network of relationships with their coworkers. They develop these networks through both chance encounters and planned meetings during shifts, and the use of smartphones for staying connected when meeting up is not possible. However, these interactions are not purely social, since they serve to transmit and reinforce knowledge about downtime, such as the example from Chapter 5, when public bathrooms' quality was the subject of lengthy discussion. Providers also discuss emergency calls during downtime, updating each other on the "frequent fliers" they have recently seen and patients they have recently treated.

The transmission and reinforcement of knowledge through war stories is part of the broader occupational community among EMS providers at Private Ambulance. At their core, occupational communities describe how shared norms, practices, and standards become accepted and reinforced among individuals in the same line of work (Van Maanen and Barley 1984). At Private Ambulance, patients' and neighborhoods' perceptions throughout the preceding chapters are not reflections of idiosyncratic beliefs or past experiences. These views are also not idiosyncratic to Private Ambulance as an organization. Instead, they are part of the fabric of EMS work in the United States. The focus of the Institute of Medicine's report on EMS (Institute of Medicine 2007), whose authors focused almost exclusively on critical care and trauma care, is one example of the more extensive orientation of EMS work in the United States. Providers' conceptions of "grunt work" and "appropriate use" are widespread constructs that are not specific to individuals or Private Ambulance. This widespread nature of their perceptions makes Van Maanen and Barley's conception of "occupational communities" (1984) particularly useful for understanding the diffusion of shared perceptions among EMS providers.

Appropriate Use of EMS Services and Institutional Stigma

The contradictions between the EMS system as we conceive it and the reality of urban EMS work are nowhere more apparent than with two groups of patients—the most critical patients and the least. The reality of urban EMS is that another group of patients is the defining clinical population. Providers define these patients at Private Ambulance as "bullshit" calls or as "abusers" of the system. No example illustrates this orientation's occupation-wide nature more than a public information campaign in Lake County, Florida. The county public-health and EMS agencies launched a public information campaign in 2007 that included billboards and a website named "When to Call 9-1-1." Among other things, the website discouraged calling 9-1-1 for "emotional upsets" (no further definition given).

At its core, the divide between so-called critical and bullshit patients is a debate within Private Ambulance and the broader EMS community over what is an appropriate use of this medical service. From a sociological perspective, providers' definitions of appropriate service use (Roth 1972) and patient labels (Brown 1989; Leiderman and Grisso 1985; Shem 2009) are critical aspects of how providers frame their interactions with patients. These preexisting conceptions of what appropriate use is and who embodies that definition of appropriate use may also have broader influences on how providers view their work and the satisfaction they take from that work (Glisson and Hemmelgarn 1998; Glisson and Durick 1988).

As with other health-care providers, appropriate use of EMS services is a social construct where definitions are shared and reinforced through EMS providers' everyday discursive practices. At Private Ambulance, these include downtime conversations with colleagues, seeing known patients in the emergency department while there on an unrelated call or errand, and treating patients they believe to be using the EMS system for "bullshit" reasons. Providers' definitions of "grunt" or "bullshit" work are foundational to their stigmatized views about health and social problems. Chapter 6's discussion of how psychiatric calls and examples like the Lake County public information campaign also point to institutionalized stigmas (Corrigan and Kleinlein 2007; Pescosolido et al. 2008) within the EMS system. These stigmas result in policies, training materials, and protocols that reinforce ideas about particular patients' validity and calls.

There have been theoretical attempts to link the varying levels at which stigma may operate. Within the context of Private Ambulance, stigmatized views at the providers' level are reinforced by and reinforce the agency's broader orientation. We can think of these connections as the "Treatment System," which links labels to individual responses to various system-level factors such as treatment modalities and institutional policies. In the case of Chapman, "37-Deltas" and "frequent fliers" generate responses from providers that are a part of an institutional context where a set of mental, behavioral, and social issues are generally stigmatized. As providers interact with individuals repeatedly, we can see the role that stigma plays not just in single interactions but in shaping patients' illness careers and life courses.

Spatializing Stigma

It is critical to recognize, however, that while stigmas toward mental illness, substance use, and homelessness shape individuals' experiences with institutions, so do stigmas of place. These stigmas of illnesses and social issues become intrinsically associated with particular neighborhoods (in the case of Chapman, it is Midtown). The connection to place provides empirical evidence for the phenomenon of neighborhood stigma, something that Besbris and colleagues (Besbris et al. 2015) have only recently established as an empirical phenomenon separate from previous work that theorized the existence of spatial stigmas. My findings suggest that one way in which neighborhood stigmas may be produced is from the explicit spatialization and aggregation of individual traits. On a micro level, Bourgois and Schonberg (2009) described a small group of homeless men living in San Francisco as a "community of addicted bodies." In Chapman, EMS providers treat Midtown as a neighborhood of homeless, addicted, and stigmatized bodies, applying the stigmas described here and by Bourgois and Schonberg (2009) to an entire neighborhood. Providers' responses to the neighborhood's physical condition reinforced their perceptions about patients; as one provider described it, Midtown and its patients were just "dirty."

Neighborhood perceptions, then, may reflect both aggregated individual characteristics and perceptions of the broader physical state of the community. These two groups of traits and responses by EMS providers (or civic-service providers more generally) result in the marking and labeling of neighborhoods as "bad," "dirty," "dangerous," and so on. By articulating the roots of neighborhood stigma in this way, we can make explicit parallels between the sociological literature on mental illness and stigma and the concept of neighborhood stigma. Indeed, by swapping the "treatment system" for "civic institutions," we can expand existing models of stigma for theorizing and framing how neighborhood stigmas are constructed and responded to by inter-neighborhood institutions. Many of the constituent characteristics of both the individual and the community that such models describe, the social-psychological context and social characteristics of individuals and media and national contexts of the community, could readily be applied to neighborhood questions of stigma.

For EMS providers in Chapman, the existence of spatial stigma is the critical connection between place and individual health outcomes. These sorts of connections are part of a broader need to seek out mechanisms that can connect individuals to place in ways that produce disparate health outcomes. At Private Ambulance, providers' stigmatized orientations to particular illnesses and patients are explicitly situated within neighborhoods. These are views that do not exist in a vacuum but are part of a larger institutional orientation toward the issues of substance use, mental illness, and homelessness. Providers' assumptions about Midtown and the types of calls frame their responses from the moment of dispatch onward, and these frames have consequences for their treatment of patients. Stigma, then, is the driving force behind how the EMS system mediates between place and individual health outcomes for patients in Chapman.

Making Space for Providers: Bridging Occupational and Spatial Marginalities in Urban Pre-Hospital Medicine

For the providers at Private Ambulance, space is not the academic exercise that I lay out in the prior section. Instead, it is something they live and breathe day in and day out. There are conflicts over specific places that emerge, such as the experience of being evicted from Eaton Plaza. There is also the effect that individuals who experience housing instability have on the Midtown neighborhood. Beyond what we can learn from these conflicts, there are ways in which pre-hospital medicine could be reconfigured to work *for* providers rather than against them.

We need to start with the ambulance itself. Ambulance design has remained static for several decades now, built on two-door trucks or van chassis with a patient compartment behind. They are utilitarian vehicles designed with a focus on how to provide care for patients. Such a focus largely ignores how they are used most frequently during shifts. They are not just a platform for providing patient care. Instead, they are an office, kitchen, and bedroom for providers.

Agencies are beginning to discover the challenges this brings. At least two in the United States, the Fire Department of New York (FDNY) and New Orleans EMS, have begun to place alternative designs into service that create the space available to providers in ambulances' cabs (EMS World 2010; Petrillo 2011). Crew-cab designs give providers more space and allow them the simple pleasure of, for example, reclining their seat. Crew cabs also allow for "third riders" to join crews while remaining belted into the cab, facilitating both communication and safety for third riders. Reconfiguring cabs to facilitate better socializing, eating, and sleeping can help make marginalized work conditions more manageable for providers.

Ideally, however, providers have a physical station to visit during shifts. In systems with high call volumes, these stations may exist, but providers may only visit them at the beginning and end of shifts. Increasing staffing levels to reduce the number of calls per shift per ambulance can help address these pressures. Doing so would also provide EMTs and paramedics the space to take scheduled breaks. These are important for the day-to-day of EMS work, increasing retention of providers and developing a more skilled workforce that struggles less with burnout and the mental and physical consequences of busy shifts, day in and day out.

Where stations are not physically and economically possible, an alternative is to formalize what providers at Private Ambulance do informally, which is to identify posts throughout a jurisdiction and reserve parking for at least two ambulances per post. Reserving street parking can make downtime more predictable for providers even if they do not have a physical station to rotate through. By reserving spaces with at least two spots for ambulances, agencies can increase the amount of social interaction between crews and provide more possibilities for managing long shifts out on the road, where finding parking or seeing colleagues is routinized rather than a luxury. Another strategy for agencies like Private Ambulance is to reduce reliance on shifts that stretch to twenty-four hours or longer. Sleep deprivation among health-care providers and first responders is a serious concern (Carey et al. 2011; Patterson et al. 2010; Patterson et al. 2012). It increases the probability of a range of adverse outcomes, including burnout, motor vehicle accidents, clinical errors, and "getting burned" by a patient.

These suggestions largely run counter to the ways jurisdictions in many parts of the United States organize first-responder work. They also chafe against the profit motives often present in for-profit EMS agencies and the very real financial pressures that nonprofit agencies face as well. Many EMS agencies have prioritized so-called lean workforces that contribute to financial stability for organizations in lieu of creating sustainable, long-term career trajectories for providers (Seim 2020). Reversing this trend is essential for addressing the marginalities that providers confront during their shifts.

COVID-19, George Floyd, Daniel Prude, and the Challenges of Pre-Hospital Medicine

At the same time, workforce retention and development within pre-hospital medicine is perhaps more challenging than ever. In early 2020, the United States began to identify cases of individuals infected with a "novel coronavirus," SARS-CoV-2, that causes a disease known as COVID-19. The pandemic that emerged was not the first infectious disease outbreak that providers at Private Ambulance had faced. As I was collecting this book's pilot data in 2009, Private Ambulance prepared for an onslaught of cases of the H1N1 strain of influenza. Public-health officials first identified this novel influenza A virus that spring. Like COVID-19 today, "swine flu" was also declared a pandemic by the World Health Organization, the first such flu epidemic in decades. Private Ambulance stockpiled large amounts of personal protective equipment (PPE) for their providers, much of it going unused. The H1N1 pandemic was severe both in the United States and regionally around Chapman, but public-health officials' worst fears did not materialize.

Likewise, in 2014, another highly infectious disease, Ebola, was identified in the United States. The case was associated with travel to West Africa, where Ebola had circulated with disastrous results in crowded urban areas since December of 2013. Public-health officials identified a total of eleven patients with Ebola in the U.S. during the fall and winter of 2014. These patients had all either traveled to West Africa, often to help treat Ebola patients, or had treated Ebola patients in American hospitals. The fear, thankfully unrealized in 2014, was that Ebola could begin to spread not just through travel and health-care exposures but within American communities. Private Ambulance again stockpiled PPE in preparation for this possibility of community spread. Like Private's experience with H1N1, the equipment went unused, as community spread of Ebola never occurred in the United States.

However, these stockpiles of PPE meant that when COVID-19 cases began to emerge in and around Chapman, Private Ambulance had the equipment to outfit their providers. After public-health officials identified cases locally, Private Ambulance quickly mandated that PPE be used widely in the headquarters and on calls. Gloves were, of course, already a part of the regular PPE providers used on calls. Surgical masks became a part of that same routine, and after a short period, safety glasses did as well. For more high-risk calls, including those that required intubations or patients who had COVID-19, providers would wear the more intensive PPE, including N-95 masks, face shields, and disposable gowns.

Unlike H1N1 and Ebola, these precautions were not theoretical. By the end of 2020, Chapman had seen well over four thousand cases and a hundred deaths. These included large shares of patients who were living in the city's nursing homes. Private Ambulance's EMTs and paramedics found the COVID-19 virus on calls and out in the community, and approximately 15 percent of the workforce at Private Ambulance became infected. The leadership at Private Ambulance quickly moved to incentivize providers to stay home when sick by continuing to pay providers who needed to call out for health reasons for the time they would work. Though leadership worried about some providers abusing this flexibility, their fears proved unfounded. Providers experienced stress about becoming sick, and anxiety within headquarters was high, but they continued to show up for shifts.

The city of Chapman integrated Private Ambulance's operations into a broader response network that spanned the public-health agency, the Mather and Muir hospitals, Chapman's fire and police departments, and other city agencies. This type of collaborative effort was the first of its kind in Chapman. However, many of these agencies had prior histories of close collaboration, including Private Ambulance and Chapman Fire Department's joint response framework described in the Introduction. Private Ambulance saw the intimate planning environment as essential to managing the COVID-19 outbreak in Chapman and keeping residents, first responders, and health-care providers safe and healthy if possible. These collaborative relationships differed from training scenarios, when everything seemed more theoretical, and laid the foundation for not just a successful response to COVID-19 but also to future events.

Like other private EMS agencies, Private Ambulance saw its call volume decline as demand for interfacility transports decreased. However, Private Ambulance's leadership quickly embraced other forms of public-health work, particularly around facilitating testing in Chapman's nursing homes and homeless shelters and pop-up testing in Chapman's neighborhoods. The testing work more than made up for lost work resulting from temporary declines in transports and 9-1-1 calls. Its success enabled Private Ambulance to expand its workforce when other private EMS agencies experienced layoffs and furloughs, during a period where the U.S. economy more broadly experienced significant contractions.

One surprise for Private Ambulance's providers was that the patients living on the street and in shelters in and around Midtown did not become a focal point of the COVID-19 outbreak. The city's recreation center, between Midtown and the Old Quarter, was converted into a temporary COVID-19 shelter for individuals who lacked stable housing. However, few individuals needed to use the shelter because there were no significant outbreaks of COVID-19 among the "37-Deltas" in the city. This low COVID-19 rate occurred despite the risks of living in shelters and high rates of comorbidities that could increase these individuals' risks. No one was sure why infection rates remained low. Perhaps it was time spent outside, or the proactive testing practices coordinated between Private Ambulance and the shelters. What did not change, however, was the frequency of contact between Private Ambulance and these patients. They remained an ever-present source of EMS calls throughout the pandemic.

A long-term challenge for Private Ambulance's continued responses with "37-Deltas" came from the protests that erupted in Minneapolis in late May 2019. After a Minneapolis police officer killed George Floyd by kneeling on his neck, protests began first in Minneapolis and then around the United States. Chapman was no exception. Unlike other cities, however, the protests did not devolve into looting and arson fires after dark, except for a small amount of vandalism one night in the city. The protests, therefore, did not require substantial engagement from Private Ambulance providers. However, the protests generated a small but committed group of "defund the police" activists in Chapman.

A supervisor at Private Ambulance I spoke with worried what defunding the police in Chapman could mean for the coordinated responses between Chapman police and Private Ambulance. As I noted in earlier chapters, CPD officers responded to many calls with Private Ambulance, particularly those involving psychiatric issues and "37-Delta" patients. They also helped transport "37-Delta" patients to shelters. What if, the supervisor wondered, defunding CPD meant that the backup these officers provide Private's crews and the transport they provide for patients who have housing instability went away? These forms of collaboration are critical in the eyes of both Private Ambulance's management and its providers.

We also need to acknowledge that EMS providers can be complicit in this process. For example, in 2021, Colorado restricted the practice of paramedics injecting patients with ketamine to control behavior at the behest of police officers.[1] In other states, EMS providers have been present for deaths of Black men at the hands of police. In one graphic example in Rochester, New York, medics on-scene explained away Daniel Prude's cardiac arrest as "excited delirium."[2] This term has a tortuous history within medicine, and clinicians do not universally agree upon its validity as a medical phenomenon. Nevertheless, as the EMS provider in Rochester did that snowy evening, it is often used to explain

African American men's deaths in police custody. Thus, it represents not just an EMS provider invoking a problematic concept but how EMS providers can reinforce socially constructed knowledge that perpetuates disparities.

At the same time, the testimony of Genevieve Hansen, a Minneapolis EMT and firefighter, was crucial during Derek Chauvin's trial. Hansen approached Chauvin, whom a jury convicted of murder in 2021 for his role in George Floyd's death, as he was restraining Floyd, and tried to intervene. However, another officer on-scene told Hansen that "if you really are a Minneapolis firefighter, you would know better than to get involved."[3] EMS providers are there to be seen and not heard, the officer implies. Understanding how these power relations evolve and how providers benefit from law-enforcement presence is essential for considering the future of pre-hospital medicine in the United States.

Toward the Future: Bridging Social and Institutional Marginalities in Urban Pre-Hospital Medicine

These experiences during the pandemic and the parallel protests over deaths at the hands of police officers suggest that EMS work does not need to continue to unfold in the same ways. For example, Private Ambulance's work during the pandemic is innovative, meaningful, and unique. Unfortunately, facilitating testing has not been a significant part of first-responder work during the COVID-19 outbreak. However, it does suggest that there are paths forward for addressing the various marginalities present in EMS work. The public-health work that Private Ambulance engaged with during the COVID-19 pandemic also illustrates possibilities for making EMS work less marginal. Beyond the changes I have recommended to ambulance configurations, shifts, and stations, we must make three additional changes to how we think about pre-hospital medicine.

Embracing the Job

One essential transition is from thinking about EMS to thinking about Pre-Hospital Health Care (PHHC) systems. Whereas we see EMS now mainly through the lens of critical care, we need to be realistic that the most pressing community health challenges that providers confront are primarily not acute. The solution is not to increase paramedic-initiated refusals, allowing providers to refuse care to patients if deemed inappropriate. These represent a logical next step beyond posting billboards exhorting patients to use 9-1-1 correctly, a development that I see as stigmatizing the most vulnerable members of the communities EMS providers serve.

Instead, we need to reorient EMS to see community health through the lens of pre-hospital medicine as *the job* rather than a distraction. Instead of seeing patient contacts for sub- or non-acute health and social issues as inappropriate, we need to see them as opportunities to connect patients with various resources. This shift means both hospital care if warranted and being able to offer other dispositions to patients. It may mean facilitating a primary-care appointment or connecting patients to mental- or behavioral health services. Perhaps it means ensuring that they know the location of the closest food pantry. Right now, all providers can typically offer is transport to the hospital or advice for patients to follow up with their primary-care provider. The menu of choices needs to change to match patients' needs rather than continuing to believe that we can make patients respect the symbolic boundaries around "real emergencies" that we have created.

For example, in Chapman, Private Ambulance relies on the Chapman Police Department to take individuals to shelters. EMS agencies cannot take patients to any facility other than an emergency department in the United States. Alternative disposition options are a critical piece of transforming EMS into truly pre-hospital medicine. Providers could eliminate the need for law enforcement to interact with individuals who have housing instability in Chapman by merely having the ability to transport individuals to shelters. Implementing such a shift requires careful planning. We cannot only expand the number of destinations to which ambulances can transport patients. Instead, we must also ensure that those transports result in effective interventions for patients.

Giving providers the training and resources needed to do that means elevating our expectations for them. I do not believe this will be an easy transition. Areas of the United States have increasingly found it hard to staff ambulances,[4] a situation that I worry COVID-19 will only exacerbate. In many areas of the U.S., especially rural areas, volunteer EMS providers are still the norm rather than the exception. These volunteers lie at the core of the EMS's amateur past and form a dual labor market alongside career providers. However, a continual struggle is our expectations for what volunteers can do in training and skills. If policymakers see additional training requirements as burdensome, it may make recruitment and retention more challenging.

Resolving these tensions and those between EMS providers and the broader health-care system means increasing expectations for what providers can do clinically and the level of care they can provide. In practical terms, if we want to raise the bar for what we expect from the PHHC system, we need to increase the compensation we provide to EMTs and paramedics. Providing living wages to pre-hospital health-care providers is necessary, but even more so if we are going to increase the clinical expectations. For volunteers, we need to reconsider whether the mid-twentieth-century organizational paradigm can still deliver the clinical care that communities need. There may not be a one-size-fits-all answer, but policymakers should not scale back this clinical evolution because of the limits to what we can ask of volunteers.

An essential corollary here is that we need to change our funding mechanisms for pre-hospital health care. The EMS system is considered an "essential service" in only a minority of states (eleven as of 2021). Not being an "essential service" means that, in most states, providing EMS services is not a statutory requirement for municipalities. Changing this would compel local municipalities to provide funding and ensure the provision of at least some pre-hospital health care. Funding must include so-called readiness costs, the capital and infrastructure needed to be on stand-by, that an essential service designation could cover. Beyond that change, EMS systems need to be allowed to bill insurance for the sub-acute care they provide and receive subsidies from states and the federal government for traditionally uncompensated work. Providers do not just need alternative dispositions, like clinics, but reimbursement for the assessment and treatment of these patients. In short, they need recognition as health-care providers and not clinical-transport services.

Creating New Career Paths

The second major shift needed in pre-hospital medicine is to create paths for upward mobility for providers. For a paramedic with field experience, there are only two current possibilities. One is to a supervisor position, or some other leadership position, within an EMS agency, though there are few of these relative to the number of practicing paramedics. The other is moving on to a more advanced practice setting, which means working with an air ambulance agency for many providers. Creating sustainable career trajectories within EMS means expanding the possibilities of what EMS work itself entails.

One possibility to address this is to institutionalize "community practice paramedicine" (CPP) around the United States, instead of in the ad hoc manner it exists right now (Bigham et al. 2013). CPP programs give additional training to paramedics in managing chronic illnesses. Agencies have used CPP providers in some areas as a means for helping break the cycle of 9-1-1 calls and hospitalizations that a small number of "frequent flier" patients would find themselves in. Instead of a patient being repeatedly transported and hospitalized for diabetic emergencies, for example, a CPP program could give EMS agencies the ability to go out to that patient proactively. Providers could ensure that they monitor their blood sugars, take their medications, and connect them with other social services. Agencies have also experimented with pairing EMS providers with advanced practice nurses to meet the same goals (Sanko et al. 2020).

These programs could be transformational not just for patients but also for providers. They create a means for them to "move up the ladder" and for communities to benefit, but EMS bureaucracies have been slow to adopt them. Private Ambulance, for example, would love to start a CPP program but cannot because of exceptionally high licensing costs and byzantine rules put in place by the state's Office of Emergency Medical Services. We need to incentivize these types of innovation and make them available systematically rather than only providing them in jurisdictions with wealthy and progressive EMS agencies.

We have also not spent time, however, envisioning a similar role for emergency medical technicians. In the few places where agencies have started CPP programs, they leave EMTs out of a similar community-oriented role. Instead, EMTs must become paramedics, develop their critical-care skill sets, and then undergo additional training to develop chronic conditions skills. Given the widespread nature of "grunt work" in Chapman, I believe this is the wrong way to develop providers' skill sets. Rather than treating these skills as a niche, Private Ambulance's providers' experience suggests that they need to be at the core of a revised pre-hospital medical curriculum. Doing so, however, requires significant transformation and change across the entire existing EMS system.

This type of work is not just about creating career paths for providers. It also can transform their work with the most marginalized patients in their jurisdictions. While agencies have typically viewed CPP as a tool for managing chronic illness, COVID-19 and George Floyd suggest other possibilities. Providers do not just need tools for helping patients manage their heart disease and diabetes, and the goal should not just be about reducing the number of EMS calls from "frequent fliers." Instead, providers need tools and options for helping connect patients to mental-health resources, quickly pivoting to address infectious disease outbreaks, and helping address chronic social problems that often bring patients into their orbits. The "defund the police" movement and COVID-19 highlight that our current health-care and first-responder systems, in their current forms, can address only a portion of their communities' needs. A re-envisioned pre-hospital medical system could serve as an alternative for police involvement.

Creating a Pre-Hospital Continuum of Care

The third major necessary shift is to develop system-wide integrations between public-health departments, hospital systems, and PHHC agencies. Currently, providers typically cannot view patients' medical histories, allergies, medications, and diagnoses. As a result, they cannot make informed decisions on the best facility to transport patients with chronic illnesses. Instead, providers rely on patients' preferences or merely take them to the closest facility. Effective pre-hospital medicine requires the same situational awareness that other health-care providers have. This shift is not just about training and labels but also structural changes that fully realize the potential of preventative medicine not just *for* the community but *in* the community. Each patient contact is a possibility to address patients' needs across a full range of issues.

Just as we talk about coordinated care in hospital systems, treating pre-hospital health-care providers as part of a coordinated team that helps disrupt patients' cycles through various institutions in Chapman and elsewhere ultimately benefits everyone. If EMS is to evolve into a full-fledged pre-hospital health-care system, placing it on equal footing and in deliberate dialogue with health-care system partners is essential. The experience of Private Ambulance during COVID-19 illustrates that this coordination is possible if we embrace it as a valuable tool.

Taking on these three shifts will require significant changes to how we talk about, fund, train, and equip EMS providers. After spending time in the field with Private Ambulance providers and then, several years later, watching the COVID-19 pandemic stress the EMS system from my home's confines, I am convinced that we need these changes both for providers and their communities. I am not naive enough to believe these changes will happen overnight, nor will they be roundly embraced within the current EMS community. Many providers remain committed to the idea of emergency medicine as their vocation, many communities remain committed to using volunteers, and many career EMS systems do not have the resources to implement change on their own. There are bright spots in this darkness, however, like the possibilities Private Ambulance has tentatively begun to explore amid a global pandemic.

The Ambulance, the City, and Urban Studies

Like other contemporary investigators of ambulance work, I believe emergency medical services is a proverbial canary in a sea of urban suffering (Seim 2020). If we listen to EMS providers, we can learn much about the state of cities. EMS providers know intimately where individuals who live on the streets camp, where people go to use drugs, and what types of alcohol-based substances people substitute for liquor. They are a jaded bunch, though I take pains to remind readers that their cynicism is born out of the daily grind of "grunt work." Were policymakers and public-health professionals to regularly and meaningfully engage with the street knowledge EMS providers develop, they would find a wealth of deep understanding for how the most marginalized individuals in society live.

The same, I should note, can be said of researchers, beginning with Engels (1984) and Mayhew (1861), who have long sought to peel back the curtains into the alleys, apartments, and dark corners of the urban experience. Since few social scientists (with several notable exceptions) have meaningfully engaged with first responders, including EMS providers, we have missed an opportunity to understand the scope of advanced marginality in the cities. Traveling with EMS providers can provide those of us interested in better understanding the urban experience the opportunity to enter many of the places we could never otherwise see and to visualize how social services, the healthcare system, and the public-safety system work together to both perpetuate the causes and relieve the consequences of structural failures in our society. Like policymakers, social scientists interested in urban life would do well to listen to our cities' EMS providers with far greater frequency.

When we do engage with EMS providers, as I have done here and others have done before me, there is also much we can learn about EMS work itself. Like both Corman (2017) and Seim (2020), I emphasize in Part I that providers have socially constructed strong definitions of what appropriate use of EMS services entails. These "real emergencies" and "bullshit calls" are not just contemporary curiosities, however. Unlike in past work, I tie them to the historical development of EMS work in the United States. I also build on the concepts of "vertical" and "horizontal" relations in EMS work that Seim (2020) introduces, but with an emphasis on how these relations are not static but rather subject to continual negotiation. This negotiation is both practical, because EMS calls are difficult to script, and exhausting, because EMS providers must continually justify their skills and role. The confusion about this role, such as the "ambulance driver" or "taxi driver" tropes, is rooted not just in misunderstandings but in the character of interfacility transfer work, another contribution that prior researchers have not discussed.

Like Perlow (1999) and later on Clawson and Gerstel (2014), I argue in Part II that time is a crucially overlooked component for understanding social life. For EMS providers, their downtime spent at work but not on calls is a crucial facet of managing what otherwise is an unmanageable patient flow. Downtime allows providers to eat and relax between calls. They can socialize, smoke, and sleep. These themes are no doubt present in other EMS researchers' notes but have not been a significant focus for them. Moreover, I focus on how downtime itself happens in place, not just in time, a finding that moves beyond the confines of this small existing literature.

Place, like downtime, is a crucial facet of EMS work. While Seim (2020) addresses the poverty rates of tracts where ambulance calls occur and he and others (Seim 2020; Jusionyte 2018; Mannon 1992; Metz 1981) have noted the precarity that patients often live with, I explicitly tie these two concepts together to understand how neighborhood stigmas are socially constructed and applied. Space is omnipresent in EMS work and becomes another ascriptive category that providers can apply to patients and use to make judgments about the moral worth of patients. Part III's findings move Seim's finding about "bullshit calls" forward in several crucial ways, emphasizing their connection to place and highlighting how this pernicious construct can harm patient care.

Shift's End

Shifts at Private Ambulance end predictably. Dispatchers exercise discretion over when and how ambulances return to headquarters in North Chapman, calling ambulances back one at a time to wrap up their shifts. On the drive back to headquarters, crews stop for gas if their ambulances need it and then drive through the industrial park full of squat metal-clad buildings to Private Ambulance's garage. There they park the ambulance inside, often marking it as temporarily out of service so that the technicians who work in the garage cleaning and restocking ambulances know to check the truck for missing supplies. Providers must return portable radios to the chargers located in the dispatch center, and some providers head to the locker rooms to change out of their uniforms and shower. Others head straight for their cars, parked either in the cavernous garage or out in the front parking lot.

These shifts also end unpredictably, however. While there is a pattern to how shifts end, the timing is always uncertain. Dispatchers may hold providers over the end of their shifts because no other ambulances are available in the city, or because they are in the middle of a call when their shift ends. Structure fires, vent transfers, and other long calls can keep providers over the official end of their shift by several hours, depending on how the individual calls unfold.

This unpredictability is yet another way EMS work is marginalizing work. Once you step into that ambulance, you never quite know when you will get to end your shift. While providers may work "eights," "twelves," or "twenty-fours" on paper, their shifts may end up being far longer. If there are call-outs, they may have the ability to pick up overtime work and extend their shifts even further. This level of unpredictability perfectly captures the challenging, unpredictable nature of pre-hospital medicine. There are undoubtedly other jobs and careers where days are unpredictable, but the constellation of boredom, unpredictability, and mobility that EMTs and paramedics face makes EMS particularly challenging work. For many providers, there are only so many shifts they can end before changing jobs is needed. Others can make it a career, though we can and should make this path more comfortable and sustainable.

My final shift at Private Ambulance ended by walking out through its headquarters' front door shortly before Christmas in 2013. It was late in the evening, and I sat in my car, sent text messages to my wife, and then to my research advisor. Texts sent, I then headed to a liquor store in North Chapman to buy some celebratory beer. The interview portion of data collection remained, and I was still cycling my way through every block of the city of Chapman, but that night felt like "goodbye" just the same. I drove further south from the liquor store through the Old Quarter, radio blasting, and beer on the passenger seat. At that moment, my time "riding third" was over, but out in Chapman, at the same time I was driving home, Private Ambulance trucks were responding to calls. In the Old Quarter, kids living on the street were busking and grinding for spare change. In Midtown, older men and women sat in the Plaza drinking from bottles inside paper bags and taking shots from "nips." That night, people called 9-1-1 for severe illnesses and not so serious issues, as well. I was leaving Private Ambulance, but at that moment and every day since, the beat of "grunt work" continued, with providers stepping out into the street saying, "Let's try this again."

Appendix

Notes on Data and Methods

Positionality

As I mention in the Preface, "riding third" was not my first time in an ambulance. By the time I stepped through the doors at Private Ambulance, I had eight years of experience in EMS, including four as an emergency medical technician. I did not go to Private Ambulance to be a full-fledged participant. I wanted to be a fly on the wall. The reality, however, is that everyone there knew I had some clinical experience. They would sometimes assume knowledge on my part, such as saying, "You know how it is." Being able to converse with providers about shared experiences using a common vernacular outweighed any drawbacks to being open about my past experiences in EMS.

It also meant that, occasionally, I helped on calls. Providing care under the direction of the providers I was with was not a regular occurrence. During the pilot phase of data collection, the crew asked me to help as we transported a pregnant woman who nearly delivered her new child in the back of our ambulance. I also helped the crews I was with during three severe trauma calls, including taking blood pressures, holding bandages, and helping backboard a patient. These were not the norm, though I regularly helped crews clean their trucks, cots, and equipment after calls. It was a small token of respect, an excuse to chat them up further, and a way to show my thanks for them taking me out on the road. Therefore, I was a participant-as-observer, someone with adjacent membership in the community I was studying, though without direct responsibilities for providing care when I was conducting fieldwork.

Pilot Work

In 2009, when I first arrived at Private Ambulance, I spent four shifts, about forty-eight hours, with different "MB" crews consisting of either two paramedics or a paramedic and an EMT. After these observations, I conducted twenty interviews to learn more about EMS work in Chapman and identify salient topics for future work. These pilot data appeared in a 2015 paper in the *American Journal of Orthopsychiatry* (Prener and Lincoln 2015). They also were used in this book, especially in Chapter 2's discussion of "real emergencies." The themes I ultimately explored with the second round of fieldwork emerged from this initial pilot data collection round. These included an interest in space, Chapman's population of street homeless persons, and the effect of sub-acute substance use and other calls on the EMS system.

Research Design

The pilot work did not just inspire thematic priorities but also solidified the methods at the core of this book. These methodological priorities included an explicit mixed-methods approach to data collection and analysis, the implementation of qualitative GIS techniques, and mobile devices for data collection.

Mixed-Methods Design

Mixed-methods research designs are not conceptually new. However, they have received limited attention in sociology (Small 2011) and pre-hospital medicine (McManamny et al. 2015) until recently. Small (2011) has argued that studies could mix methods on three axes: data, data collection, and data analysis. This broad definition includes studies that collect multiple data types using more than one mode of collecting primary data or analyzing data using two or more alternate analytical techniques. The research design presented here (see Figure 19) utilized all these approaches to mixed methods to varying degrees.

I split this project's overall research design into two distinct elements: a "core" qualitative body of data and a "supplementary" quantitative body. The distinction drawn between these two project elements is common within mixed-methods research, with "core" data intended to stand on their own (Morse 2016, 2010). "Supplementary" data are characterized by being either incomplete or somehow hampered by shortcomings, which prevent them from being used alone (Morse 2010). EMS patient data have been subject to long-standing concerns (Institute of Medicine 2007) and were ultimately unavailable for this project. Like other first-responder organizations, Private

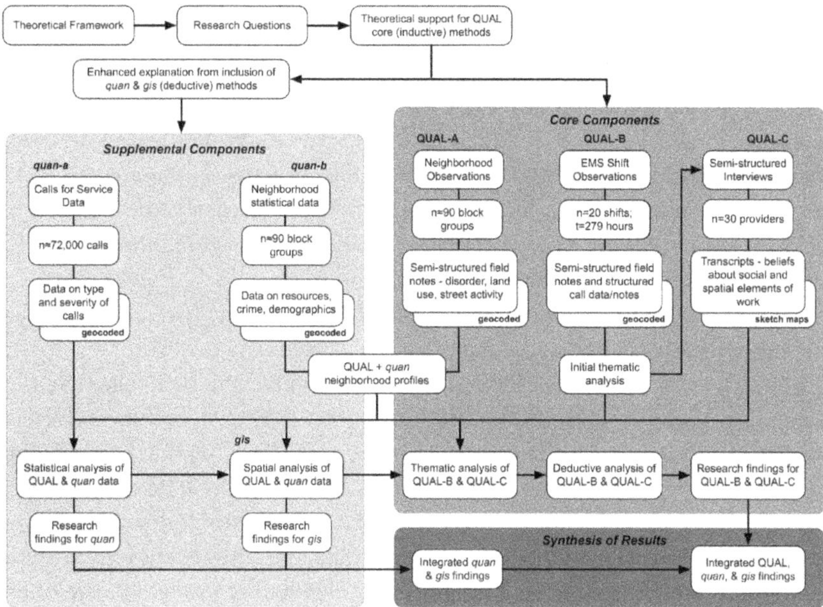

Figure 19. Research Design (graph by author)

Ambulance could not provide machine-readable outputs from its electronic health-record system. Similar data from the state's NEMSIS system was also unavailable because of data-access policies. Focusing on qualitative data, then, made the most sense for this research design.

The "core" qualitative data for this project had three "strands" (Morse 2010):

1. neighborhood observations (QUAL-A in Figure 19),
2. EMS shift observations at Private Ambulance (QUAL-B),
3. and semi-structured interviews with EMS providers at Private Ambulance (QUAL-C).

The "supplemental" quantitative data also had three strands:

1. Chapman Police Department "calls for service" data that served as a proxy for EMS demand in the absence of patient-level records (QUAN-A),
2. neighborhood statistical data from several sources including the 2010 U.S. Census, the 2008–13 American Community Survey, and a variety of publicly available local data sources (QUAN-B),
3. and a geo-database of spatial features combined with data from various qualitative and quantitative strands (GIS).

Qualitative GIS

The growing literature on mixed-methods research in the social sciences has often ignored GIS techniques regardless of their qualitative or quantitative orientation. Tashakkori and Teddlie's (2010) otherwise seminal mixed-methods handbook gave only passing attention to GIS techniques, and many researchers treat them as a means for data visualization (Dickinson 2010). However, GIS tools can provide powerful platforms for collecting qualitative data in addition to data visualization itself (Cope and Elwood 2009; Prener 2021).

Sketch mapping, the technique utilized in this study, uses a preexisting, cartographically accurate base map to guide spatial data collection where the goal is to understand the distribution of activities or perceptions of space (Boschmann and Cubbon 2014). Rather than being the only form of data collected, sketch mapping is typically a supplementary activity alongside focus group (Dongus et al. 2007; Fielding and Cisneros-Puebla 2010; Sletto 2015; Weiner and Harris 2003; Wridt 2010) or interview data (Brennan-Horley and Gibson 2009; Cieri 2003). The digitization of these data and subsequent GIS analysis is an essential part of the analytic process. Individual or group data are often aggregated into composite maps to demonstrate where perceptions or activities "cluster" in a particular place.

My use of geocoding represented a deviation from the standard approach to mixed-methods research design. Rather than GIS existing solely as a strand, geographic data in this project was a specific aspect of each data strand regardless of its overarching methodological orientation. This decision meant that I could conduct spatial analyses of data collected from any strand of the study. I enabled this by using a standard unit of analysis, the census block group. I gathered each strand's data so that I could aggregate them based on the census block group. This "spatial common denominator" meant that each spatial data element could be easily integrated with the others, ensuring a seamless analysis regardless of the source.

Mobile Data Collection

The integration of qualitative GIS data into the ethnographic strands (QUAL-A and QUAL-B) required another nascent methodological technique, mobile data collection. The growth in mobile devices in recent years allows researchers to conduct face-to-face interviews while availing themselves of the accuracy and data-entry strengths of a computer-based approach (Forster et al. 1991; Gravlee 2002; Gravlee et al. 2006; Patnaik, Brunskill, and Thies 2009; Shaw et al. 2011). Mobile computer-assisted personal interviewing ("MCAPI") techniques, however, have primarily been deployed in studies in the global South.

There has also been little use of MCAPI by sociologists, with Gravlee's (Gravlee 2002; Gravlee et al. 2006) neighborhood research in Detroit one of the only examples of sociological research using MCAPI methods.

MCAPI techniques in this study represented the key to collecting spatial data in the field. The collection of these data was enabled by the widespread integration of Global Position System (GPS) hardware into smartphones. These chips have accuracy levels roughly equivalent to consumer-grade, stand-alone GPS devices (Zandbergen 2009; Zandbergen and Barbeau 2011) and are not as accurate as commercial-grade GPS devices common in surveying applications. This study used three applications that blended commercially available mobile applications with custom data solutions to collect point (latitude/longitude), travel route, and census block group data in the field.

Human Subjects Concerns

Given the health focus of the study's data, the study site is confidential. However, confidentiality raises a challenge for spatial work. If cartographically accurate data are a core element of qualitative GIS, how could this be achieved without giving the research site away? As a solution, I employed the novel concept of "alternative cartography." This approach's goal was to faithfully represent spatial relationships while retaining a greater sense of space than other studies' denuded graphics. I transformed each census block group polygon from its distinct shape into (with a few exceptions) a quadrilateral shape that preserved the block group's size and positioning relative to its neighbors (see Figure 20). What resulted is an altered form of the city of Chapman that is faithful to its census block group's positioning but obscures its actual shape.

This process was time-consuming and, at the time I developed it, could not be automated. As I prepared this book's manuscript several years later, I experimented with several tools for creating tessellations and cartograms. None achieved the desired "alternative cartographic" effect I achieved for my research. The difficulties this approach poses are, therefore, considerable and limit its wider use. However, they allowed me to share and visualize spatial data without divulging the research site's identity.

Data Sources

Neighborhood Observations (QUAL-A)

The first core strand of qualitative data consisted of visits to each of the city of Chapman's approximately ninety census block groups between August 2013 and

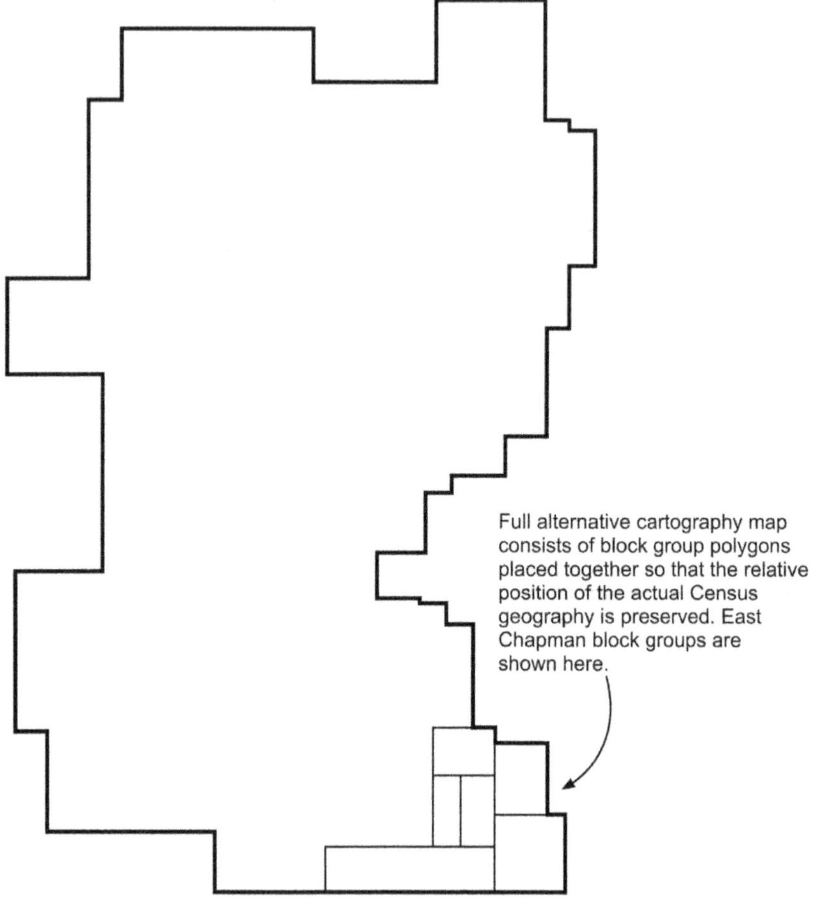

Figure 20. Example of "Alternative Cartography" Used in Mapping (graph by author)

September 2014. Visits were completed either on foot or by bicycle and included notations about each block within the block group. Fieldnotes included descriptions of the block's housing stock and any businesses visible from the street (as indicated by signs or storefronts). I also noted signs of "disorder," including graffiti, the presence of individuals who appeared to be homeless or signs of their presence (encampments, belongings), vacant buildings, and empty alcohol bottles. These observations aimed to capture these block groups as close to their conditions in December 2013 as possible. To collect these data, I used a custom iPhone-based database solution named FieldWerks to capture geocoded fieldnotes.

EMS Shift Observations (QUAL-B)

The second core strand of qualitative data consisted of observing EMS shifts at Private Ambulance over six months between July 2013 and December 2013. I spent twenty shifts, covering approximately 279 hours, as a "third rider" with Private's ambulance crews. Shifts were selected to cover a range of days of the week and times of day, including overnight shifts. In most cases (fifteen of twenty shifts), the observation periods covered most, but not all, of the ambulance crew's shift because Private Ambulance schedules many of its providers on "24s"—twenty-four-hour shifts. For example, I would arrive for a shift beginning at six in the morning and stay until late in the evening (typically ten or eleven). However, the participating crew would drop me off and continue with their shift until six the next morning. For the two overnight shifts observed, I joined crews halfway through their shift and stayed with them until the end of their shift the next morning. Combined with the pilot data collection, these observations yielded approximately 325 hours spent with Private Ambulance crews.

I selected shifts in consultation with Private Ambulance's director of operations (DO), who also assigned me to a crew working on a given shift. The DO notified crews in advance that I was conducting research. They could opt out of participation when Private Ambulance scheduled me and again when I arrived for my shift. No providers declined to participate at the beginning of shifts. Approximately half of Private Ambulance's staff participated in the data collection observation phase, including the vast majority of the paramedics regularly assigned to shifts in the city of Chapman. The final sample included twenty-eight providers, several of whom participated throughout multiple shifts. These providers included seven emergency medical technicians and twenty-one paramedics. A total of nine women and nineteen men participated; I oversampled women purposely to increase gender diversity. I had providers sign consent forms before the beginning of their first observation shift. Providers who participated in more than one observation shift could opt out of further participation, though again, none chose to do so.

During shifts, I took brief notes to outline each event. Then, during lengthy downtime periods and after completing the shift, I transcribed these notes into long-form narratives of each event. These fieldnotes described the providers' work during both emergency calls and downtime activities. I organized notes in the following manner: "Emergency" notes began when the ambulance was dispatched to a call and covered the entire course of that call until its disposition. "Disposition" referred to the result of the call. These results included dispatchers canceling the crew's response, not finding a patient, releasing the patient after treating him or her on-scene, or transporting the patient to a medical facility. Downtime notes encompassed any non-call–related activities. Downtime notes were divided based on ambulance movements, with each note beginning with the crew driving the ambulance to their destination. The note would cover the crew's activities at the destination. When the crew moved the ambulance to a new location or dispatchers sent them to a call, the note would end, and a new note would begin. I completed 478 notes during the twenty shifts, including 160 emergency calls and 318 downtime notes.

The fieldnotes included two types of data: unstructured notes describing providers' actions during emergency calls and downtime activities and structured variables of standardized data. Emergency note variables included data on response times and geographic data related to the starting location, scene location, disposition location, and driving routes. I also collected other variables, including data on the call found, the scene type, transport, and call disposition. These data were structured to match variables present in the National Emergency Medical Services Information System (NEMSIS) under the version "two standard."

Spatial data for both emergency and downtime notes were collected using two iPhone applications. Intersections and addresses relating to downtime activity locations were collected using the Google Maps web application. I used the same Google Maps application to collect census geography in the field for call locations. I created custom maps containing polygons representing each of the census block groups before beginning fieldwork. Tapping once on the appropriate polygon as we arrived on-scene revealed the appropriate census block group identification number, which I then recorded into my fieldnotes. This process ensured that detailed spatial data about call locations did not need to be collected only to be de-identified later.

I used a third tool named myTracks to record travel route data. When running, this application collected waypoints for travel routes every five seconds. These routes were displayed on a map within the application and saved until I could transcribe that travel-route data into my fieldnotes. Once transcribed, I permanently deleted these data from my phone. For routes involving emergency call scenes, I transcribed route data only when the ambulance was outside the census block group containing the call location. I used these data to add additional context to fieldnotes.

EMS Interviews (QUAL-C)

The third "core" strand of data I collected consisted of interviews with Private Ambulance providers in March and April of 2014, approximately three months after completing EMS shift observations. All twenty-eight participants in the EMS shift observations opted into the EMS interview phase of data collection by indicating a willingness to participate in interviews on their consent forms. By the beginning of the interview phase, two of the twenty-eight providers were no longer employed at Private Ambulance, leaving twenty-six original providers. I asked four additional providers who had not participated in the observations to participate in the interviews to generate the final sample. I had met and spoken with all four of these providers during downtime periods of the observation phase. The final interview sample of thirty providers included eight women and twenty-two men. Six emergency medical technicians and twenty-four paramedics participated in the interview phase. All providers, regardless of their observation participation status, consented before the beginning of the interview.

On each of the seven interview days, Private Ambulance's director of operations and I matched a list of potential participants with the roster of providers working. I then worked with Private Ambulance's dispatchers to rotate ambulances out of the field to conduct interviews. Interviews were conducted either in a private conference room or an office used by several supervisors, none of whom were present. Due to call volume, four interviews were interrupted by dispatchers so that the provider's ambulance could be returned to "the road" to respond to a call. I completed each of these four interviews later—three later the same day and one during a subsequent interview day.

All interviews, which lasted approximately an hour each, were audio-recorded with the participants' permission and then transcribed. The interviews were semi-structured, with topics selected based on an initial thematic analysis of the fieldnotes from the EMS shift observation. Several emergent themes, including downtime during shifts, the use of personal technology, and five groups of patients (homeless patients, patients with mental illnesses, patients with substance-use disorders, patients with "non-acute" illnesses, and patients with chronic illnesses) were identified for further exploration. The interview began with participants describing typical, good, and bad shifts. Providers were then asked about their downtime activities and to describe their views of Chapman City. The remaining time of the interview was spent discussing providers' views of each of the five groups of patients previously noted.

I introduced the qualitative GIS sketch map instrument to participants approximately a third of the way through each interview. All participants were given the same introduction to the landmarks labeled on the map, which included Chapman's street grid, significant bodies of water, and several locations providers were known from the observations to be familiar with as part of their daily work routines: Private Ambulance's headquarters, both hospitals in Chapman, fire stations, the police station, and major public transit hubs. I printed maps in color and large, 11″×17″ formats. Each map set included a participant map and an interview map. I used the following prompts to solicit information about areas where providers believed they (1) spent downtime and (2) could not spend downtime. I also collected data on areas where providers (3) responded "frequently" to calls as well as areas where they responded to calls for (4) patients who were homeless, (5) substance use, (6) mental-health issues, (7) "non-acute" issues, and (8) chronic illnesses.

I combined each area circled on the participant's map, termed a "cluster" here, with annotations on the interviewer's map. After completing the interviews, I digitized these map data working a "touch" rule. If the cluster touched a census block group, I included it in the digitized cluster. Once I had digitized all the maps, I was then able to generate counts for each block group with the number of clusters that included it for each prompt. Clusters could also overlap, meaning that the total count for some census block groups exceeded the interview sample size.

Calls for Service Data (QUAN-A)

I derived supplemental data on the distribution of EMS work within the city of Chapman from police data. In Chapman, the police department routinely responded to EMS calls with the fire department and Private Ambulance. Police "calls for service," therefore, represent a rough proxy for EMS demand. These data are incomplete, since not all of Private Ambulance's calls come through the 9-1-1 system. Calls made directly to Private Ambulance included requests for emergency and nonemergency transports from medical facilities; these interfacility transfer cries did not include regular police responses. Another group of calls, those made where another police agency, such as the state police, transit police, or a university police department, has jurisdiction were also missing from this database.

Given the focus of this study on EMS work in the community instead of interfacility transfer work, however, the "calls for service" data provided an approximation for EMS demand in neighborhoods. The total Chapman Police Department calls for service database, from 2011 to 2013, contained 283,811 records. Of these, 30,939 records were EMS-related incidents. I identified these based on an emergency medical dispatch code in the incident type. I aggregated these records to create frequencies for each census block group representing estimated EMS demand for 2011, 2012, 2013, and a total of those three years.

Neighborhood Statistical Data (QUAN-B)

I compiled neighborhood statistical data from several sources. The primary source was the 2008–13 American Community Survey. These included census block group estimates for various demographic, social, and economic variables. I also obtained additional neighborhood statistical data from several publicly available local and state databases. These described the presence of various civil (e.g., public housing, transit station, fire station) and health (e.g., hospitals, clinics, homeless shelters, harm-reduction programs) facilities.

Spatial Data (GIS)

Publicly available spatial data describing the city of Chapman was obtained from the city's Geographic Information Systems Office. These data included a variety of features compiled in a geodatabase. Among the features contained in this database were the data used for creating the sketch-map base maps: Chapman's street grid (centerlines), TIGER/Line data for the city including the census block group geography, water features, and the locations of a number of the social and health resources described in the previous section. These data were an essential element of the data collection process, and I used them extensively in the analysis of spatial data collected throughout the study. These spatial data refer specifically to the existing geodatabase to link spatial data from other strands.

Data Analysis

The original analysis for my research included three streams: qualitative, quantitative, and spatial. Since the quantitative data did not ultimately find their way into this book, I have not included them here. Instead, I focus on qualitative and spatial analytical methods.

Qualitative Coding

I used the analysis program Dedoose to conduct the "core" qualitative data analyses. I selected Dedoose because of its mixed-methods–oriented feature set. This analysis consisted primarily of the textual data collected during the EMS observations (QUAL-B) and the semi-structured interviews (QUAL-C). Fieldnote and interview data were de-identified in the data warehouse and then uploaded to Dedoose's servers. I selected two shifts worth of fieldnotes for initial inductive code development where emergent themes were identified

(Charmaz 1983; Glaser 1978). An initial pass was made on these fieldnotes to identify emergent themes, which I then subdivided into individual codes. After I produced a draft code list, I applied these codes to the same two shifts. As they were applied, I refined the draft code list. These codes were further refined by applying them to two additional shifts. I then used the resulting code list to code the remaining shifts' fieldnotes.

I followed a similar process with the interview transcripts, selecting two interviews for an initial round of inductive coding where codes from the fieldnotes were applied where possible. I focused on identifying themes that were not present in the fieldnotes. I applied these new codes to the two initial interviews, and then the entire code list was refined further using two additional interview transcripts. Once complete, I coded the remaining twenty-six interview transcripts. Once coding was complete, I generated code reports using Dedoose and reviewed them for overarching themes present within the fieldnotes and interview transcripts.

Beyond the generation of these inductive codes, I used several other coding strategies and categorizing qualitative data. I tagged mentions of particular neighborhoods using a set of deductive geographic codes. Discussions of the "Midtown" neighborhood (and other neighborhoods) were therefore coded both for the themes present in the discussion and a code identifying the block of text as relating to Midtown. These codes relied on providers' language choices for referring to particular neighborhoods and did not presuppose a particular spatial definition of the neighborhoods in question. Similarly, I coded particular sections of the semi-structured interview transcripts using deductive codes that referred to specific sketch-map prompts, allowing me to analyze patterns within each prompt across respondents. I made these comparisons using a code-by-code analysis technique in which codes were cross-tabulated. This process allowed me to identify emergent themes that co-occurred frequently.

Spatial Analyses

I conducted the "supplemental" spatial analyses using both ArcGIS and, for two measures of spatial autocorrelation, GeoDa (Anselin and Rey 2014). These analyses include the spatial analysis of EMS observation fieldnotes (QUAL-B), sketch-map data (QUAL-C), and data from the quantitative analytic dataset. The input feature class for all analyses was the TIGER/Line data for Chapman's census block groups obtained from the geo-database described previously. Initial analyses of data aggregated to the census block group resulted in thematic choropleth maps. The final maps selected for inclusion in my research (and this book) were then converted to the alternative cartography map using the vector editing tool OmniGraffle.

I conducted additional analyses using spatial statistics using ArcGIS and GeoDa. These included several related tests of spatial autocorrelation, all of which were variants of the Moran's I statistic (Getis and Ord 2010). Spatial autocorrelation represents the concept that like things tend to be near each other geographically, and the Moran's I statistic captures the degree to which this is the case for specific distributions. Moran's I values, like correlation coefficients, range from -1 to 1, where -1 represents perfectly non-clustered data (think of the distribution of black and white squares on a chessboard). A value of 0 for Moran's I represents randomly distributed data, and a value of 1 represents highly clustered data.

I also conducted hot-spot analyses of these data using the Getis-Ord Gi* technique (Getis and Ord 2010), which is ideal for aggregated data. The Getis-Ord Gi* test calculates z-scores and p-values for each analysis (in this case, each census block group). Larger z-scores represent a greater degree of spatial clustering among high values in the data; the smallest z-scores represent a greater degree of spatial clustering among low values in the data. These data are useful for identifying areas where a given concept occurs or does not occur. I use them to understand the degree of spatial clustering for specific calls or providers' views about their work. Hot spots, which appear in figures using shades of gray, identified areas of higher-than-average values. Cold spots, which were omitted in the book, were also part of the original output identifying areas of lower-than-average values.

Final Thoughts

As with any research project, I learned a considerable amount throughout this effort. In retrospect, I would have done some aspects of this project differently. In particular, I spent quite a long time developing relational database solutions for storing the qualitative GIS that were slow, cumbersome, and difficult to repurpose for other projects. I have since completely overhauled the sketch-map technique I used, creating a package for the programming language R that replicates the core methodology without using a relational database. I discuss the evolution of this tool in a pre-print. The software, which is named qualmap, is available on CRAN and GitHub. This library represents the most concrete methodological outgrowth of this project.

I also focused on using proprietary tools for both data storage and analysis. If I could do this project over again, I would focus on using SQL instead of FileMaker and R instead of Stata. For mapping, I would have created a "dummy" shapefile representing the alternative cartography rather than manually applying hues from the original maps. I also would have focused on using analysis tools other than ArcGIS and Geoda. Using open-source tools and focusing on reproducibility with the mapping process would have made publishing and developing this manuscript far easier. I make these self-critiques with significant hindsight and the benefit of research experiences in the intervening years since I started data collection at Private Ambulance.

Doing mixed-methods research is time-consuming but incredibly rewarding. While there are decisions I would have made differently, I would not change the mixed-methods focus of this project. I am the researcher I am today because of this, and the skills I started developing as a research student have paid off in wonderful ways.

Acknowledgments

Like working on an emergency scene, academic work is not a solitary act. There is a litany of folks to thank who have made this work possible. I would not have a book on EMS work without sitting in the back of an ambulance myself. I joined Perinton Ambulance in 2000 after my friend in middle school, David Williams, told me about it. The Explorer Program at Perinton Ambulance, led at the time by Steve Watters, gave me my first taste of patient care. Over the next eight years, I worked with many different EMS educators and partners, far too many to name here, at Perinton Ambulance, Canton Fire and Rescue, and St. Lawrence University EMS. I learned so much from them. I would have never tried to write this book without first putting on a uniform to try and help my neighbors.

I also would not have a book on EMS work without Private Ambulance's leadership team opening their agency up to me. Likewise, I am indebted to the dozens of providers I got the chance to share ambulances, meals, naps, class, and an interview room with between 2011 and 2012. Your willingness to open up to me about the joys and challenges of pre-hospital medicine made this book possible. Thank you so much for showing me a side of Chapman and EMS work I would have never otherwise experienced.

My move from EMS provider to being a researcher was unplanned and motivated by a serendipitous conversation with Alisa K. Lincoln. She quickly supported the initial pilot project that gave me my first fieldwork experience and the professional connections I developed with Private Ambulance. Over the past fourteen years, Alisa has been a constant source of inspiration and guidance, professionally and personally. Without Alisa's mentorship, I would not be half the researcher I am today.

Alisa was far from the only academic who helped shape what would eventually become *Medicine at the Margins*. Steven Vallas, Shelley Kimelberg, and Patrick Sharkey deserve enormous credit for supporting this project. Their influence appears throughout the book. Steve's was critical in shaping my view of EMS as an occupation. At the same time, Shelley and Pat were essential to developing the idea of EMS as an inter-neighborhood institution. I remain awe-inspired by Pat's methodological creativity and continue to draw inspiration from his innovative work. Likewise, Theresa Osypuck, James Connolly, and Daniel O'Brien provided guidance that helped shape the project at critical moments. Theresa introduced me to social epidemiology. Without formal training, James and Dan encouraged me to build GIS into my research design.

Dan Monti deserves special thanks for immediately catching the vision that this would be a book one day after he saw me speak in 2015. He never let go of that vision and, in doing so, inspired me to come around to the idea that maybe, just maybe, he was right. Dan made a home for the book in his Polis series and continued to advocate fiercely for *Medicine at the Margins*' publication. Likewise, I am grateful to Fred Nachbaur for shepherding the book through the publishing process at Fordham University Press.

I am also tremendously grateful for the feedback of Patricia Rieker, Tania Jenkins, and Josh Seim. Their manuscript reviews were critical, challenging, and beneficial for its development. Josh deserves special mention, not just because the club of EMS providers in sociology is tiny, but because his book inspired me. I am so glad I could benefit from his incisive observations about my theoretical arguments and view of what EMS work is and could be.

To my friends Anna Revette, Lisa Pal, and Christopher Hovey, thank you for reading very early versions of many of these chapters. Likewise, Joel Jennings, Amy Cooper, Liz Chiarello, and Bruce O'Neill, thank you for pushing me to write *Medicine at the Margins* when I was not sure I would ever make it to the finish line. The collective feedback you all provided was instrumental in shaping what this book became.

Through this adventure, my family has been there to cheer me on. I am tremendously fortunate to have benefited from their encouragement and help: my parents' untold number of trips back and forth to Perinton's ambulance base before I had a license and a car, the midnight calls I made to my wife, Johanna, from emergency room parking lots to decompress after challenging calls, and my older daughter's effusive excitement about a dad who loves ambulances and is "a new author," as she regularly reminds me with a wide grin. My youngest daughter missed the years of research and writing but gets to share in the excitement of a completed book, and I couldn't be more grateful to have her to celebrate with. It feels fitting that adding her to the acknowledgments was the last sentence of the book that I wrote. I am so lucky to have all of you in my life and would never have made it as far as writing a book without your constant patience, support, and cheerleading. Thank you.

Notes

Preface

1. Josh Seim (2020) eventually moved from researcher to practitioner as well, working at his field site partially out of necessity.

Introduction: Shit Work on Urban America's Front Lines

1. Quickly, the "B" identifies the ambulance as being staffed by "Basic Life Support"–trained personnel, otherwise known as emergency medical technicians. This is in contrast to "M" or "medic" units, which are staffed by paramedics. This is discussed in greater detail later.

2. Philippe Bourgois and Jeff Schonberg, in *Righteous Dopefiend*, discuss briefly how cleanliness and smell become essentializing elements in the lives of street homeless individuals (2009). One of their respondents reported something similar to what the EMTs experienced that night: "When I used to be next to Al, I could barely breathe. I be like, 'I'm suffocating. I need air.'" Others have also described the sensory experience of homelessness, including an account of a homeless shelter's "smell of sweat and urine hitting you like a wall" (Kozol 2011).

3. These terms have a long history in the sociology of work and occupations. Hughes (1962, 1971) invokes the term to describe work that is either discrediting or discreditable, to borrow Goffman's (2009) description of stigma. The references to "dirty work" overlap but are not entirely congruent with the idea of "shit work," work that is either literally dirty (emptying a bedpan) or otherwise dull or repetitive. The short vignette at the outset of this chapter captures the essence of "shit work": dirty, smelly, putrid. It does not necessarily follow that "shit work" becomes "dirty work," though it is entirely possible (Star 1995, 501–7).

4. Estimates of the total volume of EMS work are difficult to come by. This is driven by the balkanization described at the outset of this chapter. We know from the National Hospital Ambulatory Medical Care Survey, for example, that over 20 million patients were transported to American emergency departments in 2015. These data do not reflect patients who were treated and released by EMS providers before they ever reached a hospital, nor does it account for the number of patients who were transported by EMS providers between medical facilities.

5. There is some precarity in this status, however. In most states, there is not a legal requirement to offer EMS services, since it is not legally enshrined as an "essential service" like fire and public safety. Some rural parts of the United States are struggling to continue to offer constantly available 9-1-1 services.

6. Though they were published in the 1980s and early 1990s, the data in both Mannon (1992) and Metz (1981) reflected fieldwork conducted years earlier.

7. Much of the more recent work by social scientists has focused on the relationship between EMS providers and health-care practitioners. Several accounts have shown how providers have attempted to carve out an occupational niche for themselves with varying degrees of success (Palmer 1989; Palmer and Gonsoulin 1990), largely inhibited by the trappings of EMS work's amateur past (Whalley and Barley 1997). Negotiation between paramedics and other health-care providers has been documented as a key part of this process (Mellinger 1992, 1994; Palmer 1989). Negotiation between paramedics and others at emergency scenes, including law enforcement, families, and bystanders, has also been described in a recent study of scene management by Canadian EMS providers (Campeau 2008).

8. In addition to Seim's 2020 book, see also Seim 2017.

9. These three overarching types of marginality are rooted in Billson's (2005) typology of marginality.

10. Sociology's emphasis, for example, on the experiences of individuals living in poverty, suffering from housing instability, or being disenfranchised from the political levers of society are all examples for Billson (2005) of structural marginality. Billson (2005) writes that this is perhaps the focus of much of the contemporary literature on marginality and has intellectual roots that go further back than Park's 1928 essay. Rather, she argues, sociology draws upon the work of Marx and Engels for its root inspiration on issues of structural marginality.

11. This sense of "lack of fit" is key for Billson (2005). We can see this in a variety of modern contexts, such as Adia Harvey Wingfield's (2013) analyses of the struggles African American men face in entering largely white, male work contexts. Similarly, the constraints women face in the workplace, captured by Roseabeth Moss Kanter in her classic *Men and Women of the Corporation* (2008) and a bevy of more recent studies, captures the same "lack of fit" Billson describes as typifying social role marginality.

12. This is the first of Billson's (2005) ideal types of marginality. Noel Gist and Roy Wright (1973) made a classic study of this "out-group" devaluation, focusing their research on the marginality experienced by individuals living in post-independence India who identified with a number of European nationalities. Marginality here

comes to represent a cultural gap between these anachronistic holdovers of colonialism, who practice Christianity, speak English, and follow Western cultural customs, and the far more numerous communities of Hindus, Muslims, Sikhs, and others. The fissures that Gist and Wright observed are emblematic of the relative marginality of those they describe as "Anglo-Indians" in this new, modern, postcolonial India.

13. This is a common observation in the public-health literature on EMS from Europe, in particular, that has focused on the range of patients that access EMS services for non- or sub-acute issues and injuries. This literature often frames these patients' use of EMS as "misuse" (Ruger, Richter, and Lewis 2006; Snooks et al. 1998; Snooks et al. 2004; Hjalte et al. 2007).

14. A significant literature captures the barriers that exist for individuals living with mental illness in America (Link and Phelan 2001; Link et al. 1997).

15. As much as they are products of physical construction—the brick, concrete, and steel that prop up contemporary cities—urban spaces are socially constructed, as well. Though Wacquant does not cite him in *Urban Outcasts*, the work of Henri Lefebvre is particularly relevant for this discussion. In *The Production of Space*, Lefebvre leans on the proposition that "(social) space is a (social) product" (Lefebvre and Nicholson-Smith 1991). Space therefore has meaning and symbolism imbued in it, meaning that social construction is a process producing and reproducing our understandings of space itself. This notion that space can embody social meaning and is, itself, a product of the division of labor and social relations of production in a given society is critical for understanding the meaning of space for contemporary urban sociology generally and EMS work specifically.

16. There is a strong parallel here to the ways in which EMS work unfolds and the broader interest in neighborhoods that has existed within urban sociology since the Chicago School's rise (Bloom 2002). The nineteenth-century interest in the variation of crime, health, and demographic factors across cities in France and England is epitomized by Snow's (1855) mapping of London cholera outbreaks as well as early studies of crime (Guerry 2002) and urban social problems (Mayhew 1861). Though the role of mapping in some of these early analyses has perhaps been overstated (McLeod 2000), this early emphasis on spatial context makes Snow and others early pioneers of the "ecological" paradigm emphasized by Park and Burgess (1967).

17. Among other things, neighborhoods serve as labels applied to individuals (Lalli 1992; Macintyre, Ellaway, and Cummins 2002; Uzzell, Pol, and Badenas 2002). Neighborhood labels are applied in ways that are generalized to most residents (i.e., stereotypes) and lead to the acts of individual and institutional discrimination (Bauder 2001, 2002; Dean and Hastings 2000; Newman 2000; Taylor 1998; Wacquant 1993, 2008). Extending discussions of stigma to place therefore appears theoretically justified (Chaix 2009; Galster 2012). Indeed, if Lefebvre is correct and the social meaning of space is itself a product of the relations of production, any inequality or stigma embedded in those larger social relations will be reflected in the way space is produced, understood, and reproduced.

18. Such spatial or "territorial stigmatization" (Wacquant 1993), however, has received little empirical assessment (Besbris et al. 2015; Chaix 2009; Galster 2012), particularly in terms of widespread studies designed to estimate the effect of neighborhood on behavior. The paper by Besbris et al. (2015), for example, which found individuals are less likely to respond to online advertisements from disadvantaged neighborhoods, is one of few such studies. Furthermore, no studies have analyzed neighborhood stigma and health (Chaix 2009), even though the concept provides a vehicle for understanding how institutional actors may respond to neighborhoods, perpetuating place-based disadvantage and inequalities in health outcomes (Macintyre, Ellaway, and Cummins 2002).

19. The model that has often been used to describe service work is based on the dyadic relationship between workers on the shop floor and the managers who oversee this work. The fundamental difference between manufacturing and service work is the addition of a third constituency, the customer. With three constituent groups, managers, employees, and customers, participating to varying degrees in the provision of services, our understanding of the scope of interactions must necessarily be expanded from the dyadic to the triadic. Known as the "service triangle," triadic models for visualizing key constituents have become popular features of the service-work literature (Lopez 2010). These models' popularity and wide application is due in part to their ability to summarize the scope and scale of workplace interactions using an intuitive heuristic and have been broadly applied (Leidner 1993; Brown and Korczynski 2010; Korczynski 2009; Fine 2008; Orr 2016; Sallaz 2009). A fundamental strength of these models is their focus on the key constituents involved in work relationships between customers, employees, and managers.

The simplicity of these models is also a weakness. Much of the service-work literature has focused on the various ways power is distributed between management, workers, and employees, what Lopez (2010) calls "three-way interest alliances." Yet it may not be appropriate to include customers as "coproducers" of a product so explicitly (Belanger and Edwards 2013). Furthermore, the categories of manager, customer, and employee are themselves reductive (Hanser 2012), and the connections between the three groups are not, in reality, as equilateral as the triangular model implies.

In their excellent overview of these limitations, Belanger and Edwards (2013) argue that labor-process theory may help to overcome such shortcomings. They also note that "both agency and structure both have to be considered seriously" (436) in studies of service work. While such an emphasis may be possible using labor-process theory, the concept of "street-level bureaucracy" (Lipsky 1980) also draws attention to such issues. For EMS providers and other front-line service workers working in civil or public-service environments, it may have more relevance because of its emphasis on the provision of social services where ethnical decision-making is required (Korczynski 2009).

The Scene

1. The National Registry of EMS Providers includes two additional levels of certification. The first, the Emergency Medical Responder or "EMR," is a Basic Life

Support certification aimed particularly at police officers, firefighters, and other first responders. In some states, the driver of the ambulance may also be an Emergency Medical Responder as opposed to an EMT, though this was not the case at Private Ambulance. The other level of certification providers can obtain through the National Registry is the Advanced EMT or "AEMT" level. This exists in a space between BLS and ALS, with AEMTs having access to some additional skills that are traditionally seen as Advanced Life Support skills. These additional skills are limited in nature, however.

1. Dial 9-1-1 for Emergencies

1. "Working up" is the term used by paramedics to describe providing a full set of diagnostic measures, including cardiac monitoring, and taking other precautionary steps like obtaining IV access.

2. This is the type of system described in Seim's work (2017, 2020)

3. National Registry of Emergency Medical Technicians.

4. This is a consistent theme in the key historical (Metz 1981; Mannon 1992) and contemporary (Corman 2017; Seim 2020) ethnographies of EMS work.

5. There is a strong parallel here to two literatures. The first comes from medical sociology, where there have been discussions of "deserving" versus "undeserving" patients. There are also connections to the sociology of work, where there has long been interest in "dirty work" (Hughes 1951) or "shit work" (Emerson and Pollner 1976). These two interests have strong crossover—for instance, in the study of mental- and behavioral health care (Emerson and Pollner 1976; Lincoln 2006) or occupations like nursing (Allen 2002).

2. The Ambulance Drivers Are Here!

1. The term "division of labor" can be traced back to classical sociology theory, including work by Marx and Durkheim. In its contemporary context, there is a long tradition of its use in both the sociology of medicine (Freidson 1988) and the sociology of work (Strauss 1985).

2. This framing was used in Whalley and Barley's (1997) classic text on technicians.

3. The literature on street-level bureaucracy has focused largely on public servants who are involved in controlling access to or the provision of services (Lipsky 1980). Police officers, teachers, and social workers are all classical examples (Maynard-Moody and Musheno 2009). It has also been used in Seim's recent monograph on EMS work. As with the service-work literature, there is an emphasis within the street-level bureaucracy literature on internal forces that shape work (Vinzant, Denhardt, and Crothers 1998), such as the effect of managers on work (May and Winter 2009) and organizational culture (Kelly 1994; Isett, Morrissey, and Topping 2006).

There is also a focus on external forces, however, such as the political climate street-level bureaucrats operate in (Gilboy 1992; May and Winter 2009) and the identities of the clients that bureaucrats serve (Henderson 2013; Scott 1997). This last point is critical because it is a contrasting bridge between the service-work literature and the empirical work on street-level bureaucrats. Whereas customers in the service-work literature are often framed as coproducers, Henderson (2013) frames clients and patients as external actors. More generally, the acknowledgment of external forces represents a major strength relative to the service-work literature's treatment of social structure (Belanger and Edwards 2013).

4. Discretion is a critical facet of the work of street-level bureaucrats (Vinzant, Denhardt, and Crothers 1998). It is so important because street-level bureaucrats often work in situations where a client's individual circumstances do not clearly fall into a procedural category (Loyens and Maesschalck 2010). The ambiguity inherent in this discretion is both "a curse and an opportunity" (Vinzant, Denhardt, and Crothers 1998, 19) for service providers because it gives them flexibility while also leaving them in a procedural gray area. Thus, while the service-work literature often emphasizes deskilled work and routinization (Leidner 1993), the street-level bureaucracy literature focuses on more complex work environments where both structure and agency are important, influential factors.

5. The emphasis that the street-level bureaucracy literature has placed on discretion is one facet of a more general interest in the ways workers navigate the workplace. This is particularly important with occupations where there are higher degrees of mobility and autonomy. Policing, a classic example of street-level bureaucracy work, relies on negotiation between officers to compensate for the lack of structure that being constantly available for emergency responses requires (Klinger 1997). Such a view of work is known as negotiated order, which describes the shared, sometimes tacit agreements among participants in a social organization (Strauss 2008, 1988). The order is understood as "negotiated" because it is constantly in flux; participants frequently reevaluate and restructure the rules that constitute the order (Hall 1987). Negotiated order, therefore, occurs in situations where the social order inadequately or incompletely dictates action or where additional flexibility is required. Such negotiated orders may occur on a small scale between individuals or on a larger scale between organizations or groups within organizations (Maines 1977), though the degree to which negotiated orders operate varies (Hall and Spencer-Hall 1982).

6. This is a long-standing area of interest for sociology, including classic works like *Men and Women of the Corporation* (Kanter 2008) as well as more recent work (e.g., Wingfield 2009, 2013). Among first responders, there has been some investigation of it in the fire service (Chetkovich 1997).

7. Karen Levy's recent work in this area on truck drives (2015) equates such surveillance with scientific management strategies and more general attempts at governance inside and outside of institutions (Foucault 1980, 2012; Espeland and Stevens 1998; Sauder and Espeland 2009). She also notes that information technology has a long tradition as a vector for exercising managerial control (Ball 2010; Beniger 2009;

Kling 1996; Yates 1993) and has particular relevance for occupations that are highly mobile (see also Rolland and Monteiro 2002).

8. Loyens and Maesschalck (2010) point to a greater need to understand the process through which street-level bureaucrats exercise discretion.

3. The Twenty-Four: The Rhythm of EMS Shifts

1. In my fieldnotes, this shift was labeled "Shift 99," which is how I will refer to it here. I was not present for a full twenty-four-hour shift for any of the providers—this was one of the most extended shifts I observed during my six months of fieldwork.

2. Seim (2020) mentions this briefly, and others have observed a similar culture around storytelling in EMS (Tangherlini 1998). The idea of "war stories" has strong parallels, for example, with the stories told in other occupations about clients or machines (see Orr 2016).

3. Few other notes were taken on this call because of human subjects' concerns.

4. There is a very limited literature on time spent at work. Perlow's (1999) sociology of work time provides both theoretical framing and empirical support for the ways in which work is temporally structured. She purposes a triangular model that connects both the social and temporal contexts of work to the structure of interdependent work patterns. In doing so, she draws upon Giddens's (2013) theory of structuration and his discussion of institutional time (or institutional durée). Giddens describes this as the wider trajectory of institutions within which individual experiences and time patterns are situated (see also Bryant and Jary 2014). A more recent take on this is from Clawson and Gerstel (2014), who use the term "web of time" to describe the ways in which institutions shape individuals' abilities to schedule themselves and their families.

4. Hurry Up and Wait: Passing Time and Avoiding Conflict

1. This is an underacknowledged area of first-responder work. Ethnographies of EMS work tend to emphasize calls themselves (Mannon 1992; Metz 1981; Seim 2020; Corman 2017). Desmond (2008) does spend time describing how wildland firefighters spend their time when not on-duty at remote fire camps, for example. By and large, however, there are few discussions of how first responders manage their time between calls.

2. The term "spatial turn" has been used in a variety of disciplines to denote a gradual acknowledgment of the role that both place and space have on sociological phenomena (Fuller and Löw 2017). There is a rich tradition of sociospatial thinking from Simmel (1950) and DuBois (Battle-Baptiste and Rusert 2018) through Lefebvre (1991, 1996), Löw (2016), and Logan (2012). However, the spatial turn has come to symbolize a transition in the 1970s and 1980s toward questions of space within sociology (Fuller and Löw 2017).

3. For a survey of spatial sociology, see Fuller and Löw (2017).

4. As I have noted previously, the idea of "interdependent work routines" is a nod to Perlow's (1999) concepts of work time.

5. This is similar to the challenge that Giddens (2013) describes as bridging space and time.

6. While there has been development of sociological understandings of space more generally (Fuller and Löw 2017), the sociology of work in particular has seen little spatially grounded research.

7. My conceptualization of "focal points" is roughly parallel to Giddens's concept of "stations" (2013). Bryant and Jary (2014) describe these "places" as locations that bind time and space for individuals—"stations" provide meaning for social interactions as well as both enabling and constraining individuals' actions. Stations, according to Giddens, can be something as simple as rooms within a house or the home itself. I do not use the term "station" here in part because it also has a specific meaning in the context of Emergency Medical Services, where it refers to the locations where ambulance users are based or "stationed." Another reason to part with Giddens's term is that any space is a station, meaning that no distinction exists between spaces that may be more or less important in a particular context.

8. This quote also offers a glimpse into the distinction between individual time and institutional time (Giddens 2013; Perlow 1999). Individual shifts began and ended throughout the day, with providers continually churning in and out of Private's headquarters. A single provider's shift occurs within a larger institution operating around the clock, a cycle that evokes Giddens's (1984) notion of individual and institutional time.

9. Occupational communities, also called communities of practice (Duguid 2012; Fox 2000; Kellogg, Orlikowski, and Yates 2006; Osterlund and Carlile 2005) or communities of knowledge (Boland and Tenkasi 1995), describe the process of knowledge transmission within the workplace (Bechky 2003; Peltonen 2007; Van Maanen and Barley 1984). Through occupational communities, employees "acquire a particular community's subjective viewpoint and learn to speak its language" (Brown and Duguid 1991). These viewpoints structure not only how employees view the work that they do, but also the wider world that work occurs within (Bechky 2003; Orr 2016). The occupational community perspective is therefore ideal for developing an understanding of how employees make meaning out of their work and the context within which this work occurs. Further, it provides an explanation about how these meanings become shared throughout a workplace or profession.

Occupational communities have been identified in a wide variety of occupations and workplaces. In addition to Orr's (2016) seminal study of copier-repair technicians, occupational community has been used to analyze manufacturing plants (Bechky 2003), web design firms (Kellogg, Orlikowski, and Yates 2006), middle managers in a variety of settings (Peltonen 2007), and software developers (Marschall 2014). It has also been applied in health-care settings, including with various nursing specialties (Aydin 1989; Bolton 2005; Wooten and Crane 2004) and pharmacists (Aydin 1989). In these health-care settings, occupational communities have been used to describe how professional norms related to the practice of medicine become shared values.

10. In elaborating his idea of "stations," space, and time for individuals and institutions, Giddens (2013) relied heavily on Erving Goffman's theories of social life. He made use, with some critique, of Goffman's (1990) concepts of "frontstage" and "backstage." Giddens termed some "stations" or "regions" as "front regions" (i.e., "frontstage") because they required "actors" to place a public persona forward. Other "regions" were "back regions" (i.e., "backstage"), since actors could obscure particular behaviors.

11. While I rely heavily on Giddens (2013) for his work on institutional time, it is important to note that he does little to offer an analysis of space and the ways it is socially constructed. However, the urban literature generally (Lefebvre and Nicholson-Smith 1991; Logan and Molotch 2007) and literature on urban homelessness more specifically offer a language for understanding such sociospatial exclusion. The concepts of "primary" and "marginal" space (DeVerteuil, May, and Mahs 2009; Stuart 2014, 2016) have been typically used to describe differences in how urban space is viewed with respect to use by the homeless. "Prime" spaces are those "that are primarily used and valued by domiciled and 'mainstream' society" (Stuart 2014, 2), as opposed to "marginal" spaces to where homeless individuals are pushed or expelled (Stuart 2014, 2016). The quintessential marginal space, according to Stuart (2014), is the Skid Row neighborhood in Los Angeles. We can adapt this distinction here for EMS providers by defining prime spaces as public arenas constructed as commercial or residential spaces where the long-term presence of EMS providers is seen as an unwanted distraction. Marginal spaces, for EMS providers, are those where their presence is not a distraction or could otherwise be defined as "backstage" from the providers' standpoint.

5. The Daily Grind of Grunt Work

1. Labeling theory is a particular area of emphasis within the sociology of mental health (Link et al. 1987; Link 1987; Link et al. 1989; Rosenfield 1997; Brown 1989) in part because of a "package deal" (Link et al. 1997) whereby individuals labeled as patients may receive access to medical care (Link et al. 1997; Corrigan 2004). However, for individuals who have a label such as a diagnosis or the status as "patient" applied to them, it may be a double-edged sword. While the label itself may open doors to care, these individuals may also face stigmatized responses from medical providers (Desai et al. 2002; Druss et al. 2002; Link, Mirotznik, and Cullen 1991). Labels can also be used to identify specific categories of patients that are not explicitly clinical. For example, identifying patients as "gomers"—"get out of my emergency room"—can serve to identify a group of individuals regardless of a specific diagnosis (Shem 2009; Leiderman and Grisso 1985).

2. The sociological literature on homelessness is wide and varied (Lee, Tyler, and Wright 2010; Meanwell 2012; Shlay and Rossi 1992) and includes a number of seminal

qualitative works, particularly Gowan (2010) and Bourgois and Schonberg (2009). Meanwell (2012) breaks the literature down into a number of major categories, including those on the stigmatization of homelessness, the experience of homelessness, and the interactions individuals who are homeless have with shelters and other social-service agencies.

3. The experience of homelessness in the United States is paradoxically framed both by pity (Link et al. 1995; Meanwell 2012; Phelan et al. 1995; Phelan et al. 1997; Toro et al. 2007) and stigmatization (Link et al. 1995; Meanwell 2012; Phelan et al. 1997). This stigmatization spills into everyday interactions between homeless individuals and peers, service providers, and members of the public (Anderson, Snow, and Cress 1994; Roschelle and Kaufman 2004; Snow et al. 1986; Snow and Anderson 1993). One complicating factor with these interactions is the assumption that homeless individuals have either mental-health or substance-use issues (or both), a common belief (Fischer and Breakey 1991) that many have argued is overstated (Lyon-Callo 2000; Snow et al. 1986), though these are certainly issues for some individuals who are street homeless (Bourgois and Schonberg 2009).

4. For assessments of the deinstitutionalization movement in the United States, see Mechanic and Rochefort (1990) as well as Lamb and Bachrach (2001).

6. Stigma and Space in Midtown

1. The disciplinary history's dominant narrative tends to only acknowledge W. I. Thomas, despite the contributions of Dorothy Thomas to the development of this idea (Smith 1995).

2. For more on the label "frequent flier" as it is applied to patients in emergency medicine contexts, see Billings et al. 2013.

3. Just as "37-Delta" is a label providers apply to patients, so too can place be a label that individuals apply to others (Lalli 1992; Macintyre, Ellaway, and Cummins 2002; Uzzell, Pol, and Badenas 2002). Given that neighborhood labels are applied in ways that are generalized to most residents (i.e., stereotypes) and lead to the acts of individual and institutional discrimination (Bauder 2001, 2002; Dean and Hastings 2000; Newman 2000; Taylor 1998; Wacquant 1993, 2008), extending discussions of stigma to place appears theoretically justified (Chaix 2009; Galster 2012). Such spatial or "territorial stigmatization" (Wacquant 1993), however, has received little empirical assessment (Besbris et al. 2015; Chaix 2009; Galster 2012), particularly in terms of widespread studies designed to estimate the effect of neighborhood on behavior. Furthermore, no studies have analyzed neighborhood stigma and health (Chaix 2009), even though the concept provides a vehicle for understanding how institutional actors may respond to neighborhoods, perpetuating place-based disadvantage and inequalities in health outcomes (Macintyre, Ellaway, and Cummins 2002).

4. I refer to this as "informal" exclusion because enforcing unwritten prohibitions on the use of particular spaces is not a part of the occupational mandate for EMS

providers. They have no responsibility to undertake this work in Chapman or elsewhere in the United States.

Marginality, Stigma, and the Future of Pre-Hospital Medicine

1. Elise Schmelzer, "Colorado Paramedics Inject Agitated People with Ketamine Without Their Consent. How Should the Practice Be Regulated?," *Denver Post*, June 13, 2021.

2. "Excited delirium" is a term embraced by some health-care providers to describe "aggressive behavior, altered sensorium, and a host of other signs that may include hyperthermia, 'superhuman' strength, diaphoresis, and lack of willingness to yield to overwhelming force" (Vilke et al. 2012). This has been critiqued as an overly broad definition that some organizations, like the American Psychiatric Association and the World Health Organization, do not recognize (Gonin et al. 2018). Moreover, it is seen relatively rarely by pre-hospital providers (Stratton et al. 2001) but is assigned as a cause for about 10 percent of deaths in police custody (Gonin et al. 2018), suggesting that the term itself has become a way to explain in-custody mortality in pseudo-scientific terms. Much of what we know about Daniel Prude's death comes from media reports, including a local TV station's timeline of events (WHEC-TV 2020), as well as body camera footage from officers who responded to the scene (10 Tampa Bay 2020).

3. Vanessa Romo, "Firefighter Testifies: 'I Was Desperate to Help . . . and This Human Was Denied That,'" *NPR*, Mar. 31, 2021.

4. In an October 11, 2021, letter to Congress, the American Ambulance Association and the National Association of Emergency Medical Technicians warned of "crippling" shortages of EMS providers because of low pay and high turnover.

Works Cited

10 Tampa Bay. 2020. "Body Cam Footage Released of Daniel Prude's Encounter with Rochester Police." https://www.youtube.com/watch?v=NxQ3klqpoOg.

Abbott, Andrew. 2014. *The System of Professions: An Essay on the Division of Expert Labor.* Chicago: University of Chicago Press.

Alejandro, Arroliga. 2015. "'Frequent Fliers' Do Not Receive a Free Trip in the Emergency Department." *CHEST* 128 (6): 4051–52.

Allen, Davina. 2002. *The Changing Shape of Nursing Practice: The Role of Nurses in the Hospital Division of Labour.* London and New York: Routledge.

Anderson, Leon, David A. Snow, and Daniel Cress. 1994. "Negotiating the Public Realm: Stigma Management and Collective Action among the Homeless." *Research in Community Sociology* 1 (1): 121–43.

Anselin, Luc, and Sergio Joseph Rey. 2014. *Modern Spatial Econometrics in Practice: A Guide to GeoDa, GeoDaSpace and PySAL.* Chicago: GeoDa Press.

Austin, Daniel. 2014. "Medical Debt as a Cause of Consumer Bankruptcy." *Maine Law Review* 67: 1.

Aydin, Carolyn E. 1989. "Occupational Adaptation to Computerized Medical Information Systems." *Journal of Health and Social Behavior* 30 (2): 163–79. https://doi.org/10.2307/2137011.

Bain, Peter, and Phil Taylor. 2000. "Entrapped by the 'Electronic Panopticon'? Worker Resistance in the Call Centre." *New Technology, Work and Employment* 15 (1). https://doi.org/10.1111/1468-005X.00061.

Ball, Kirstie. 2010. "Workplace Surveillance: An Overview." *Labor History* 51 (1): 87–106. https://doi.org/10.1080/00236561003654776.

Barley, Stephen R., and Julian Edgerton Orr. 1997. *Between Craft and Science: Technical Work in U.S. Settings.* Ithaca, N.Y.: Cornell University Press.

Battle-Baptiste, Whitney, and Britt Rusert, eds. 2018. *W. E. B. Du Bois's Data Portraits: Visualizing Black America.* New York: Princeton Architectural Press.

Bauder, Harald. 2001. "Work, Young People and Neighbourhood Representations." *Social & Cultural Geography* 2 (4): 461–80.

———. 2002. "Neighbourhood Effects and Cultural Exclusion." *Urban Studies* 39 (1): 85–93.

Bechky, Beth A. 2003. "Sharing Meaning across Occupational Communities: The Transformation of Understanding on a Production Floor." *Organization Science* 14 (3): 312–30. https://doi.org/10.1287/orsc.14.3.312.15162.

Belanger, Jacques, and Paul Edwards. 2013. "The Nature of Front-Line Service Work: Distinctive Features and Continuity in the Employment Relationship." *Work, Employment and Society* 27 (3): 433–50. https://doi.org/10.1177/0950017013481877.

Beniger, James. 2009. *The Control Revolution: Technological and Economic Origins of the Information Society*. Cambridge, Mass.: Harvard University Press.

Bergman, Abraham B., David C. Grossman, Angela M. Erdrich, John G. Todd, and Ralph Forquera. 1999. "A Political History of the Indian Health Service." *Milbank Quarterly* 77 (4): 571–604. https://doi.org/10.1111/1468-0009.00152.

Besbris, Max, Jacob William Faber, Peter Rich, and Patrick Sharkey. 2015. "Effect of Neighborhood Stigma on Economic Transactions." *Proceedings of the National Academy of Sciences* 112 (16): 4994–98.

Bigham, Blair L., Jan L. Jensen, Walter Tavares, Ian R. Drennan, Humaira Saleem, Katie N. Dainty, and Glenn Munro. 2014. "Paramedic Self-Reported Exposure to Violence in the Emergency Medical Services (EMS) Workplace: A Mixed-Methods Cross-Sectional Survey." *Prehospital Emergency Care* 18 (4): 489–94. https://doi.org/10.3109/10903127.2014.912703.

Bigham, Blair L., Sioban M. Kennedy, Ian Drennan, and Laurie J. Morrison. 2013. "Expanding Paramedic Scope of Practice in the Community: A Systematic Review of the Literature." *Prehospital Emergency Care* 17 (3): 361–72.

Billings, John, and Maria C. Raven. 2013. "Dispelling an Urban Legend: Frequent Emergency Department Users Have Substantial Burden of Disease." *Health Affairs* 32 (12): 2,099–108.

Billson, Janet Mancini. 2005. "No Owner of Soil: Redefining the Concept of Marginality." In *Marginality, Power, and Social Structure: Issues in Race, Class, and Gender Analysis*, edited by R. Dennis, 29–47. Amsterdam and Boston: Elsevier.

Bloom, Samuel. 2002. *The Word as Scalpel: A History of Medical Sociology*. New York: Oxford University Press.

Bluestone, Barry, and Bennett Harrison. 1982. *The Deindustrialization of America: Plant Closing, Community Abandonment, and the Dismantling of Basic Industry*. New York: Basic Books.

Bobo, Lawrence D. 2001. "Racial Attitudes and Relations at the Close of the Twentieth Century." In *America Becoming: Racial Trends and Their Consequences*, edited by Neil J Smelser, William Julius Wilson, and Faith Mitchell, 1–19. Washington, D.C.: National Academies Press.

Boland, Richard J., and Ramkrishnan V. Tenkasi. 1995. "Perspective Making and Perspective Taking in Communities of Knowing." *Organization Science* 6 (4): 350–72. https://doi.org/10.1287/orsc.6.4.350.

Bolton, Sharon C. 2005. "Women's Work, Dirty Work: The Gynaecology Nurse as 'Other.'" *Gender, Work & Organization* 12 (2): 169–86. https://doi.org/10.1111/j.1468-0432.2005.00268.x.

Boschmann, E. Eric, and Emily Cubbon. 2014. "Sketch Maps and Qualitative GIS: Using Cartographies of Individual Spatial Narratives in Geographic Research." *Professional Geographer* 66 (2): 236–48. https://doi.org/10.1080/00330124.2013.781490.

Bourdieu, Pierre. 1979. "Symbolic Power." *Critique of Anthropology* 4 (13–14): 77–85. https://doi.org/10.1177/0308275X7900401307.

———. 1984. *Distinction: A Social Critique of the Judgement of Taste*. Cambridge, Mass.: Harvard University Press.

———. 1998. *On Television*. New York: New Press.

Bourgois, Philippe, and Jeffrey Schonberg. 2009. *Righteous Dopefiend*. Berkeley: University of California Press.

Boyle, Malcolm, Stella Koritsas, Jan Coles, and Janet Stanley. 2007. "A Pilot Study of Workplace Violence towards Paramedics." *Emergency Medicine Journal: EMJ* 24 (11): 760–63. https://doi.org/10.1136/emj.2007.046789.

Boyle, Maree V. 2002. "'Sailing Twixt Scylla and Charybdis': Negotiating Multiple Organisational Masculinities." *Women in Management Review* 17 (3/4). https://doi.org/10.1108/09649420210425273.

Brennan-Horley, Chris, and Chris Gibson. 2009. "Where Is Creativity in the City? Integrating Qualitative and GIS Methods." *Environment and Planning A: Economy and Space* 41 (11): 2,595–2,614. https://doi.org/10.1068/a41406.

Brown, John Seely, and Paul Duguid. 1991. "Organizational Learning and Communities-of-Practice: Toward a Unified View of Working, Learning, and Innovation." *Organization Science* 2 (1): 40–57.

Brown, Kenneth, and Marek Korczynski. 2010. "When Caring and Surveillance Technology Meet: Organizational Commitment and Discretionary Effort in Home Care Work." *Work and Occupations* 37: 404–32.

Brown, Phil. 1989. "Psychiatric Dirty Word Revisited: Conflicts in Servicing Nonpsychiatric Agencies." *Journal of Contemporary Ethnography* 18 (2): 182–201.

Bryant, Christopher, and David Jary. 2014. *Giddens' Theory of Structuration: A Critical Appreciation*. London and New York: Routledge.

Buckner, John C. 1988. "The Development of an Instrument to Measure Neighborhood Cohesion." *American Journal of Community Psychology* 16 (6): 771–91.

Bulmer, Martin. 1986. *The Chicago School of Sociology: Institutionalization, Diversity, and the Rise of Sociological Research*. Chicago: University of Chicago Press.

Burawoy, Michael. 1982. *Manufacturing Consent: Changes in the Labor Process under Monopoly Capitalism*. Chicago: University of Chicago Press.

Burns, Eric. 2004. *The Spirits of America: A Social History of Alcohol*. Philadelphia: Temple University Press.

Campeau, Anthony G. 2008. "The Space-Control Theory of Paramedic Scene-Management." *Symbolic Interaction* 31 (3): 285–302.

Carey, Mary G., Salah S. Al-Zaiti, Grace E. Dean, Loralee Sessanna, and Deborah S. Finnell. 2011. "Sleep Problems, Depression, Substance Use, Social Bonding, and Quality of Life in Professional Firefighters." *Journal of Occupational and Environmental Medicine* 53 (8): 928.

Cavan, Ruth S. 1928. *Suicide.* New York: Russell & Russell.

Chaix, Basile. 2009. "Geographic Life Environments and Coronary Heart Disease: A Literature Review, Theoretical Contributions, Methodological Updates, and a Research Agenda." *Annual Review of Public Health* 30 (1): 81–105.

Charmaz, Kathy. 1983. "The Grounded Theory Method: An Explication and Interpretation." In *Contemporary Field Research: A Collection of Readings*, edited by Robert Emerson, 109–28. Boston: Little, Brown.

Chetkovich, Carol A. 1997. *Real Heat: Gender and Race in the Urban Fire Service.* New Brunswick, N.J.: Rutgers University Press.

Chibber, Vivek. 2017. "Why We Still Talk about the Working Class." https://www.jacobinmag.com/2017/03/abcs-socialism-working-class-workers-capitalism-power-vivek-chibber/.

Cieri, Marie. 2003. "Between Being and Looking Queer: Tourism Promotion and Lesbian Social Space in Greater Philadelphia." *ACME* 2: 147–66.

Clawson, Dan, and Naomi Gerstel. 2014. *Unequal Time: Gender, Class, and Family in Employment Schedules.* New York: Russell Sage Foundation.

Cohen, Patricia, and Jacob Cohen. 1984. "The Clinician's Illusion." *Archives of General Psychiatry* 41 (12): 1,178–82.

Collins, Pamela Y., Hella von Unger, and Adria Armbrister. 2008. "Church Ladies, Good Girls, and Locas: Stigma and the Intersection of Gender, Ethnicity, Mental Illness, and Sexuality in Relation to HIV Risk." *Social Science & Medicine* 67 (3): 389–97.

Committee on Shock, and Committee on Trauma. Division of Medical Sciences, National Academy of Sciences, and National Research Council. 1966. *Accidental Death and Disability: The Neglected Disease of Modern Society.* Washington, D.C.: National Academies Press.

Connelly, Joe. 1999. *Bringing Out the Dead.* New York: Vintage.

Coontz, Phyllis, Charles Lidz, and Edward Mulvey. 1994. "Gender and the Assessment of Dangerousness in the Psychiatric Emergency Room." *International Journal of Law and Psychiatry* 17: 369–76.

Cope, Meghan, and Sarah Elwood. 2009. *Qualitative GIS: A Mixed Methods Approach.* New York: SAGE.

Corman, Hope, and Nanci Mocan. 2005. "Carrots, Sticks, and Broken Windows." *Journal of Law and Economics* 48 (1): 235–66.

Corman, Michael. 2017. *Paramedics On and Off the Streets: Emergency Medical Services in the Age of Technological Governance.* Toronto: University of Toronto Press.

Corrigan, Patrick. 2004. "How Stigma Interferes with Mental Health Care." *American Psychologist* 59 (7): 614–25. https://doi.org/10.1037/0003-066X.59.7.614.

Corrigan, Patrick, and P. Kleinlein. 2007. "The Impact of Mental Illness Stigma." In *On the Stigma of Mental Illness: Practical Strategies for Research and Social Change*, edited by Patrick Corrigan, 11–44. Washington, D.C.: American Psychological Association.

Crandall, Christian S. 1991. "Multiple Stigma and AIDS: Illness Stigma and Attitudes toward Homosexuals and IV Drug Users in AIDS-related Stigmatization." *Journal of Community Applied Social Psychology* 1: 165–72.

Davis, Kenneth Culp. 1969. *Discretionary Justice: A Preliminary Inquiry*. Baton Rouge: LSU Press.

Dean, Jo, and Annette Hastings. 2000. *Challenging Images: Housing Estates, Stigma and Regeneration*. Bristol: Policy Press.

Dennis, Rutledge M. 2005. *Marginality, Power and Social Structure: Issues in Race, Class and Gender Analysis*. Vol. 12. Amsterdam: Elsevier.

Desai, Mayur M., Robert A. Rosenheck, Benjamin G. Druss, and Jonathan B. Perlin. 2002. "Mental Disorders and Quality of Diabetes Care in the Veterans Health Administration." *American Journal of Psychiatry* 159 (9): 1584–90.

Desmond, Matthew. 2008. *On the Fireline: Living and Dying with Wildland Firefighters*. Chicago: University of Chicago Press.

DeVerteuil, Geoffrey, Jon May, and Jürgen von Mahs. 2009. "Complexity Not Collapse: Recasting the Geographies of Homelessness in a 'Punitive' Age." *Progress in Human Geography* 33 (5): 646–66. https://doi.org/10.1177/0309132508104995.

Dickinson, Wendy B. 2010. "Visual Displays for Mixed Methods Findings." In *SAGE Handbook of Mixed Methods in Social & Behavioral Research*, 469–504. New York: SAGE. https://doi.org/10.4135/9781506335193.n19.

Dongus, Stefan, Dickson Nyika, Khadija Kannady, Deo Mtasiwa, Hassan Mshinda, Ulrike Fillinger, Axel W. Drescher, Marcel Tanner, Marcia C. Castro, and Gerry F. Killeen. 2007. "Participatory Mapping of Target Areas to Enable Operational Larval Source Management to Suppress Malaria Vector Mosquitoes in Dar Es Salaam, Tanzania." *International Journal of Health Geographics* 6 (1): 37. https://doi.org/10.1186/1476-072X-6-37.

Druss, Benjamin G., Robert A. Rosenheck, Mayur M. Desai, and Jonathan B. Perlin. 2002. "Quality of Preventive Medical Care for Patients with Mental Disorders." *Medical Care* 40 (2): 129–36.

Du Bois, William Edward Burghardt, and Isabel Eaton. 1996. *The Philadelphia Negro: A Social Study*. Philadelphia: University of Pennsylvania Press.

Duguid, Paul. 2012. "'The Art of Knowing': Social and Tacit Dimensions of Knowledge and the Limits of the Community of Practice." In *The Knowledge Economy and Lifelong Learning: A Critical Reader*. Knowledge Economy and Education 4. Leiden: Brill Sense.

Dunham, Warren H. 1959. *Sociological Theory and Mental Disorder*. Detroit: Wayne State University Press.

Dunne, Robert J. 2004. "Marginality: A Conceptual Extension." In *Marginality, Power and Social Structure: Issues in Race, Class and Gender Analysis*, 11–27. Amsterdam: Elsevier.

Edwards, Matthew L. 2019. "Pittsburgh's Freedom House Ambulance Service: The Origins of Emergency Medical Services and the Politics of Race and Health." *Journal of the History of Medicine and Allied Sciences* 74 (4): 440–66.

Emerson, Robert M., and Melvin Pollner. 1976. "Dirty Work Designations: Their Features and Consequences in a Psychiatric Setting." *Social Problems* 23 (3): 243–54. https://doi.org/10.2307/799771.

EMS World. 2010. "Medtec Delivers 10 Type I Ambulances to City of New Orleans EMS." *EMS World*. https://www.emsworld.com/news/10336968/medtec-delivers-10-type-i-ambulances-city-new-orleans-ems.

Engels, Friedrich. 1984. *The Condition of the Working Class in England: From Personal Observation and Authentic Sources*. Chicago: Academy Chicago.

Espeland, Wendy Nelson, and Mitchell L. Stevens. 1998. "Commensuration as a Social Process." *Annual Review of Sociology* 24 (1): 313–43. https://doi.org/10.1146/annurev.soc.24.1.313.

Evans, Tony. 2015. "Professionals and Discretion in Street-Level Bureaucracy." In *Understanding Street-Level Bureaucracy*, edited by Peter Hupe, Michael Hill, and Aurélien Buffat. Bristol: Policy Press.

Evans, Tony, and John Harris. 2004. "Street-Level Bureaucracy, Social Work and the (Exaggerated) Death of Discretion." *British Journal of Social Work* 34 (6). https://doi.org/10.1093/bjsw/bch106.

Faris, Robert E., and Warren H. Dunham. 1939. *Mental Disorders in Urban Areas: An Ecological Study of Schizophrenia and Other Psychoses*. Chicago: University of Chicago Press.

Fielding, Nigel, and César A. Cisneros-Puebla. 2010. "CAQDAS-GIS Convergence: Toward a New Integrated Mixed Method Research Practice?" *Journal of Mixed Methods Research* 3 (4): 349–70. https://doi.org/10.1177/1558689809344973.

Fine, Gary Alan. 2008. *Kitchens: The Culture of Restaurant Work*. Berkeley: University of California Press.

Fischer, Pamela, and William R. Breakey. 1991. "The Epidemiology of Alcohol, Drug, and Mental Disorders among Homeless Persons." *American Psychologist* 46 (11): 1,115–28.

Flood, Joe. 2010. *The Fires: How a Computer Formula, Big Ideas, and the Best of Intentions Burned Down New York City–and Determined the Future of Cities*. New York: Penguin.

Ford, Matt. 2015. "America's Largest Mental Hospital Is a Jail—*The Atlantic*." *Atlantic*, June. https://www.theatlantic.com/politics/archive/2015/06/americas-largest-mental-hospital-is-a-jail/395012/.

Forster, D., R. H. Behrens, H. Campbell, and P. Byass. 1991. "Evaluation of a Computerized Field Data Collection System for Health Surveys." *Bulletin of the World Health Organization* 69 (1): 107–11.

Foucault, Michel. 1980. *Power/Knowledge: Selected Interviews and Other Writings, 1972–1977*. New York: Pantheon.

——. 2012. *Discipline and Punish: The Birth of the Prison.* New York: Knopf Doubleday.

Fox, Stephen. 2000. "Communities of Practice, Foucault and Actor-Network Theory." *Journal of Management Studies* 37 (6): 853–68. https://doi.org/10.1111/1467-6486.00207.

Freidson, Eliot. 1988. *Profession of Medicine: A Study of the Sociology of Applied Knowledge.* Chicago: University of Chicago Press.

Freudenburg, William R. 1986. "The Density of Acquaintanceship: An Overlooked Variable in Community Research?" *American Journal of Sociology* 92 (1): 27–63.

Friedman, Steve, Donald Feinsilver, Geri Davis, Ruben Margolis, Oliver David, and Martin Kesselman. 1981. "Decision to Admit in an Inner-City Psychiatric Emergency Room: Beyond Diagnosis—The Psychosocial Factors." *Psychiatric Quarterly* 53: 259–74.

Fuller, Martin G., and Martina Löw. 2017. "Introduction: An Invitation to Spatial Sociology." *Current Sociology* 65 (4): 469–91.

Galster, George C. 2012. "The Mechanism(s) of Neighbourhood Effects: Theory, Evidence, and Policy Implications." In *Neighbourhood Effects Research: New Perspectives*, 23–56. Dordrecht: Springer Netherlands.

Gans, Herbert J. 1972. "The Positive Functions of Poverty." *American Journal of Sociology* 78 (2): 275–89.

Getis, Arthur, and J. Keith Ord. 2010. "The Analysis of Spatial Association by Use of Distance Statistics." In *Perspectives on Spatial Data Analysis*, edited by Luc Anselin and Sergio J. Rey, 127–45. Advances in Spatial Science. Berlin and Heidelberg: Springer. https://doi.org/10.1007/978-3-642-01976-0_10.

Giddens, Anthony. 2013. *The Constitution of Society: Outline of the Theory of Structuration.* Hoboken, N.J.: John Wiley & Sons.

Gilboy, Janet A. 1992. "Penetrability of Administrative System: Political Casework and Immigration Inspections." *Law & Society Review* 26: 273.

Gist, Noel Pitts, and Roy Dean Wright. 1973. *Marginality and Identity: Anglo-Indians as a Racially Mixed Minority in India.* Vol. 3. Leiden: Brill.

Glaser, Barney G. 1978. *Theoretical Sensitivity: Advances in the Methodology of Grounded Theory.* Mill Valley, Calif.: Sociology Press.

Glisson, Charles, and Mark Durick. 1988. "Predictors of Job Satisfaction and Organizational Commitment in Human Service Organizations." *Administrative Science Quarterly* 33 (1): 61–81. https://doi.org/10.2307/2392855.

Glisson, Charles, and Anthony Hemmelgarn. 1998. "The Effects of Organizational Climate and Interorganizational Coordination on the Quality and Outcomes of Children's Service Systems." *Child Abuse & Neglect* 22 (5): 401–21.

Goffman, Erving. 1990. *The Presentation of Self in Everyday Life.* New York: Penguin.

——. 2009. *Stigma: Notes on the Management of Spoiled Identity.* New York: Simon and Schuster.

Gonin, Philippe, Nicolas Beysard, Bertrand Yersin, and Pierre-Nicolas Carron. 2018. "Excited Delirium: A Systematic Review." *Academic Emergency Medicine* 25 (5): 552–65.

Gowan, Teresa. 2010. *Hobos, Hustlers, and Backsliders: Homeless in San Francisco.* Minneapolis: University of Minnesota Press.

Granovetter, Mark. 1973. "The Strength of Weak Ties." *American Journal of Sociology* 78 (6): 1,360–80.

Gravlee, Clarence. 2002. "Mobile Computer-Assisted Personal Interviewing with Handheld Computers: The Entryware System 3.0." *Field Methods* 14 (3): 322–36.

Gravlee, Clarence C., Shannon N. Zenk, Sachiko Woods, Zachary Rowe, and Amy J. Schulz. 2006. "Handheld Computers for Direct Observation of the Social and Physical Environment." *Field Methods* 18 (4): 382–97.

Greenberg, Amy S. 2016. "The Origins of the American Municipal Fire Department: Nineteenth-Century Change from an International Perspective." In *Municipal Services and Employees in the Modern City*, 47–65. London: Routledge.

Gresham, R. 1994. "Does EMS Belong in the Fire Service?" *Emergency Medical Services* 23 (3): 47–48.

Griswold, Sharon K., Carla R. Nordstrom, Sunday Clark, Theodore J. Gaeta, Michelle L. Price, and Carlos A. Camargo Jr. 2015. "Asthma Exacerbations in North American Adults." *CHEST* 127 (5): 1,579–86.

Guerry, Andre-Michel. 2002. *Essai sur la Statistique Morale de La France* [Essay on the Moral Statistics of France]. Lewiston, N.Y.: Edwin Mellen.

Hall, Peter M. 1987. "Presidential Address: Interactionism and the Study of Social Organization." *Sociological Quarterly* 28 (1): 1–22. https://doi.org/10.1111/j.1533-8525.1987.tb00280.x.

Hall, Peter M., and Dee Ann Spencer-Hall. 1982. "The Social Conditions of the Negotiated Order." *Urban Life* 11 (3): 328–49. https://doi.org/10.1177/089124168201100305.

Haller, John S. 1990. "The Beginnings of Urban Ambulance Service in the United States and England." *Journal of Emergency Medicine* 8 (6): 743–55. https://doi.org/10.1016/0736-4679(90)90289-8.

———. 2011. *Battlefield Medicine: A History of the Military Ambulance from the Napoleonic Wars through World War I.* Carbondale, Ill.: SIU Press.

Hanser, Amy. 2012. "Class and the Service Encounter: New Approaches to Inequality in the Service Workplace." *Sociology Compass* 6 (4): 293–305.

Henderson, Alexander. 2013. "Patient Assessment in Emergency Medical Services: Complexity and Uncertainty in Street-Level Patient Processing." *Journal of Health and Human Services Administration* 35 (4): 505–42.

Himmelstein, David U., Deborah Thorne, Elizabeth Warren, and Steffie Woolhandler. 2009. "Medical Bankruptcy in the United States, 2007: Results of a National Study." *American Journal of Medicine* 122 (8): 741–46.

Hjalte, Lena, Bjorn-Ove Suserd, Johan Herlitz, and Karlberg Ingvar. 2007. "Why Are People Without Medical Needs Transported by Ambulance? A Study of

Indications for Pre-Hospital Care." *European Journal of Emergency Medicine* 14: 151–56.

Hughes, Everett C. 1951. "Work and the Self." In *Social Psychology at the Crossroads*, edited by J. Rohrer and M. Sherif, 313–23. New York: Harper and Brothers.

———. 1962. "Good People and Dirty Work." *Social Problems* 10 (1): 3–11.

———. 1971. *The Sociological Eye: Selected Papers*. New Brunswick, N.J.: Transaction.

Institute of Medicine. 2007. *Emergency Medical Services at the Crossroads*. Future of Emergency Care. Washington, D.C.: National Academies Press.

Isett, Kimberly Roussin, Joseph P. Morrissey, and Sharon Topping. 2006. "Systems Ideologies and Street-Level Bureaucrats: Policy Change and Perceptions of Quality in a Behavioral Health Care System." *Public Administration Review* 66 (2): 217–27. https://doi.org/10.1111/j.1540-6210.2006.00574.x.

Ivory, Danielle, Ben Protess, and Kitty Bennett. 2016. "When You Dial 911 and Wall Street Answers." *New York Times*, June. https://www.nytimes.com/2016/06/26/business/dealbook/when-you-dial-911-and-wall-street-answers.html.

Jeffery, Roger. 1979. "Normal Rubbish: Deviant Patients in Casualty Departments." *Sociology of Health & Illness* 1 (1): 90–107. https://doi.org/10.1111/1467-9566.ep11006793.

Jenkins, Thomas H. 2004. "The Marginal Man: Evolution of a Concept." In *Marginality, Power and Social Structure: Issues in Race, Class and Gender Analysis*, 49–67. Amsterdam: Elsevier.

Jones, Nikki, and Christina Jackson. 2011. "'You Don't Go Down There': Learning to Avoid the Ghetto in San Francisco." In *The Ghetto: Contemporary Global Issues and Controversies*, 83–10. Boulder, Colo.: Westview.

Joyce, Steven M., Douglas E. Brown, and Elizabeth A. Nelson. 1996. "Epidemiology of Pediatric EMS Practice: A Multistate Analysis." *Prehospital and Disaster Medicine* 11 (3): 180–87.

Jusionyte, Ieva. 2018. *Threshold: Emergency Responders on the US-Mexico Border*. Berkeley: University of California Press.

Kanter, Rosabeth Moss. 2008. *Men and Women of the Corporation*. New ed. New York: Basic Books.

Kelling, George L., and Catherine M. Coles. 1996. *Fixing Broken Windows: Restoring Order and Reducing Crime in Our Communities*. New York: Free Press.

Kelling, George L., and William H. Sousa. 2001. *Do Police Matter? An Analysis of the Impact of New York City's Police Reforms*. New York: CCI Center for Civic Innovation at the Manhattan Institute, 2001.

Kelling, George L., and James Q. Wilson. 1982. "Broken Windows: The Police and Neighborhood Safety." *Atlantic*, March.

Kellogg, Katherine C., Wanda J. Orlikowski, and JoAnne Yates. 2006. "Life in the Trading Zone: Structuring Coordination across Boundaries in Postbureaucratic Organizations." *Organization Science* 17 (1): 22–44. https://doi.org/10.1287/orsc.1050.0157.

Kelly, Marisa. 1994. "Theories of Justice and Street-Level Discretion1." *Journal of Public Administration Research and Theory* 4 (2): 119–40. https://doi.org/10.1093/oxfordjournals.jpart.a037201.

Kling, Rob. 1996. *Computerization and Controversy: Value Conflicts and Social Choices.* Amsterdam: Elsevier.

Klinger, David A. 1997. "Negotiating Order in Patrol Work: An Ecological Theory of Police Response to Deviance." *Criminology* 35 (2): 277–306. https://doi.org/10.1111/j.1745-9125.1997.tb00877.x.

Knight, Louise W. 2010. *Jane Addams: Spirit in Action.* New York: W. W. Norton.

Knowlton, Amy, et al. 2013. "Patient Demographic and Health Factors Associated with Frequent Use of Emergency Medical Services in a Midsized City." *Academic Emergency Medicine* 20 (11): 1,101–11.

Korczynski, Marek. 2009. "The Mystery Customer: Continuing Absences in the Sociology of Service Work." *Sociology* 43 (5): 952–67.

Koritsas, Stella, Malcolm Boyle, and Jan Coles. 2009. "Factors Associated with Workplace Violence in Paramedics." *Prehospital and Disaster Medicine* 24 (5): 417–21. https://doi.org/10.1017/S1049023X0000724X.

Kozol, Jonathan. 2011. *Rachel and Her Children: Homeless Families in America.* New York: Broadway.

Krieger, Nancy. 1999. "Embodying Inequality: A Review of Concepts, Measures, and Methods for Studying Health Consequences of Discrimination." *International Journal of Health Services* 29 (2): 295–352.

Krysan, Maria. 2002. "Whites Who Say They'd Flee: Who Are They, and Why Would They Leave?" *Demography* 39 (4): 675–96.

Krysan, Maria, Mick P. Couper, Reynolds Farley, and Tyrone A Forman. 2009. "Does Race Matter in Neighborhood Preferences? Results from a Video Experiment." *American Journal of Sociology* 115 (2): 527–59.

LaCalle, Eduardo, and Elaine Rabin. 2010. "Frequent Users of Emergency Departments: The Myths, the Data, and the Policy Implications." *Annals of Emergency Medicine* 56 (1): 42–48.

Lalli, Marco. 1992. "Urban-Related Identity: Theory, Measurement, and Empirical Findings." *Journal of Environmental Psychology* 12 (4): 285–303.

Lamb, H. Richard, and Leona L. Bachrach. 2001. "Some Perspectives on Deinstitutionalization." *Psychiatric Services* 52 (8): 1039–45.

Lee, Barrett A., Kimberly A. Tyler, and James D. Wright. 2010. "The New Homelessness Revisited." *Annual Review of Sociology* 36: 501–21.

Lefebvre, Henri. 1991. *The Production of Space.* Translated by Donald Nicholson-Smith. Vol. 142. Oxford: Blackwell.

———. 1996. *Writings on Cities.* Hoboken, N.J.: John Wiley & Sons.

Leiderman, Deborah B., and Jean-Anne Grisso. 1985. "The Gomer Phenomenon." *Journal of Health and Social Behavior* 26 (3): 222–32. https://doi.org/10.2307/2136754.

Leidner, Robin. 1993. *Fast Food, Fast Talk: Service Work and the Routinization of Everyday Life.* Berkeley: University of California Press.

Levy, Karen E. C. 2015. "The Contexts of Control: Information, Power, and Truck-Driving Work." *Information Society* 31 (2): 160–74. https://doi.org/10.1080/01972243.2015.998105.

Lincoln, Alisa K. 2006. "Psychiatric Emergency Room Decision-Making, Social Control and the 'Undeserving Sick.'" *Sociology of Health & Illness* 28 (1): 54–75.

Lincoln, Alisa K., Andrew White, Casandra Aldsworth, Peggy Johnson, and Lee Strunin. 2010. "Observing the Work of an Urban Safety-Net Psychiatric Emergency Room: Managing the Unmanageable." *Sociology of Health & Illness* 32 (3): 437–51.

Lindsey, Kenneth, and Gordon Paul. 1989. "Involuntary Commitments to Public Mental Institutions: Issues Involving the Overrepresentation of Blacks and Assessment of Relevant Functioning." *Psychological Bulletin* 106: 171–83.

Link, Bruce G. 1982. "Mental Patient Status, Work, and Income: An Examination of the Effects of a Psychiatric Label." *American Sociological Review* 47 (2): 202–15. https://doi.org/10.2307/2094963.

———. 1987. "Understanding Labeling Effects in the Area of Mental Disorders: An Assessment of the Effects of Expectations of Rejection." *American Sociological Review* 52 (1): 96–112. https://doi.org/10.2307/2095395.

Link, Bruce G., Francis T. Cullen, J. Frank, and J. Wozniak. 1987. "The Social Rejection of Former Mental Patients: Understanding Why Labels Matter." *American Journal of Sociology* 92 (6): 1,461–500.

Link, Bruce G., Francis T. Cullen, Elmer Struening, Patrick E. Shrout, and Bruce P. Dohrenwend. 1989. "A Modified Labeling Theory Approach to Mental Disorders: An Empirical Assessment." *American Sociological Review* 54 (3): 400. https://doi.org/10.2307/2095613.

Link, Bruce G., Jerrold Mirotznik, and Francis T. Cullen. 1991. "The Effectiveness of Stigma Coping Orientations: Can Negative Consequences of Mental Illness Labeling Be Avoided?" *Journal of Health and Social Behavior*, 302–20.

Link, Bruce G., and Jo [C.] Phelan. 1995. "Social Conditions as Fundamental Causes of Disease." *Journal of Health and Social Behavior*, 80–94. https://doi.org/10.2307/2626958.

———. 2001. "Conceptualizing Stigma." *Annual Review of Sociology* 27: 263–85.

———. 2013. "Labeling and Stigma." In *Handbook of the Sociology of Mental Health*, edited by Carol S. Aneshensel, Jo C. Phelan, and Alex Bierman, 525–41. Handbooks of Sociology and Social Research. Dordrecht: Springer Netherlands. https://doi.org/10.1007/978-94-007-4276-5_25.

Link, Bruce G., Sharon Schwartz, Robert Moore, Jo Phelan, Elmer Struening, Ann Stueve, and Mary Ellen Colten. 1995. "Public Knowledge, Attitudes, and Beliefs about Homeless People: Evidence for Compassion Fatigue?" *American Journal of Community Psychology* 23 (4): 533–55. https://doi.org/10.1007/BF02506967.

Link, Bruce G., Elmer L. Struening, et al. 1997. "On Stigma and Its Consequences: Evidence from a Longitudinal Study of Men with Dual Diagnoses of Mental Illness and Substance Abuse." *Journal of Health and Social Behavior* 38: 177–90.

Link, Bruce G., and Heather Stuart. 2017. "On Revisiting Some Origins of the Stigma Concept as It Applies to Mental Illnesses." In *The Stigma of Mental Illness—End of the Story?*, edited by Wolfgang Gaebel, Wulf Rössler, and Norman Sartorius, 3–28. Cham: Springer. https://doi.org/10.1007/978-3-319-27839-1_1.

Lipsky, Michael. 1980. *Street-Level Bureaucracy: The Dilemmas of the Individual in Public Service.* New York: Russell Sage Foundation.

Logan, John R. 2012. "Making a Place for Space: Spatial Thinking in Social Science." *Annual Review of Sociology* 38: 507–24.

Logan, John R., and Harvey Luskin Molotch. 2007. *Urban Fortunes: The Political Economy of Place.* Berkeley: University of California Press.

Logie, Carmen H., Llana James, Wangari Tharao, and Mona R. Loutfy. 2011. "HIV, Gender, Race, Sexual Orientation, and Sex Work: A Qualitative Study of Intersectional Stigma Experienced by HIV-Positive Women in Ontario, Canada." *PLoS Medicine* 8 (11): e1001124-12.

Lopez, Steven Henry. 2010. "Workers, Managers, and Customers: Triangles of Power in Work Communities." *Work and Occupations* 37 (3): 251–71. https://doi.org/10.1177/0730888410375683.

Löw, Martina. 2016. *The Sociology of Space: Materiality, Social Structures, and Action.* New York: Palgrave Macmillan.

Loyens, Kim, and Jeroen Maesschalck. 2010. "Toward a Theoretical Framework for Ethical Decision Making of Street-Level Bureaucracy: Existing Models Reconsidered." *Administration & Society* 42 (1): 66–100. https://doi.org/10.1177/0095399710362524.

Lyon-Callo, Vincent. 2000. "Medicalizing Homelessness: The Production of Self-Blame and Self-Governing within Homeless Shelters." *Medical Anthropology Quarterly* 14 (3): 328–45. https://doi.org/10.1525/maq.2000.14.3.328.

Macintyre, Sally, Anne Ellaway, and Steven Cummins. 2002. "Place Effects on Health: How Can We Conceptualise, Operationalise and Measure Them?" *Social Science & Medicine* 55 (1): 125–39.

Maines, D. R. 1977. "Social Organization and Social Structure in Symbolic Interactionist Thought." *Annual Review of Sociology* 3 (1): 235–59. https://doi.org/10.1146/annurev.so.03.080177.001315.

Major, Brenda, and Laurie T. O'Brien. 2005. "The Social Psychology of Stigma." *Annual Review of Psychology* 56 (1): 393–421.

Mancini Billson, Janet. 2004. "No Owner of Soil: Redefining the Concept of Marginality." In *Marginality, Power and Social Structure: Issues in Race, Class and Gender Analysis*, 29–47. Amsterdam: Elsevier.

Mannon, James M. 1992. *Emergency Encounters: EMTs and Their Work.* Boston: Jones and Bartlett.

Marschall, Daniel. 2014. *The Company We Keep: Occupational Community in the High-Tech Network Society*. Philadelphia: Temple University Press.

Mathieu, Arline. 1993. "The Medicalization of Homelessness and the Theater of Repression." *Medical Anthropology Quarterly* 7 (2): 170–84. https://doi.org/10.1525/maq.1993.7.2.02a00030.

May, Peter J., and Soren C. Winter. 2009. "Politicians, Managers, and Street-Level Bureaucrats: Influences on Policy Implementation." *Journal of Public Administration Research and Theory* 19 (3): 453–76. https://doi.org/10.1093/jopart/mum030.

Mayhew, Henry. 1861. *London Labour and the London Poor: The Condition and Earnings of Those That Will Work, Cannot Work, and Will Not Work*. London: C. Griffin.

Maynard-Moody, Steven Williams, and Michael Craig Musheno. 2009. *Cops, Teachers, Counselors: Stories from the Front Lines of Public Service*. Ann Arbor: University of Michigan Press.

McLeod, Kari S. 2000. "Our Sense of Snow: The Myth of John Snow in Medical Geography." *Social Science & Medicine* 50 (7–8): 923–35.

McManamny, Tegwyn, Jade Sheen, Leanne Boyd, and Paul A Jennings. 2015. "Mixed Methods and Its Application in Prehospital Research: A Systematic Review." *Journal of Mixed Methods Research* 9 (3): 214–31.

Meanwell, Emily. 2012. "Experiencing Homelessness: A Review of Recent Literature." *Sociology Compass* 6 (1): 72–85. https://doi.org/10.1111/j.1751-9020.2011.00432.x.

Mechanic, David, and David A. Rochefort. 1990. "Deinstitutionalization: An Appraisal of Reform." *Annual Review of Sociology* 16 (1): 301–27.

Mellinger, Wayne M. 1992. "Talk-as-Work: The Case of Paramedic Calls for Emergency Orders." *Current Research on Occupations and Professions* 7: 79–109.

———. 1994. "Negotiated Orders: The Negotiation of Directives in Paramedic-Nurse Interaction." *Symbolic Interaction* 17 (2): 165–85.

Merton, Robert K. 1995. "The Thomas Theorem and The Matthew Effect." *Social Forces* 74 (2): 379–422.

Metz, Donald L. 1981. *Running Hot: Structure and Stress in Ambulance Work*. Cambridge, Mass.: Abt.

Meyer, Ilan H. 2007. "Prejudice and Discrimination as Social Stressors." In *The Health of Sexual Minorities*, edited by Ilan H. Meyer and Mary E. Northridge, 242–67. Dordrecht: Springer.

Milbrett, Pat, and Margo Halm. 2009. "Characteristics and Predictors of Frequent Utilization of Emergency Services." *Journal of Emergency Nursing* 35 (3): 191–98.

Monkkonen, Eric H. 2004. *Police in Urban America, 1860–1920*. Cambridge and New York: Cambridge University Press.

Morris, Aldon. 2017. *The Scholar Denied: W. E. B. Du Bois and the Birth of Modern Sociology*. Berkeley: University of California Press.

Morse, Janice (M.). 2010. "Procedures and Practice of Mixed Method Design: Maintaining Control, Rigor, and Complexity." In *SAGE Handbook of Mixed Methods in Social & Behavioral Research*, 339–52. New York: SAGE. https://doi.org/10.4135/9781506335193.n14.

———. 2016. *Mixed Method Design: Principles and Procedures*. London and New York: Routledge.

National Center for Health Statistics. 2018. "National Hospital Ambulatory Medical Care Survey: 2015 Emergency Department Summary Tables," 1–34.

"National Registry of Emergency Medical Technicians." n.d. Accessed February 17, 2021. https://nremt.org.

Newman, Katherine S. 2000. *No Shame in My Game: The Working Poor in the Inner City*. New York: Vintage.

Nichol, Graham, Allan S. Detsky, Ian G. Stiell, Keith O'Rourke, George Wells, and Andreas Laupacis. 1996. "Effectiveness of Emergency Medical Services for Victims of Out-of-Hospital Cardiac Arrest: A Meta-analysis." *Annals of Emergency Medicine* 27 (6): 700–710. https://doi.org/10.1016/S0196-0644(96)70187-7.

Norman, Chenelle, Michael Mello, and Bryan Choi. 2016. "Identifying Frequent Users of an Urban Emergency Medical Service Using Descriptive Statistics and Regression Analyses." *Western Journal of Emergency Medicine* 17 (1): 39–45.

Oakes, J. Michael. 2004. "The (Mis) Estimation of Neighborhood Effects: Causal Inference for a Practicable Social Epidemiology." *Social Science & Medicine* 58 (10): 1929–52.

O'Brien, Daniel Tumminelli, and David Sloan Wilson. 2011. "Community Perception: The Ability to Assess the Safety of Unfamiliar Neighborhoods and Respond Adaptively." *Journal of Personality and Social Psychology* 100 (4): 606–20.

O'Neill, Bruce. 2017. *The Space of Boredom: Homelessness in the Slowing Global Order*. Durham, N.C.: Duke University Press.

Orr, Julian E. 2016. *Talking about Machines: An Ethnography of a Modern Job*. Ithaca, N.Y.: Cornell University Press.

Osterlund, Carsten, and Paul Carlile. 2005. "Relations in Practice: Sorting through Practice Theories on Knowledge Sharing in Complex Organizations." *Information Society* 21 (2): 91–107.

Palmer, C. Eddie. 1983. "'Trauma Junkies' and Street Work: Occupational Behavior of Paramedics and Emergency Medical Technicians." *Urban Life* 12 (2): 162–83.

———. 1989. "Paramedic Performances." *Sociological Spectrum* 9 (2): 211–25.

Palmer, C. Eddie, and Sheryl M. Gonsoulin. 1990. "Paramedics, Protocols, and Procedures: 'Playing Doc' as Deviant Role Performance." *Deviant Behavior* 11 (3): 207–19.

Pantridge, J. F., and J. S. Geddes. 1967. "A Mobile Intensive-Care Unit in the Management of Myocardial Infarction." *Lancet* 290 (7510): 271–73.

Park, Robert E. 1928. "Human Migration and the Marginal Man." *American Journal of Sociology* 33 (6): 881–93.

Park, Robert E., and Ernest W Burgess. 1967. *The City: Suggestions for Investigation of Human Behavior in the Urban Environment*. Chicago: University of Chicago Press.

Patnaik, S., E. Brunskill, and W. Thies. 2009. "Evaluating the Accuracy of Data Collection on Mobile Phones: A Study of Forms, SMS, and Voice." In *2009 International Conference on Information and Communication Technologies and Development (ICTD)*, 74–84. https://doi.org/10.1109/ICTD.2009.5426700.

Patrick, William B. 2005. *Saving Troy: A Year with Firefighters and Paramedics in a Battered City*. Troy, N.Y.: Hudson Whitman.

Patterson, P. Daniel, Brian P. Suffoletto, Douglas F. Kupas, Matthew D. Weaver, and David Hostler. 2010. "Sleep Quality and Fatigue among Prehospital Providers." *Prehospital Emergency Care* 14 (2): 187–93.

Patterson, P. Daniel, Matthew D. Weaver, David Hostler, Francis X. Guyette, Clifton W. Callaway, and Donald M. Yealy. 2012. "The Shift Length, Fatigue, and Safety Conundrum in EMS." *Prehospital Emergency Care* 16 (4): 572–76.

Paul, David A. 2020. "The Death of Daniel Prude—Reflections of a Black Neurosurgeon." *New England Journal of Medicine* 383 (24): e135.

Peck, Jamie. 2012. "Austerity Urbanism." *City* 16 (6): 626–55. https://doi.org/10.1080/13604813.2012.734071.

Peltonen, Tuomo. 2007. "In the Middle of Managers' Occupational Communities, Global Ethnography and the Multinationals." *Ethnography* 8 (3): 346–60.

Perlow, Leslie. 1999. "The Time Famine: Toward a Sociology of Work Time." *Administrative Science Quarterly* 44 (1): 57–81.

Pescosolido, Bernice A. 2013. "The Public Stigma of Mental Illness: What Do We Think; What Do We Know; What Can We Prove?" *Journal of Health and Social Behavior* 54 (1): 1–21. https://doi.org/10.1177/0022146512471197.

Pescosolido, Bernice A., Jack K. Martin, Annie Lang, and Sigrun Olafsdottir. 2008. "Rethinking Theoretical Approaches to Stigma: A Framework Integrating Normative Influences on Stigma (FINIS)." *Social Science & Medicine, Stigma, Prejudice, Discrimination and Health* 67 (3): 431–40. https://doi.org/10.1016/j.socscimed.2008.03.018.

Pescosolido, Bernice A., Jack K. Martin, J. Scott Long, Tait R. Medina, Jo C. Phelan, and Bruce G. Link. 2010. "'A Disease Like Any Other'? A Decade of Change in Public Reactions to Schizophrenia, Depression, and Alcohol Dependence." *American Journal of Psychiatry* 167 (11): 1321–30. https://doi.org/10.1176/appi.ajp.2010.09121743.

Petrillo, Adam. 2011. "Ambulance Makers Offer Roomier, Larger Rigs." *Fire Apparatus*. May. https://www.fireapparatusmagazine.com/ems/ambulance-makers-offer-roomier-larger-rigs/.

Phelan, Jo, Bruce G. Link, Robert E. Moore, and Ann Stueve. 1997. "The Stigma of Homelessness: The Impact of the Label 'Homeless' on Attitudes Toward Poor Persons." *Social Psychology Quarterly* 60 (4): 323–37. https://doi.org/10.2307/2787093.

Phelan, Jo, Bruce G. Link, Ann Stueve, and Robert E. Moore. 1995. "Education, Social Liberalism, and Economic Conservatism: Attitudes Toward Homeless People." *American Sociological Review* 60 (1): 126–40. https://doi.org/10.2307/2096349.

Phelan, Jo C., Bruce G. Link, Ann Stueve, and Bernice A. Pescosolido. 2000. "Public Conceptions of Mental Illness in 1950 and 1996: What Is Mental Illness and Is It to Be Feared?" *Journal of Health and Social Behavior* 41 (2): 188–207. https://doi.org/10.2307/2676305.

Poteat, Tonia, Danielle German, and Deanna Kerrigan. 2013. "Managing Uncertainty: A Grounded Theory of Stigma in Transgender Health Care Encounters." *Social Science & Medicine* 84 (May): 22–29.

Pourshaikhian, Majid, Hassan Abolghasem Gorji, Aidin Aryankhesal, Davood Khorasani-Zavareh, and Ahmad Barati. 2016. "A Systematic Literature Review: Workplace Violence against Emergency Medical Services Personnel." *Archives of Trauma Research* 5 (1). https://doi.org/10.5812/atr.28734.

Powell, Walter W., and Kaisa Snellman. 2004. "The Knowledge Economy." *Annual Review of Sociology* 30: 199–220.

Pozner, Charles N., Richard Zane, Stephen J. Nelson, and Michael Levine. 2004. "International EMS Systems: The United States: Past, Present, and Future." *Resuscitation* 60 (3): 239–44. https://doi.org/10.1016/j.resuscitation.2003.11.004.

Prener, Christopher. 2021. "Digitizing and Visualizing Sketch Map Data: A Semi-Structured Approach to Qualitative GIS." *Cartographica: International Journal for Geographic Information and Geovisualization* 56 (4): 267–83.

Prener, Christopher, and Alisa K. Lincoln. 2015. "Emergency Medical Services and 'Psych Calls': Examining the Work of Urban EMS Providers." *American Journal of Orthopsychiatry* 85 (6): 612–19.

President's Committee for Traffic Safety. 1965. *Health, Medical Care and Transportation of the Injured: A Section of the Action Program for Highway Safety*. Washington, D.C.: U.S. Government Printing Office.

Quillian, Lincoln, and Devah Pager. 2001. "Black Neighbors, Higher Crime? The Role of Racial Stereotypes in Evaluations of Neighborhood Crime." *American Journal of Sociology* 107 (3): 717–67.

Rolland, Knut H., and Eric Monteiro. 2002. "Balancing the Local and the Global in Infrastructural Information Systems." *Information Society* 18 (2): 87–100. https://doi.org/10.1080/01972240290075020.

Roschelle, Anne R., and Peter Kaufman. 2004. "Fitting In and Fighting Back: Stigma Management Strategies among Homeless Kids." *Symbolic Interaction* 27 (1): 23–46. https://doi.org/10.1525/si.2004.27.1.23.

Rosenfield, Sarah. 1997. "Labeling Mental Illness: The Effects of Received Services and Perceived Stigma on Life Satisfaction." *American Sociological Review* 62 (4): 660–72. https://doi.org/10.2307/2657432.

Ross, Catherine E., and John Mirowsky. 2001. "Neighborhood Disadvantage, Disorder, and Health." *Journal of Health and Social Behavior* 42 (3): 258–76.

Roth, Julius A. 1972. "Some Contingencies of the Moral Evaluation and Control of Clientele: The Case of the Hospital Emergency Service." *American Journal of Sociology* 77 (5): 839–56. https://doi.org/10.1086/225227.

Ruger, Jennifer Prah, Christopher J. Richter, and Lawrence M. Lewis. 2006. "Clinical and Economic Factors Associated with Ambulance Use to the Emergency Department." *Academic Emergency Medicine* 13 (8): 879–85.

Rush, Ladonna. 1998. "Affective Reactions to Multiple Social Stigmas." *Journal of Social Psychology* 138 (4): 421–30.

Sallaz, Jeff. 2009. *The Labor of Luck: Casino Capitalism in the United States and South Africa*. Berkeley: University of California Press.

Sampson, Robert J. 1988. "Local Friendship Ties and Community Attachment in Mass Society: A Multilevel Systemic Model." *American Sociological Review* 53 (5): 766–79.

———. 2012. *Great American City: Chicago and the Enduring Neighborhood Effect*. Chicago: University of Chicago Press.

———. 2013. "The Place of Context: A Theory and Strategy for Criminology's Hard Problems." *Criminology* 51 (1): 1–31.

Sampson, Robert J., and Stephen W. Raudenbush. 2004. "Seeing Disorder: Neighborhood Stigma and the Social Construction of 'Broken Windows.'" *Social Psychology Quarterly* 67 (4): 319–42.

Sampson, Robert J., Stephen W. Raudenbush, and Felton Earls. 1997. "Neighborhoods and Violent Crime: A Multilevel Study of Collective Efficacy." *Science* 277 (5328): 918–24.

Sanko, Stephen, Saman Kashani, Terrance Ito, Aaron Guggenheim, Shangnon Fei, and Marc Eckstein. 2020. "Advanced Practice Providers in the Field: Implementation of the Los Angeles Fire Department Advanced Provider Response Unit." *Prehospital Emergency Care* 24 (5): 693–703.

Sauder, Michael, and Wendy Nelson Espeland. 2009. "The Discipline of Rankings: Tight Coupling and Organizational Change." *American Sociological Review* 74 (1): 63–82. https://doi.org/10.1177/000312240907400104.

Schrack, Dan. 2020. "Daniel Prude's Death Raises Concerns about Police Response to Mental Health Cases." *WHAM*, September. https://13wham.com/news/local/daniel-prudes-death-raises-concerns-about-police-response-to-mental-health-calls.

Scott, James C. 2008. *Weapons of the Weak: Everyday Forms of Peasant Resistance*. New Haven, Conn.: Yale University Press. Originally published in 1985.

Scott, Patrick G. 1997. "Assessing Determinants of Bureaucratic Discretion: An Experiment in Street-Level Decision Making." *Journal of Public Administration Research and Theory* 7 (1): 35–58. https://doi.org/10.1093/oxfordjournals.jpart.a024341.

Seim, Josh. 2017. "The Ambulance: Toward a Labor Theory of Poverty Governance." *American Sociological Review* 82 (3): 451–75.

———. 2020. *Bandage, Sort, and Hustle: Ambulance Crews on the Front Lines of Urban Suffering*. Berkeley: University of California Press.

Seim, Josh, Joshua English, and Karl Sporer. 2017. "Neighborhood Poverty and 9-1-1 Ambulance Contacts." *Prehospital Emergency Care* 21 (6): 722–28.

Seim, Josh, Melody J. Glenn, Joshua English, and Karl Sporer. 2018. "Neighborhood Poverty and 9-1-1 Ambulance Response Time." *Prehospital Emergency Care* 25 (1): 1–9.

Shah, Manish N. 2006. "The Formation of the Emergency Medical Services System." *American Journal of Public Health* 96 (3): 414–23.

Shah, Manish N., Jeffrey J. Bazarian, E. Brooke Lerner, Rollin J. Fairbanks, William H. Barker, Peggy Auinger, and Bruce Friedman. 2007. "The Epidemiology of Emergency Medical Services Use by Older Adults: An Analysis of the National Hospital Ambulatory Medical Care Survey." *Academic Emergency Medicine* 14 (5): 441–47.

Shah, Manish N., Jeremy T. Cushman, Colleen O. Davis, Jeffrey J. Bazarian, Peggy Auinger, and Bruce Friedman. 2008. "The Epidemiology of Emergency Medical Services Use by Children: An Analysis of the National Hospital Ambulatory Medical Care Survey." *Prehospital Emergency Care* 12 (3): 269–76.

Shah, Manish N., Cai Glushak, Theodore G. Karrison, Robert Mulliken, James Walter, Peter D. Friedmann, Deon C. Hayley, and Marshall H. Chin. 2003. "Predictors of Emergency Medical Services Utilization by Elders." *Academic Emergency Medicine* 10 (1): 52–58.

Sharkey, Patrick T. 2006. "Navigating Dangerous Streets: The Sources and Consequences of Street Efficacy." *American Sociological Review* 71 (5): 826–46.

Shaw, Arthur, Lena Nguyen, Ulrike Nischan, and Herschel Sy. 2011. "Comparative Assessment of Software Programs for the Development of Computer-Assisted Personal Interview (CAPI) Applications." *IRIS Center.*

Shaw, Clifford R., and Henry D. McKay. 1969. *Juvenile Delinquency and Urban Areas.* Chicago: University of Chicago Press.

Shem, Samuel. 2010. *House of God.* New York: Berkley.

Shlay, Anne B., and Peter H. Rossi. 1992. "Social Science Research and Contemporary Studies of Homelessness." *Annual Review of Sociology* 18 (1): 129–60.

Simmel, Georg. 1950. *The Sociology of Georg Simmel.* New York: Simon and Schuster.

Sletto, Bjørn. 2015. "Inclusions, Erasures and Emergences in an Indigenous Landscape: Participatory Cartographies and the Makings of Affective Place in the Sierra de Perijá, Venezuela." *Environment and Planning D: Society and Space* 33 (5): 925–44. https://doi.org/10.1177/0263775815604927.

Small, Mario L(uis). 2004. *Villa Victoria: The Transformation of Social Capital in a Boston Barrio.* Chicago: University of Chicago Press.

——. 2011. "How to Conduct a Mixed Methods Study: Recent Trends in a Rapidly Growing Literature." *Annual Review of Sociology* 37: 57–86.

Smith, R. S. 1995. "Giving Credit Where Credit Is Due: Dorothy Swaine Thomas and the 'Thomas Theorem.'" *American Sociologist* 26 (4): 9–28.

Snooks, Helen, J. Dale, C. Hartley-Sharpe, and M. Halter. 2004. "On-Scene Alternatives for Emergency Ambulance Crews Attending Patients Who Do Not Need to Travel to the Accident and Emergency Department: A Review of the Literature." *Emergency Medicine Journal* 21: 212–15.

Snooks, Helen, Hannah Wrigley, Steve George, Eileen Thomas, Helen Smith, and Alan Glasper. 1998. "Appropriateness of Use of Emergency Ambulances." *Journal of Accident and Emergency Medicine* 15: 212–18.

Snow, David A., and Leon Anderson. 1993. *Down on Their Luck: A Study of Homeless Street People*. Berkeley: University of California Press.

Snow, David A., Susan G. Baker, Leon Anderson, and Michaei Martin. 1986. "The Myth of Pervasive Mental Illness Among the Homeless." *Social Problems* 33 (5): 407–23. https://doi.org/10.2307/800659.

Snow, David A., and Michael Mulcahy. 2001. "Space, Politics, and the Survival Strategies of the Homeless." *American Behavioral Scientist* 45 (1): 149–69. https://doi.org/10.1177/00027640121956962.

Snow, John. 1855. *On the Mode of Communication of Cholera*. London: John Churchill.

Soja, Edward W. 1996. *Thirdspace: Journeys to Los Angeles and Other Real-and-Imagined Places*. Hoboken, N.J.: John Wiley & Sons.

Squires, Peter, and John Lea. 2012. *Criminalisation and Advanced Marginality: Critically Exploring the Work of Loïc Wacquant*. Bristol: Policy Press.

Stafford, Mai, Mel Bartley, Amanda Sacker, Michael Marmot, Richard Wilkinson, Richard Boreham, and Roger Thomas. 2003. "Measuring the Social Environment: Social Cohesion and Material Deprivation in English and Scottish Neighbourhoods." *Environment and Planning* 35 (8): 1459–75.

Star, Susan Leigh. 1995. "Epilogue: Work and Practice in Social Studies of Science, Medicine, and Technology." *Science, Technology, & Human Values* 20 (4): 501–7.

Storper, Michael. 2013. *Keys to the City: How Economics, Institutions, Social Interaction, and Politics Shape Development*. Princeton: Princeton University Press.

Stratton, Samuel J., Christopher Rogers, Karen Brickett, and Ginger Gruzinski. 2001. "Factors Associated with Sudden Death of Individuals Requiring Restraint for Excited Delirium." *American Journal of Emergency Medicine* 19 (3): 187–91.

Strauss, Anselm (L.). 1985. "Work and the Division of Labor." *Sociological Quarterly* 26 (1): 1–19. https://doi.org/10.1111/j.1533-8525.1985.tb00212.x.

———. 1988. *Negotiations: Varieties, Contexts, Processes, and Social Order*. San Francisco: Jossey-Bass.

———. 2008. *Continual Permutations of Action*. New Brunswick, N.J.: Aldine Transaction.

Stuart, Forrest. 2014. "From 'Rabble Management' to 'Recovery Management': Policing Homelessness in Marginal Urban Space." *Urban Studies* 51 (9): 1909–25.

———. 2016. *Down, Out, and Under Arrest: Policing and Everyday Life in Skid Row*. Chicago: University of Chicago Press.

Tangherlini, Timothy. 1998. *Talking Trauma: Paramedics and Their Stories*. Jackson: University Press of Mississippi.

Tashakkori, Abbas, and Charles Teddlie. 2010. *SAGE Handbook of Mixed Methods in Social & Behavioral Research*. New York: SAGE.

Taylor, Marilyn. 1998. "Combating the Social Exclusion of Housing Estates." *Housing Studies* 13 (6): 819–32.

Taylor, Phil, and Peter Bain. 2003. "'Subterranean Worksick Blues': Humour as Subversion in Two Call Centres." *Organization Studies* 24 (9): 1,487–509.

Timmermans, Stefan. 2010. *Sudden Death and the Myth of CPR*. Philadelphia: Temple University Press.

Toro, Paul A., et al. 2007. "Homelessness in Europe and the United States: A Comparison of Prevalence and Public Opinion." *Journal of Social Issues* 63 (3): 505–24. https://doi.org/10.1111/j.1540-4560.2007.00521.x.

University of Rochester. n.d. "News & Archives—Equity & Anti-Racism Action Plan—University of Rochester Medical Center." Accessed February 9, 2021. https://www.urmc.rochester.edu/equity-antiracism-action-plan/news.aspx.

URochesterWC4BL. n.d. "An Open Letter to the University of Rochester Following the Murder of Daniel Prude." Accessed February 9, 2021. https://medium.com/@urochesterwc4bl/an-open-letter-to-the-university-of-rochester-following-the-murder-of-daniel-prude-9b5684d0c677.

Uzzell, David, Enric Pol, and David Badenas. 2002. "Place Identification, Social Cohesion, and Environmental Sustainability." *Environment and Behavior* 34 (1): 26–53.

Van Maanen, John, and Stephen R. Barley. 1984. "Occupational Communities: Culture and Control in Organizations." *Research in Organizational Behavior* 6: 287–365.

Venkatesh, Sudhir Alladi. 2009. *American Project: The Rise and Fall of a Modern Ghetto*. Cambridge, Mass.: Harvard University Press.

Vilke, Gary M., et al. 2012. "Excited Delirium Syndrome (ExDS): Defining Based on a Review of the Literature." *Journal of Emergency Medicine* 43 (5): 897–905.

Vinzant, Janet Coble, Janet Vinzant Denhardt, and Lane Crothers. 1998. *Street-Level Leadership: Discretion and Legitimacy in Front-Line Public Service*. Washington, D.C.: Georgetown University Press.

Wacquant, Loïc. 1993. "Urban Outcasts: Stigma and Division in the Black American Ghetto and French Urban Periphery." *International Journal of Urban and Regional Research* 17 (3): 366–83.

——. 2008. *Urban Outcasts: A Comparative Sociology of Advanced Marginality*. Walden, Mass.: Polity.

——. 2009. *Punishing the Poor: The Neoliberal Government of Social Insecurity*. Durham, N.C.: Duke University Press.

——. 2016. "Territorial Stigmatization in the Age of Advanced Marginality." *Thesis Eleven* 91 (1): 66–77.

Weimann, Gabriel. 1982. "On the Importance of Marginality: One More Step into the Two-Step Flow of Communication." *American Sociological Review* 47 (6): 764–74.

Weiner, Dan, and Trevor Harris. 2003. "Community-Integrated GIS for Land Reform." *URISA Journal* 15 (2).

Weisberger, Adam. 1992. "Marginality and Its Directions." *Sociological Forum* 7 (3): 425–46.

Whalley, Peter, and Stephen R. Barley. 1997. "Technical Work in the Division: Stalking the Wily Anomaly." In *Between Craft and Science: Technical Work in the U.S. Settings*, edited by Stephen R. Barley and Julian E. Orr, 24–52. Ithaca, N.Y.: ILR Press.

Whyte, William Foote. 1993. *Street Corner Society: The Social Structure of an Italian Slum*. Chicago: University of Chicago Press.

Wilson, William Julius. 2011. *When Work Disappears: The World of the New Urban Poor*. New York: Knopf Doubleday.

——. 2012. *The Truly Disadvantaged: The Inner City, the Underclass, and Public Policy*. 2nd ed. Chicago: University of Chicago Press.

Wingfield, Adia Harvey. 2009. "Racializing the Glass Escalator: Reconsidering Men's Experiences with Women's Work." *Gender & Society* 23 (1): 5–26.

——. 2013. *No More Invisible Man: Race and Gender in Men's Work*. Philadelphia: Temple University Press.

Wooten, Lynn Perry, and Patricia Crane. 2004. "Generating Dynamic Capabilities through a Humanistic Work Ideology: The Case of a Certified-Nurse Midwife Practice in a Professional Bureaucracy." *American Behavioral Scientist* 47 (6): 848–66. https://doi.org/10.1177/0002764203260213.

Wridt, Pamela. 2010. "A Qualitative GIS Approach to Mapping Urban Neighborhoods with Children to Promote Physical Activity and Child-Friendly Community Planning." *Environment and Planning B: Planning and Design* 37 (1): 129–47. https://doi.org/10.1068/b35002.

Yates, JoAnne. 1993. *Control Through Communication: The Rise of System in American Management*. Baltimore: Johns Hopkins University Press.

Zandbergen, Paul A. 2009. "Accuracy of IPhone Locations: A Comparison of Assisted GPS, WiFi and Cellular Positioning." *Transactions in GIS* 13 (s1): 5–25. https://doi.org/10.1111/j.1467-9671.2009.01152.x.

Zandbergen, Paul A., and Sean J. Barbeau. 2011. "Positional Accuracy of Assisted GPS Data from High-Sensitivity GPS-Enabled Mobile Phones." *Journal of Navigation* 64 (3): 381–99. https://doi.org/10.1017/S0373463311000051.

Zink, Brian J. 2005. *Anyone, Anything, Anytime: A History of Emergency Medicine*. Philadelphia: Elsevier Health Sciences.

Index

Christopher G. Prener was Assistant Professor in the Department of Sociology and Anthropology at Saint Louis University from 2015 until 2022. In addition to researching stigma, mental health, and neighborhood disorder in a variety of settings, his research explored the consequences of historical segregation for contemporary life in St. Louis, Missouri. He is also a former Emergency Medical Technician and EMS dispatcher. He is now working as a research scientist outside of academia.

POLIS: Fordham Series in Urban Studies
Edited by Daniel J. Monti, Saint Louis University

Tom Hare, *Zonas Peligrosas: The Challenge of Creating Safe Neighborhoods in Central America*
Maria Francesca Piazzoni, *The Real Fake: Authenticity and the Production of Space*
David Faflik, *Urban Formalism: The Work of City Reading*
Ron Nerio and Jean Halley, *The Roads to Hillbrow: Making Life in South Africa's Community of Migrants*
Christopher Prener, *Medicine at the Margins: EMS Workers in Urban America*

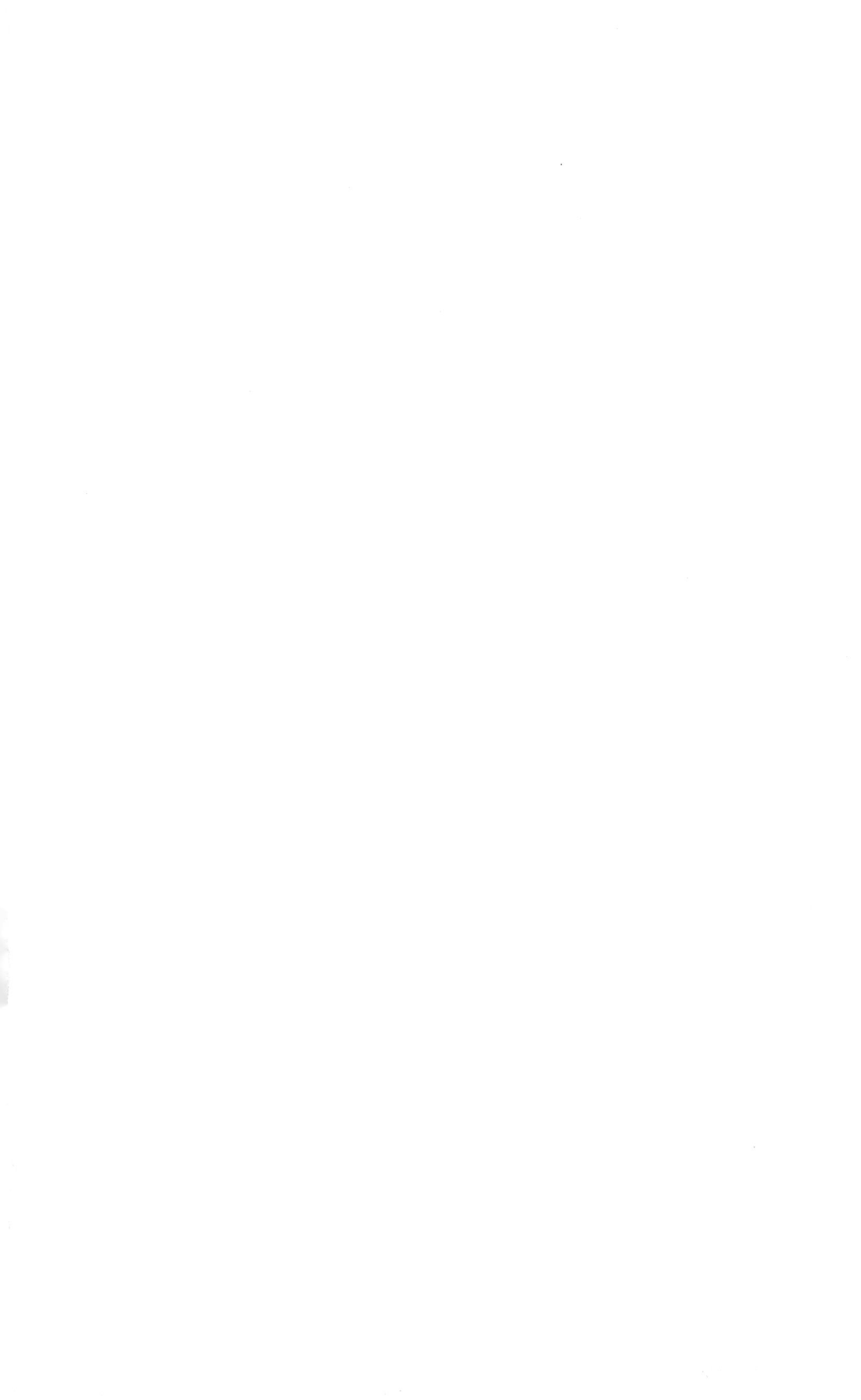

www.ingramcontent.com/pod-product-compliance
Lightning Source LLC
Chambersburg PA
CBHW020247030426
42336CB00010B/655

9781531501082